THE LIBRARY
ST. MARY'S COLLEGE OF MARYLAND
ST. MARY'S CITY, MARYLAND 20686

S0-CTU-819

ALIVE MAN!

The Physiology of Physical Activity

ALIVE MAN!

The Physiology of Physical Activity

By

ROY J. SHEPHARD, M.D., Ph.D.

Professor of Applied Physiology
School of Hygiene
University of Toronto
Toronto, Ontario, Canada

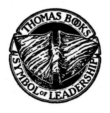

CHARLES C THOMAS • PUBLISHER
Springfield • Illinois • U.S.A.

Published and Distributed Throughout the World by
CHARLES C THOMAS · PUBLISHER
Bannerstone House
301–327 East Lawrence Avenue, Springfield, Illinois, U.S.A.
Natchez Plantation House
735 North Atlantic Boulevard, Fort Lauderdale, Florida, U.S.A.

This book is protected by copyright. No
part of it may be reproduced in any manner
without written permission from the publisher.

© 1972, by CHARLES C THOMAS · PUBLISHER

ISBN 0–398–02410–3

Library of Congress Catalog Card Number: 70–175086

With THOMAS BOOKS *careful attention is given to all details of manufacturing and design. It is the Publisher's desire to present books that are satisfactory as to their physical qualities and artistic possibilities and appropriate for their particular use.* THOMAS BOOKS *will be true to those laws of quality that assure a good name and good will.*

Printed in the United States of America

BB-14

PREFACE

Motion is characteristic of animal life. There are notable exceptions to this generalization, such as the much maligned British workman, and (more seriously) collections of bacterial spores. Nevertheless, the animal world is "designed" for action. The ability to move briskly was essential in the evolutionary struggle, a necessary "response" to the challenge of survival in a hostile world. Now, the struggle has ended. For the moment, at least, man has conquered his natural environment. A propensity for brisk movement no longer has adaptive value; indeed, automation restricts activity to the hours of leisure, and the well-adapted variant of *homo sapiens* seems the machine-minding cabbage.

But this is recent history. Over the centuries, movement has played a fundamental role throughout the animal kingdom. It is thus surprising that physiology is normally taught as a science of inactivity. Problems are illustrated by reference to anaesthetized or heavily sedated animals, with occasional distasteful glances at a "basal" man, lying supine on a couch, deprived of food and activity for much of the previous day.

A case can be made for such an approach. A baseline must be established in order to judge responses to exercise and environmental variables. Nevertheless, many courses of physiology spend so much time on the baseline that they miss the opportunity to examine responses to the challenges of everyday life. One of the objectives of the present book is to redress this balance, to consider how a healthy man meets the physical demands of work and leisure as he is active in a variety of environments.

Some knowledge of basic physiology is assumed. However, those features of normal function that are essential to an understanding of responses to exercise and an adverse environment are briefly recapitulated. The text is patterned quite closely on a didactic course entitled "The Physiology of Physical Activity." The course was originally developed for fourth-year students of physical and health education, but has grown to attract students from other disciplines within the Division of Health Sciences, individuals seeking a dynamic approach to human physiology. The prime appeal of the book may be to the physical health educator, but it is hoped that the material presented has sufficient breadth to interest also students of physiology, medicine, industrial hygiene, nursing, physiotherapy and rehabilitation.

A few comments should be made about the organization of the book. It is directed mainly to the undergraduate or recent graduate, and for this reason I have succumbed to several temptations. The occasional direct four-letter word is used in place of a much more impressive twenty-four-letter technical term. Illustrations may seem Spartan—they are simple line reproductions of chalk-board drawings, the work of my good friend Mr. John Horwood. Glossy photographs and multicoloured charts look exciting on a bookstore shelf, but add greatly to the cost of a text, often without helping the learning process. References are sparse, and I have directed the reader to review articles rather than original research communications. An average student must choose between studying a few topics in depth and obtaining an overview of a particular discipline. Both approaches have their merits in applied physiology. But I would warn the reference-seeking scholar to buy some other book—preferably *Frontiers of Fitness* or *Endurance Fitness*—rather than *Alive Man*. This latter book is intended for the type of student who likes to hear one teacher's (inevitably) biassed opinions before he embarks on the more precarious task of making his own independent decisions. A short selection of multiple-choice questions is appended to permit self-assessment when the book has been read.

Lastly, I turn to the important matter of acknowledgments. A writer incurs many debts. Sometimes they are financial! But even if a book is a financial success (and few scientific texts achieve this distinction), it is rare that proper repayment can be made. A didactic work such as this inevitably draws upon thoughts, ideas, figures and tables prepared by many of the author's colleagues, and I would like to acknowledge with sincere thanks the generous help and cooperation I have received from numerous scientists in many parts of the world; often, they have made most helpful comments on the use to be made of their data, and some have even been willing to furnish original illustrations of their work.

Where possible, their names have been cited in the text. But inevitably, it has been impossible to trace all who have contributed to this work. Some, such as Professor Horslev and Dr. DuBois are now deceased. Others, I am sure have moulded my thinking with such modesty that their names have failed to register in my consciousness. And to all such, I would pay especial tribute; this more subtle leavening of forcefully stated ideas plays a vital role in the advancement of knowledge.

How, also, can one reward the family who watch in silence, night after night, as pen is committed to paper? How can one measure the feedback of knowledge from successive generations of students, bright, alert, enthusiastic, and full of perplexing questions? And what of other staff members, who loyally maintain the routine affairs of laboratory and department, leaving the author to his cloistered search for noble phrase? Family, students, staff, my own teachers, a host of colleagues, a loyal and hard-working secretary—all have contributed to this book, and I thank them very sincerely for their respective roles in its appearance. Many have given in charity, not knowing whether the end-product would justify the gift. This is indeed generosity.

Roy J. Shephard

INTRODUCTION

Physiology has been defined as the "science of normal function," or the "study of phenomena of living things." We all understand the concept of life, yet if we attempt to characterise it, we immediately encounter a problem. A wide range of states are compatible with normal function not only in different species, but even within a given species. Most living organisms exhibit motion, growth, reproduction and a number of other common characteristics. Yet we can readily think of exceptions to these characteristics; a bacterial spore, for instance, may show no evidence of motion, growth or reproduction over a long period.

Motion is essential to the survival of most animals. Let us consider a humble unicellular amoeba, living peacefully in a pleasant aqueous environment. An enquiring physiologist takes a micropipette, and introduces a very small quantity of acid into the water. The amoeba is irritated, and responds by the liberation of energy. This causes it to move in the direction of the chemical stimulus. The physiologist now introduces a second and larger drop of acid into the water. The acidity rises dangerously, or in the terminology of the physical chemist, the pH falls. The amoeba is further irritated, and again liberates energy, allowing it to retreat from the threatening situation. If the response to the irritant is appropriately graded, the amoeba escapes, but if movement is too sluggish the irritant may induce irreversible and fatal changes in the structure of the organism.

The outcome of such an episode is more likely to be favourable in a multicellular animal than in an amoeba. Through a process of specialization, functions have been allocated firstly to specific cells, and then to specific organs. Thus the skin minimizes the influence of the external environment upon more delicate internal tissues, and the relative constancy of the internal environment (the "milieu intérieur," discussed by the famous French physiologist, Claude Bernard) is assured by a variety of specialized organs devoted to excretion, temperature regulation, and so on. Furthermore, the development of locomotor organs and of the intellect greatly enhance the possible range of response, should either a fight or flight seem appropriate.

A close control of the internal environment not only protects the organism from dangerous external changes, it also gives a more predictable response to a given stimulus. Consider the virtues of temperature regulation. The frog is a poikilothermic animal—its body temperature varies closely with that of the immediate environment. On the other hand, man is homiothermic; his body temperature is closely regulated about a mean value of 98.6°F, and it changes only slightly in response to large variations in external environment and internal heat production. Now it has been known for many years that the rate of many biochemical reactions is doubled by a 10°C rise of temperature. Thus, if a frog were to learn the force of muscle contraction needed to jump from his pond in the summer months, and attempted the same feat in the cooler days of the fall, the energy released in the latter situation would be inadequate to lift him onto the bank. Man is better placed in this respect, although even in the human the limb temperature is less well-regulated than that of the body "core." The argument can be extended to a control over other aspects of the internal environment—the precise regulation of acidity, sugar content and other blood constituents contributes to the predictable "automatic" responses that are a feature of higher life.

However, it would be dangerous to conclude that specialization is entirely advantageous. The constancy of internal environment achieved thereby is at best an unstable equilibrium. It can be upset by either a gross change in the external environment or a sudden upsurging of metabolism within the body, as in very vigorous exercise. Further, if the disturbance exceeds certain bounds, the situation becomes less favourable than in a poorly regulated organism. To take one specific instance, if a man carries out hard physical work in a hot and humid environment such as a deep coal mine, the core temperature rises briskly, and if it is allowed to exceed 104°F (only 5.4°F above the mean normal value) death may occur.

Here, in essence, are the several themes of this book—the challenges to homeostasis presented by physical activity and an adverse environment, and the limitations of man's adaptive responses, acute and chronic. We shall look at the acute disturbances of normal function induced by physical activity, the limits of adjustment that are possible, and the manner in which human performance is thereby circumscribed. We shall also evaluate the chronic effects of exercise, and will consider the manner in which responses, both acute and chronic, are altered by an abnormal external environment.

References

Harrison, G.A. *et al.: Human Biology: An Introduction to Human Evolution, Variation and Growth.* Oxford, Clarendon Press, 1964.

Baker, P.T., and Weiner, J.S.: *The Biology of Human Adaptability.* Oxford, Clarendon Press, 1966.

Books by the Same Author:

Proceedings of International Symposium on Physical Activity and Cardiovascular Health (Ed.), 1967.

Endurance Fitness, 1969.

Frontiers of Fitness (Ed.), 1971.

Fundamentals of Exercise Testing (with others), 1971.

CONTENTS

Contents

PART FOUR

SPECIAL TOPICS

ALIVE MAN!

The Physiology of Physical Activity

PART ONE

EXERCISE IN A NORMAL ENVIRONMENT

1

A "NORMAL" ENVIRONMENT

If physiology is the science of normal function, it follows that most experiments should be conducted in a "normal" or "neutral" environment, under conditions that pose no threat to the constancy of the milieu intérieur. It is doubtful how far this ideal is achieved in the harsh reality of an animal experiment or a human laboratory study; further even if a research worker were successful in creating a completely "normal" environment, it is debatable whether this concept would have much relevance to life in the natural world. Nevertheless, it is a widely used concept; we must therefore examine it, note the points of departure from reality, and suggest the possible merits of an alternative approach based on the study of free-living populations.

The Experimental Animal

Many "pure" physiologists prefer to work with an experimental animal, rather than with man. Their reasoning is that the responses of man are often distorted by anxiety and other activities of the mind, and that such problems are largely overcome by the use of a lower animal such as a cat or a dog.

The Anaesthetized Preparation

Until recently, the great majority of animal experiments have been conducted on anaesthetized or decerebrate preparations, thereby overcoming problems of discomfort and pain. Often, the anaesthetic has been administered by a rather crude technique, and in consequence the level of anaesthesia has fluctuated widely, with corresponding alterations in the responses of the animal; it is only in the last few years that the skilled methods of anaesthesia developed for human surgery have been applied to animal studies. Older methods of induction, such as the ether box, led to a wildly struggling animal, with a massive release of adrenaline and noradrenaline into the circulation; now, anaesthesia is in-

5

duced by the intraperitoneal or intravenous injection of a graded
dose of sodium thiopentone,* or some similar barbiturate, and the
animal falls gently asleep. The volatile anaesthetics such as ether
commonly stimulated a gross overproduction of mucus by the
glands lining the trachea and bronchi, and an emergency trache-
otomy was often required to relieve complete obstruction of the
airway. Nowadays, it is usual to maintain a suitably constant level
of anaesthesia by continued intravenous injection of small doses
of barbiturate, but if for any reason a gaseous anaesthetic is desired, hypersecretion of mucus is avoided by giving a small dose
of an anticholinergic drug such as atropine (0.1 mg/kg). An overdose of anaesthetic and complete arrest of breathing was not infrequent with the cruder methods of anaesthesia; the usual remedy
was to ventilate the lungs by means of a constant volume pump.
Gross overinflation of the chest was likely, and the volume of air exchanged bore no more than an accidental resemblance to normal
respiration. Often, the pulmonary blood flow was severely impeded,
and the animal suffered from either overventilation (and CO_2 lack)
or underventilation (with oxygen lack and accumulation of CO_2);
further, the normal air-conditioning mechanism of the nose was by-
passed by a trachectomy tube, and the air presented to the bronchi
was unduly cold and dry. The present generation of animal physiologists are more aware of these problems: if artificial ventilation
is needed, the air is suitably conditioned before introduction into
the pump, and the rate and depth of respiration are adjusted to
maintain the constancy of the internal environment (sampled by
recording the oxygen tension, carbon dioxide tension, and pH of
arterial blood).

However, with all the improvements in anaesthetic technique during the past decade, it is still hard to regard an anaesthetized preparation as "normal." Most anaesthetics tend to depress reflexes, and
this is particularly true of barbiturates. The systemic blood pressure
often falls, due to the action of the anaesthetic on the vasoregulatory centres of the brain, the inactivity of the animal with pooling of
blood in the extremities, and blood loss during any necessary
surgery. The body temperature is unstable, heat production is
reduced by anaesthesia, and heat loss is increased at surfaces
exposed for surgery, hence, body temperature must be maintained
by external means such as a heating pad under the animal or
exposure to infrared heaters. Finally, in the context of exercise,
no voluntary activity is possible, although muscular contraction
can be induced by a suitable frequency and intensity of motor
nerve stimulation.

---

* A suitable initial dose is 1.5 ml/kg of a solution 45 mg/ml in 10% ethanol.

The Decerebrate Preparation

Decerebration was commonly used before recent advances in anaesthesia, however, it still has important applications, both as a simple means of abolishing sensitivity to pain in lower animals such as the frog, and as a technique for studying levels of organization within the central nervous system of higher animals. Once the operation has been completed, the effects of the preliminary anesthetic can be allowed to wear-off, and responses can then be studied independently of the depressant action of anaesthetics.

The main disadvantage of the decerebrate preparation is its instability. Unless the surgeon has considerable experience, the initial level of brain transection may be higher or lower than is intended; further, over the next few hours, the effective level of transection may rise (as initially damaged brain tissue recovers), or it may fall (due to continued haemorrhage and oedema formation in the brain stem). In general, the operation is quite bloody (in the proper sense of the word), and the condition of the circulatory system progressively deteriorates as haemorrhage continues from the cut surfaces of bone and brain.

Use of Conscious Animals

For many years, occasional investigators have carried out experiments on conscious animals. Interest in this approach has been particularly strong in Eastern Europe, where studies are still framed in the context of the conditioned responses described by the famous Russian physiologist Pavlov.

Use of trained animals has permitted fascinating experiments on such topics as the interaction of conscious thought and the secretion of intestinal juices. More recently, we have seen voyages of dogs and monkeys far into space. Occasionally, also, we read of dogs and animals running on special designs of treadmill. In one experiment, the objective was to test whether animals could be exercised to the point of death, and greyhounds were persuaded to continue running until several fatalities occurred. Other animal studies have examined responses to exercise after drastic surgical intervention such as the removal of both the sympathetic and vagal innervation of the heart.

If an animal has been "conditioned" to accept an experimental laboratory and the various pieces of apparatus therein, it may be possible to conduct an experiment with less emotional response than would be the case if similar observations were made on man. On the other hand, a poorly conditioned animal is often under greater emotional stress than a human subject. In such an animal, a gross increase of pulse rate and respiratory minute volume may arise as a response to a facemask or some other simple restraint, thus obscuring the direct effect of a superimposed exercise load.

The Role of Animal Experiments in Applied Physiology

With these various strictures on the use of anaesthetized, decerebrate, and conscious animals, what is the proper role of animal experimentation in a laboratory of applied physiology?

One immediate justification of animal work is in the conduct of experiments that would be dangerous for human subjects. The exploration of space has proved a relatively safe adventure. But before man was sent on such an unknown exploit, it was undoubtedly proper to chart the course, firstly by instrument-carrying probes, and then by craft carrying suitable experimental animals. Again, it is rare for man to meet his death through running to exhaustion; but rather than test this point directly, it is advisable to review information on the mortality of animals under similar experimental conditions. Unfortunately, there are such wide differences between most animals and man that no animal test can establish the categoric safety of a given procedure; on the other hand, useful pointers to possible hazards are frequently obtained. Thus, in the specific case of running to exhaustion, death is more likely in the dog than in man. The dog is habitually a runner, and has little means of protesting his exhaustion; in contrast, the average human subject complains bitterly long before he is exhausted, and even if his pleas are ignored the experiment is halted by the assumption of a prone position long before dangerous circulatory embarassment has occurred. The differences attributable to man's erect body position might have been uncovered if a sufficient range of animal species had been studied, or if the theoretical implications of an upright posture had been considered; in any event, it is important before extrapolating to man both to study several species, and to examine how these differ physiologically from the human.

A second area where animals can be very useful is in an experiment that involves the sampling of body tissues or other relatively drastic procedures. To cite one recent example, much has been learned by biopsy of the human calf during and following sustained exercise; a very large needle is inserted into the vastus lateralis muscle and a fine cylinder of muscle tissue is removed for analysis of glycogen content and other biochemical parameters. Normally, the subject has no more than a sore calf for the next few hours, but since the needle is inserted blindly, there have been occasional episodes when it has hit a major blood vessel. The risks involved may be acceptable if the investigator is studying himself and a few medically qualified colleagues, or if the information is essential to clinical treatment. But the widespread application of such a drastic procedure is not justified. A risk of even one unfortunate episode in one thousand cases is not acceptable when dealing with normal, healthy volunteers. Experiments of this type must either be conducted on animals, or replaced by alternative and less direct methods of investigation.

The Typical Human Laboratory Experiment

The aim of a typical human laboratory experiment is to ensure the initial constancy of the internal environment by achieving a "basal" (completely resting) state. Subsequent variations of state extraneous to the purpose of the experiment are kept to a minimum by working in what the investigator hopes is a "neutral" external environment.

The "Basal" State

Unaccustomed exertion, overindulgence in food or alcohol, lack of sleep, exposure to heat, prolonged standing and minor infections all modify human performance for quite long periods. The preparation of the subject should thus begin at least one day before his visit to the laboratory. This preliminary day is free of any unusual stress, and includes a minimum of eight hours sound sleep. On the test day, the subject is brought to the laboratory prior to breakfast, having taken his last meal at least twelve hours earlier. Hair-raising car journeys and fevered sprints for the train are both avoided, if necessary, by previous admission to the institution. Early morning stimulants such as tea and coffee are forbidden, and smoking is also prohibited. After arrival, the subject lies supine on a couch for thirty minutes, and it is then judged that the "basal" state has been reached.

Although it may seem desirable from the experimental point of view, the achievement of a "basal" state is often impractical. Volunteers may submit to the necessary preparation on one occasion, but their loyalty is severely taxed by repeated experiments. Further, it can be argued that the results obtained from "basal" studies are far-removed from real life. What relevance do they have to a man who smokes every fifteen minutes, drinks a cup of black coffee every hour, and likes to work on a full stomach? Many exercise studies are thus conducted on "resting," rather than "basal" subjects; tests are conducted perhap 1½ to 2 hours after a light meal, and one hour after a drink or cigarette, with a minimum of fifteen minutes rest in a chair prior to exercise. The physiological changes induced by exercise are in general quite large, and any errors introduced by the use of a "resting" rather than a "basal" state are correspondingly small and unimportant.

Many bodily functions show a pronounced daily rhythm. This is in part a response to the periodic nature of work, play, feeding and sleeping, and in part an expression of cyclic changes in the external environment—illumination, temperature, humidity, air pollution, and the like. During a typical day, almost a half of mankind take an increasing total dose of tobacco particles and nicotine into the body, and a physiological protest is registered in terms of spasm of the airways, an increase of heart rate, a reduction of blood flow to many tissues, and an increasing conversion of the red cell pigment to a functionally useless form (carboxyhaemoglobin). In some industries, such as mining and cotton-spinning, an additional burden of dust is inhaled during the period of work. In other types of employment, prolonged standing may be necessary; this leads to a peripheral pooling of fluid, with an increase in the water content of the extracellular space (commonly reported as a swelling of the ankles), and a reduction in the "central" blood volume (the blood content of the heart and lungs). If measurements are made in the "resting" rather than the "basal" state, it is thus important to note the time of day, and to hold this constant from one experiment to another.

The "Neutral" External Environment

The main problem presented by the average laboratory is its forbidding nature. The subject is confronted by many unfamiliar and seemingly menacing pieces of equipment. The investigator must thus take time to answer questions, explain procedures, and where possible allay unwarranted fears. It is helpful if equipment and personnel not essential to the experiment are kept from the test area, and the investigation is conducted in a calm, orderly, and unhurried manner. However, if all suspicion of an interaction between mind and environment is to be avoided, we must adopt the technique of negative conditioning, as suggested for experiments on conscious animals. The subject is "habituated" to both the laboratory and the required procedures by a simple repetition of the entire routine on two or more successive days, and reliance is placed only on information collected during the final test.

A "neutral" environmental temperature neither warms nor cools the body. The temperature required depends in part on human factors (the intensity of activity and the extent of clothing), and in part on environmental considerations (humidity and wind speed, or in the swimmer water-movement). An increase of relative humidity reduces the evaporation of sweat at any given temperature, thereby increasing the effective warmth of the environment; on the other hand, a brisk wind disturbs the thin layer of still air covering the skin surface, thereby increasing the convection of heat and also removing air that is saturated with water vapour. Engineers have devised a number of scales of "effective temperature" that take into account the opposing influences of humidity and wind speed. An example is shown in Fig. 65. If the air is still and not too humid, and the subject is lightly clothed, a comfortable sitting temperature is 70°–75°F; however, in the United Kingdom much lower domestic temperatures are endured by increasing the weight of clothing, and in most countries a lower temperature (65°–70°F) is preferred if body heat production is increased by sustained physical activity. The convection of heat proceeds much more readily in water than in air, and the average person soon becomes chilled in the usual lake or stream; the "neutral" temperature for water exposure is commonly about 33.5°C, 92°F.

The main objection to the "neutral" environment is its artificiality. The subject is free of the natural stimulation provided by sunlight, a fresh breeze, the song of the birds, and the chatter of children; all who have worked in an artificial and closely controlled environment can testify that although initially comfortable, it soon becomes bland and boring, and in consequence the arousal of the higher centres of the brain is decreased. This modifies physiological responses to many stimuli and for this reason the patterns of function observed in a "neutral" environment are not necessarily applicable to the free-living organism.

The Epidemiological Approach

In an attempt to meet objections to a "neutral" environment, some applied physiologists have recently resorted to the epidemiological methods long used in studying the spread of human disease. Let us suppose we wish to investigate the possible influence of air pollutants on the vital capacity of elderly patients with chronic cardiorespiratory disease. We could build a gas chamber in which all conditions apart from the concentration of a specific pollutant were kept "neutral." We might then proceed to measure the vital capacity before and at various times during exposure to a known concentration of the supposedly toxic gas or vapour; however, even if we shut our eyes to the bland nature of the "neutral" environment, the deliberate exposure of frail and elderly patients to toxic material is not morally justified. The alternative is to follow the normal life of those citizens who live in the polluted areas of a metropolis. This can be done on a retrospective basis, relating the vital capacity when interviewed to the pattern of gas exposure as gleaned from municipal and other records. However, it is more satisfactory to carry out a prospective experiment, enrolling a population and seeking a parallel between changes in vital capacity and simultaneously measured changes in the concentration of air pollutants.

In exploring such relationships, it is important to eliminate the influence of other variables known to affect the measurement under study (vital capacity). Thus in an animal experiment, we would probably select creatures of uniform age, sex, and size, and in a human population, suitable allowance must be made for each of these factors. Environmental variables, other than air pollution (for instance, temperature and humidity) show cyclical changes, and these also can affect vital capacity. In order to define the influence of air pollution independent of extraneous variables, it is usual to calculate what is termed a multiple regression equation. This would have the general format

$$\text{Vital Capacity} = K_1 (\text{Age}) + K_2 (\text{Sex}) + K_3 (\text{Size}) + K_4 (\text{Temperature}) + K_5 (\text{Humidity}) + K_6 (\text{Pollutant}) + \text{error}$$

An equation of this sort is readily solved by a large computer, and the significance of the individual constants K_1 to K_6 can then be determined relative to the final error term. If K_6 proves significant from a statistical point of view, then we may assume that our pollutant *or* some unmeasured quantity varying in parallel with it has an effect on vital capacity.

The problem of physiological responses to air pollutants is particularly difficult in that there seems a threshold concentration below which no measurable physiological change occurs (in other words, vital capacity is a nonlinear function of the concentration of pollutant). There is also a substantial time lag between exposure and the full development of any physiological response; a series of equations must thus be calculated in order to identify the time lapse giving the largest and most significant value of K_6. Fortunately, many epidemiological problems are simpler than air pollution, and can be resolved by the use of a single equation of the type illustrated above.

The Changing Environment

One final problem of the "normal" environment is its changing nature. This in turn reacts upon members of the animal kingdom, and adaptations occur. The required "neutral" conditions are thus by no means constant. Let us consider first regional disparities. It is mid-May. A physiologist is working in the humid heat of Cincinnati. Appropriate adjustments have occurred to his temperature regulating mechanisms, including alterations in the patterns of sweating and of basal energy expenditure. The "neutral" temperature is 78°F. He now flies to Liverpool to attend a scientific meeting. The weather is cool, and the hotel is a brisk unheated 60°F; most of the English guests are tolerably comfortable, but the American is 18°F below his "neutral" temperature. He loses heat rapidly, and suffers acute discomfort. But if the meeting is long, he undergoes a progressive adaptation to cold, and his "neutral" temperature gradually drops towards that of his English colleagues.

A bigger problem is presented by irreversible changes in the environment, such as may occur with the transition from a rural to a metropolitan society. One of the goals of the International Biological Programme has been to study primitive peoples such as the Eskimo and the Kalahari Bushman, as yet unaffected by this process of acculturation, to examine in depth both the very hostile environment in which they live, and the patterns of adaptation which have developed. But in a sense, the International Biological Programme is too late. In many communities, the traditional role of the hunter has already been lost. Expeditions are made by skidoo and power boat rather than by sledge and canoe. Animal furs are collected in ever increasing numbers but the natural diet of meat and oils is increasingly supplanted by carbohydrates such as sugar, with a parallel deterioration in dental health. The primitive shelter of tent and igloo has been replaced by a warm and comfortable three bedroom bungalow. Welfare payments in many instances have removed the stimulus to traditional active pursuits. Such profound cultural and environmental changes have undoubtedly left their mark on the "neutral" environment of people such as the Eskimo.

Technically more advanced cultures have also experienced rapid environmental change during the present century; this has been associated with a migration from the village to the city, the development of the motor car, the automation of most forms of work, the control of macro- and microclimate, and gains in personal income with attendant problems of overnutrition and reliance upon service industries.

The pattern of urban life has forced adaptation to polluted atmospheres. There is now little opportunity for physical activity or recreation except in highly organized groups. Inactivity is accentuated by both the widespread availability of cars and also the progressive reduction in the physical demands of industry. Few North American factories now require a man to work at more than two or three times his basal rate of energy expenditure; thus if personal fitness is to be maintained, this must be through deliberate active leisure pursuits. Even young children, restricted to high-rise apartments and driven through crowded streets by anxious parents, are increasingly inactive. We have no knowledge of the long-term implications of inactivity during the period of growth, but we must suspect both an alteration of the "neutral" environment and a threat to cardiovascular health.

Climatic control is particularly obvious in North America. Homes possess central heating and refrigeration, equipment for humidification and dehumidification and electrostatic dust precipitators, while cars, buses, offices and shopping malls are increasingly air-conditioned. It is becoming progressively less necessary for urban man to test his capacity to adapt to the thermal environment. The same phenomenon is apparent even in more remote areas, due to improvements in protective clothing and the development of well-insulated prefabricated housing. On one recent expedition to the South Pole, a metallic suit was used to record the temperature over a large part of the body, and to the surprise of the investigators, the integrated surface temperature differed little from the figure found in a temperate climate. The combination of well-designed clothing and modern building technology gave almost complete protection against Antarctica.

Overnutrition is a significant problem in North America. The current generation are heavier than their predecessors, and by the time they reach the age of forty, they may carry a burden of 10 kg of excess tissue, largely fat. The adverse effect of excess weight is well-documented in the tables of the life-insurance companies, and is seen also in the static or decreasing life expectancy of the North American at a time when many of the major diseases are being conquered. Overnutrition alters the insulating properties of the skin, and in consequence we find a decrease of "neutral" temperature, particularly during water immersion.

The changing nature of our world limits the possibility of temporal comparisons, even if experiments are carried out under carefully standardized conditions. Men of 1972 who are asked to run on a laboratory treadmill are not the same as the men of 1902 and if their response to exercise differs, it is difficult to pinpoint which of the many changes in environment is responsible. However, there is little argument that the performance of the average 1972 man is poorer than that of his predecessor, and it is thus important that we continue to seek the reasons for the loss of performance, in order that these deleterious changes may be arrested. —

References

DuBois, E.: *Basal Metabolism in Health and Disease*. Philadelphia, Lea & Febiger, 1936.

Anderson, L.A. *et al.*: Environmental specifications and preparation for testing. In *Fundamentals of Exercise Testing*. Geneva, WHO Monograph, 1971.

Glaser, E.M.: *The Physiological Basis of Habituation*. London, Oxford University Press, 1966.

Lawther, P.J. *et al:*. *Epidemiology of Air Pollution*. Geneva, WHO, 1962.

Westlund, K.B. (Rapporteur). Epidemiological methods in the study of chronic diseases. *WHO Tech Rep*, 365, 1967.

Edholm, O.G., and Bacharach, A.L.: *The Physiology of Human Survival*. London, Academic Press, 1965.

2

THE MEASUREMENT OF HUMAN ACTIVITY

Purpose of Measurement

There are many reasons for measuring physical activity. In the acute sense, we can use the activity itself as a unit of physiological performance that would otherwise be more difficult to document (for instance, anaerobic or aerobic power). We may also wish to specify the energy demands of an industrial task, to predict the "fitness" of an individual, or to assess the performance of competitors in an athletic event. Patterns of chronic activity are of interest to the epidemiologist who seeks to relate the habitual energy expenditures of a community with its fitness, obesity, and liability to disease. The trainer, also, compares various patterns of habitual activity to determine which is the most effective in improving the performance of an athlete, while the pharmacologist and the behavioural scientist examine the effects of drugs and surgically-induced brain damage upon the movement patterns of laboratory animals.

Characterization of Activity

Activity is characterized according to the intensity, duration, and frequency of effort that is undertaken. The nature of the three variables and their interrelationships may be expressed as follows:

Intensity

Intensity is essentially a rate of performing work. If we consider an infinitely short interval of time ∂t, then the work performed in this time is ∂W, and the intensity of effort is $\dfrac{\partial W}{\partial t}$. Intensity has the physical dimensions of power, and is thus expressed either in units of power (watts, horsepower) or as a quantity of work performed in unit time (kilogram-metres per minute, foot pounds per minute). Those readers with a background in physics will recall that work is usually expressed in dyne-centimetres rather

17

than kilogram-metres; the dyne is an absolute unit, and takes account of variations in the earth's gravitational field. Some physiologists prefer to use an absolute measurement of work intensity (kilopond-metre per minute); in unit gravitational field, one kilopond-metre is exactly equal to one kilogram-metre. Small differences of gravitational acceleration occur with altitude and latitude. However, the difference between absolute and relative units of work only becomes important when gravitational forces are grossly disturbed, as when walking on the moon, or operating the controls of an aircraft during a tight turn.

The concept of intensity implies a reference point, usually zero activity. If the activity is being measured in terms of the external work performed, then the zero point is easily established. However, if the level of activity is assessed in terms of its oxygen cost, the approach is more complex. It is usual for the subject to perform exercise at a constant intensity for several minutes, and to measure the oxygen consumption during the final minute of effort, when it is hoped that a "steady-state" has been achieved. In the "steady state," the oxygen consumption measured at the mouth is equal to the oxygen consumed in the tissues, and this in turn is proportional to the work performed. Unfortunately, the oxygen consumption is not zero even if no external work is performed. In the "basal" state (see p. 9), a subject consumes some 7 percent of his maximum oxygen intake, and if he is sitting quietly on a machine such as a bicycle ergometer, he may be using 10% to 12% of his maximum oxygen intake. Thus, if activity is expressed in terms of its oxygen cost, it is important to distinguish the gross cost from the net value which has been corrected for "basal" or "resting" energy expenditure. Sometimes, instead of assuming that a "steady-state" has been reached, oxygen consumption is measured both during and following activity, and the intensity of effort is assessed from the total oxygen usage in excess of the "resting" or "basal" figure (Fig. 1). Since the external oxygen consumption is still increasing slightly after five or six minutes of exercise, the "total cost" method indicates a somewhat higher oxygen cost than the "steady-state" method. However, unless there is a slowing of the circulation due to some problem such as cardiovascular disease, the two methods agree to within about 5 percent.

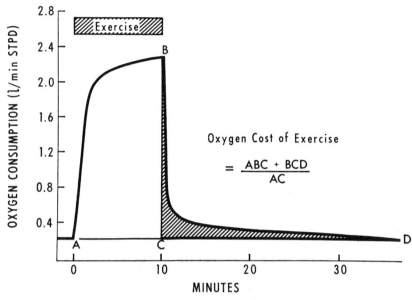

Figure 1. Illustration of calculation of the total oxygen cost of activity. The subject commences to exercise at point A, and oxygen consumption rises from the resting value along the curve AB. At point B, he stops exercising, and oxygen consumption declines along the curve BD. The total net cost of the exercise is given by the areas ABC + BCD, and the increase in oxygen consumption attributable to the exercise is given by $\dfrac{(ABC + BCD)}{AC}$.

Occasionally, the reference point is off-set, and it is noted when the intensity of activity exceeds some arbitrary threshold value. Thus Karvonen has suggested that cardiorespiratory training will not result unless intensity of activity is such that the oxygen consumption reaches at least 60 percent of the individual's aerobic power.

Duration

The total duration of activity T is easily measured and understood. If the intensity of effort is integrated over this period, $\int_{0}^{T} \dfrac{\partial W}{\partial t}$, a figure is obtained for the total quantity of work performed. As we have noted above, the units are kg-m or more precisely dyne-cm; some laboratories describe it as a "capacity," but this is dimensionally incorrect: work is the product of pressure and change of volume ($g/cm^2 \times cm^3$), while capacity expresses the relationship between change of volume and change of pressure ($cm^3 \times cm^2/gm$). If a subject is run to exhaustion, we are measuring not his "capacity" but a combination of stored energy and power; when the rate of release of stored energy and the continuing power production are no longer equal to the demands of the task, the subject is exhausted.

Frequency

The frequency of activity is commonly expressed per day or per week. Thus, the keen athlete may make as many as twenty repetitions of his favoured event in one day, while the middle-aged businessman may repeat his "work-out" three or five times per week. Where an irregular schedule is involved, and especially where weekend activity differs from weekday activity, it is desirable to calculate the total activity in terms of the number of repetitions N per week $\left(\sum_{0}^{N.} \int_{0}^{T} \frac{\partial W}{\partial t} \right)$. The total weekly effort has some relevance to training schedules, and is of particular interest when calculating either normal nutritional requirements or special diets for the control of obesity.

Procedure for the Measurement of Physical Activity

Acute Activity

Work Measurements. The observer may measure the work output of the subject directly, using some form of "ergometer," or he may estimate the work performed from displacements of the body weight against gravity.

In the usual *bicycle ergometer*, the rear wheel of a standard bicycle is replaced by a large and relatively heavy flywheel, and a friction belt is applied to the outer edge of the flywheel. The inertia of the wheel permits the subject to develop a relatively even force throughout a complete pedal revolution. The work performed is calculated from the product of the frictional force F, (shown as a decrease in belt tension) and the distance traversed by the outer rim of the flywheel. If the radius of the wheel is r, then its circumference is $2\pi r$, and the distance traversed in one minute is $(2\pi r)$ N $\overline{A}^{a}$, where N is the number of pedal revolutions per minute, a is the number of teeth on the pedal sprocket, and A the number of teeth on the rear sprocket. The intensity of working is thus given by $(2\pi r)$ N $\dfrac{a}{A}$. In the simplest types of bicycle, F is shown either as the difference in reading of two spring balances attached to opposite ends of the belt, or (in the popular Von Döbeln machine) as rotation of a weighted level about a vertical axis. There are several practical difficulties in the operation of such machines: (a) The system of springs, weights and levers forms a compound pendulum, and oscillations are such that it may become impossible to read the spring balance or the lever position accurately. This problem can be overcome by enclosing the weights in a loosely fitting metal sleeve; air resistance then damps out oscillations. (b) After several minutes of cycling, the belt becomes hot; this progressively diminishes the frictional force, and in consequence the loading screw requires repeated tightening. In one mechanical bicycle (the Fleisch "ergostat"), a servo-mechanism alters the angle of contact between the flywheel and the belt so that the frictional force is independent of temperature. (c) With all mechanical designs, the work performed depends upon the number of pedal revolutions N; this number must therefore be measured accurately. A counter can be attached directly to the pedal bearing, or alternatively the drive can be linked to a synchronous motor through a differential gear. In the latter case, if the subject pedals at the speed set by the synchronous motor, a large pointer remains in the vertical position; deviations of the pointer indicate variations of speed to within a small fraction of a pedal revolution. (d) Part of the force applied to the pedals is dissipated in the chain drive and bearings. The unmeasured frictional work can amount to 20 percent of the total effort. Some machines are calibrated to allow for this error, or actually measure the torque (turning force) generated at the pedals; however, most simpler machines ignore the problem. For accurate work, they should be calibrated by a device that applies a known torque to the pedal bearings.

In some bicycles, the mechanical source of friction is replaced by an electrical generator. An electrically-braked bicycle is an expensive addition to an exercise laboratory, and we shall thus examine the principle of its operation. In the simplest form of generator, a single coil (or armature) is rotated between the poles of a permanent magnet. However, in most modern generators there are a large number (z) of armature elements, and the permanent magnet is replaced by an electromagnet with more than one pair of poles. If Φ is the flux per pole, and there are P poles, then the total magnetic flux cut by each element is ΦP per revolution; half of the armature elements are usually arranged in parallel with the other half, so that if the generator makes $\frac{N}{60}$ revolutions per second, the total electrical force generated E is given by

$$E = \frac{\Phi ZN}{60} \times \frac{P}{2} \times 10^{-8} \text{ volts*}$$

Thus, if the magnetic flux Φ is held constant by applying a fixed external voltage, the electromotive force that is generated depends simply on the number of armature revolutions per second. Alternatively, by a suitable "feedback" device, the flux Φ can be made to vary inversely with N, so that the electromotive force becomes relatively independent of armature speed. Unfortunately, the work performed by the subject is less constant than our simplified equation suggests. As in the mechanical ergometer, frictional losses occur in the chain and bearings, and electrical energy is lost in heating of the armature, in hysteresis and in eddy currents. Hysteresis varies with N, and eddy currents with N^2; both also vary with the state of the iron core of the magnet, which is affected by vibration. The calibration of the electrically-braked ergometer thus needs to be carried out rather frequently.

Whether a mechanical or an electrically-braked bicycle is used, the work is performed with a net mechanical efficiency of approximately 23 percent. Let us suppose that a subject performs 600 kg-m of work per minute, and we wish to estimate the corresponding oxygen consumption. We know that 427 kg-m = 1 kcal; thus the rate of working of our subject may be written as 1.4 kcal/min. Assuming an average mechanical efficiency, the metabolic cost of this effort is $1.4 \times \frac{100}{23} = 6.1$ kcal/min. Further, we know that 5 kcal of energy expenditure is approximately equal to 1 litre of oxygen consumption; † thus the net oxygen cost of activity is 1.22 litre/min. In order to obtain the gross cost, we must add the oxygen consumption while sitting at rest on the bicycle, perhaps 0.30 litre/min in an average man.

In the usual form of *step test*, the subject climbs up and down a flight of one, two, or three steps, at a rate of N ascents per minute. He is paced by a metronome or a flashing signal. Account

---

* The factor 10^{-8} serves to convert absolute units of electromotive force to volts.

† The relationship of oxygen consumption to energy expenditure varies slightly according to the relative proportions of fat and carbohydrate that are consumed.

is taken simply of the work W performed against gravity; this is calculated from the step height H (metres) and the body mass (M, kg) when the subject is clothed as for the test:

$$W = MHN \text{ (kg-m/min)}$$

It is important in making this calculation to ensure that the subject maintains the intended rhythm, and lifts the centre of gravity of the body through the full step height at each cycle. No account is taken of the work performed in checking the fall of the body during descent of the staircase. The efficiency of effort is thus rather lower than for the bicycle ergometer, averaging about 16 percent at a comfortable rate of climbing.

> Occasionally, escalators are used so that work can be performed simply in an upward or a downward direction. Margaria has suggested placing photo-cells on a long flight of stairs, so that the rate of ascent from (say) the third to the twenty-third step can be measured; this is particularly useful when studying the maximum energy released in the first few seconds of exercise. A similar system of photo-cells is sometimes used to measure the horizontal speed and accelerations of a sprinter.

Work can be performed on an *inclined treadmill*. To a first approximation, the rate of working W is given by $W = V(A + \theta B) + K$ where V is the treadmill speed, θ is the slope, and A, B, and K are constants.

> If V is expressed in miles per hour, the constants appropriate to an average young man are $A = 4.6$ ml O_2/kg min, $B = 0.37$ ml/kg min, and $K = 7.7$ ml/kg min. Unless the slope is steep (greater than 12%), more work is performed in horizontal than in vertical progression. The equation can be used to specify the oxygen cost of running; in young men, the accuracy is about 10 percent.

Cinematography is currently being applied to obtain a more accurate estimate of the mechanical work involved in various types of activity. Movement of the centre of gravity of the trunk and of the arms and legs is followed frame by frame; it is then possible to calculate not only the work performed in lifting against gravity, but also energy lost in accelerating and decelerating individual body parts.

Similar information can be obtained by fitting *accelerometers* at various points on the body surface; an accelerometer is a sensing device that produces a signal proportional to the acceleration of the element; if the output of the sensor is coupled to suitable integrating devices, velocity and displacement may also be recorded.

Simple track measurements of the *time* required to run a specific distance (300 yards, 600 yards), or the *distance* covered in a specified time (12 minutes, 15 minutes) have been proposed for the field testing of fitness (pp. 405, 406). In general, the objective has been to test endurance, and three hundred and six hundred yard events are too short for this purpose. The success of the twelve and fifteen minute runs depends largely on the motivation of the group under test; more consistent results are usually obtained with men than with women. Furthermore, it may be risky to expose older adults to a maximum effort test of this duration, particularly under field conditions; there is some danger of both local tendon injuries and death from ventricular fibrillation (p. 509).

Measurements of Oxygen Consumption. For some purposes, it is convenient to measure not the external work performed, but the body's reaction to this work in terms of an increased oxygen consumption.

Two types of portable respirometer are available for field use. The *Kofranyi-Michaelis meter* is mechanical. The flow of expired gas actuates a small reciprocating pump, and this is linked to a counter that records the total volume expired. A small percentage (0.3% or 0.6%) of gas is diverted to a balloon for subsequent chemical analysis. The entire apparatus weighs about 2 kg. It is provided with a harness so that it can be strapped to the back. The machine is rugged, and it has a very consistent calibration factor if moving parts and rubber tubing are well-maintained. However, it is intended primarily for industrial surveys, and the maximum flow rate (about 60 litre/min) is not adequate for vigorous forms of athletic activity.

The *Wolff IMP* (integrating motor pneumotachograph) is a similar device, but is operated by an electrical mechanism. The flow of expired gas moves a slide wire along a potentiometer, and the voltage thus tapped is used to drive a small electric motor and counter. Again, a small percentage of the expired stream is diverted, in this case to a balloon enclosed in a metal storage can.

Again, the system is designed for military and industrial surveys, and the maximum flow rate is inadequate for most athletic studies.

The only system suited to gas collection on athletes is a low resistance box-valve, a short length of tubing, and a broad-necked *meteorological balloon*. It is cumbersome for an athlete to carry this on his back, and often it is supported in an open truck driven slowly at the side of the contestant. Care must then be taken to avoid influencing performance by the "slip-stream" of the vehicle. Samples of expired gas are taken in glass syringes for subsequent analysis, and the volume of individual bags are determined by transferring their contents to a large Tissot gasometer.

Indices of Oxygen Consumption. Sometimes, instead of measuring oxygen consumption directly, an investigator may record a simple index of oxygen consumption. The principal candidates are pulse rate and respiratory minute volume.

We know from the conductance equation (p. 108)[*] that the two main determinants of gas conductance $\dot{U}$ are alveolar ventilation ($\dot{V}_A$) and the product of blood solubility (λ) and cardiac output ($\dot{Q}$):

$$\frac{1}{\dot{U}} = \frac{1}{\dot{V}_A} + \frac{1}{\lambda\dot{Q}}$$

In young and healthy men, the maximum values of $\dot{V}_A$ and $\dot{Q}$ are, respectively, about 80 and 25 litre/min. Furthermore, λ_{O_2} is close to one, while λ_{CO_2} is about 5. Thus we may write

$$\frac{1}{\dot{U}_{O_2}} = \frac{1}{80} + \frac{1}{1(25)}$$

$$\frac{1}{\dot{U}_{CO_2}} = \frac{1}{80} + \frac{1}{5(25)}$$

The transfer of oxygen is dependent mainly on the second term, while the transfer of carbon dioxide depends more on the first than on the second term. Oxygen consumption is thus closely related to cardiac output, and the cardiac output is in turn directly related to pulse rate, providing that the stroke volume re-

[*] Readers unfamiliar with the concept of gas conductance may find it helpful to study page 108 in conjunction with;this section.

mains constant. In practice, (Fig. 2), the pulse/oxygen consumption relationship is linear between 50% and 90% of maximum oxygen consumption. However, at lower work loads, part of the oxygen demand of the tissues is met by an increased arteriovenous oxygen difference, and part by an increased stroke volume. What happens between 90% and 100% of maximum oxygen intake is still debated. Often, the individual has reached his maximum pulse rate, and the increased oxygen may be met in part by a further increase of stroke volume, in part by a further widening of the arteriovenous oxygen difference, and in part by anaerobic work. Associated hyperventilation may cause a spurious increase of oxygen consumption due to a rise in the oxygen content of alveolar gas.

Ventilation is related more to $\dot{U}_{CO_2}$ than $\dot{U}_{O_2}$. Any relationship between respiratory minute volume and oxygen consumption is thus indirect, depending upon a constant respiratory gas exchange

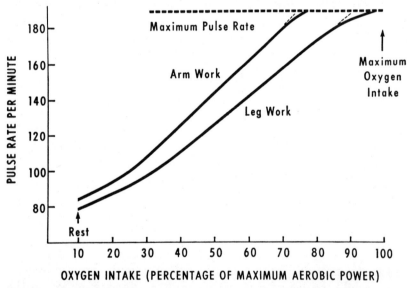

Figure 2. The relationship between pulse rate and oxygen consumption, the latter being expressed as a percentage of the aerobic power of the individual. Note: 1. the relationship conforms closely to a straight line between 50% and 90% of aerobic power. 2. the relationship is fairly consistent for different types of leg work (bicycle, step test, treadmill), but the curve is displaced markedly to the left for arm work.

ratio (CO_2 output/O_2 intake) and a constant ratio of alveolar to total ventilation. Both conditions are reasonably well-maintained in moderate work, but during more intense effort, lactate production occurs, and in an attempt to restore the pH of arterial blood, ventilation becomes disproportionate to oxygen consumption (Fig. 3). Ventilatory predictions of oxygen consumption are thus best used between 10% and 50% of maximum oxygen intake, and at higher work loads pulse predictions are more useful.

Whether ventilation or heart rate is used as the metabolic index, the relationship is fairly consistent for different forms of leg exercise (bicycle, step test, treadmill), but differs markedly for arm work. The curve is displaced to the left if tension is developed in the active muscles (as in weight lifting and iso-

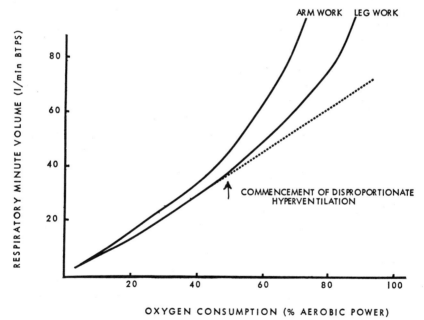

Figure 3. The relationship between respiratory minute volume and oxygen consumption, the latter being expressed as a percentage of the aerobic power of the individual. Note: 1. The relationship conforms closely to a straight line between 10% and 50% of aerobic power, but there is a disproportionate increase of ventilation at higher work loads. 2. The relationship is displaced to the left if work is performed with the arms rather than the legs.

metric exercise), and errors also arise if the subject is anxious, hot, in poor health, or has been standing for a long period. Under optimal conditions, pulse and ventilatory predictions of oxygen consumption have an accuracy of 5% to 10%.

> The choice of technique for recording the pulse rate depends on the mobility of the subject. If he is working at a factory bench, it is possible to attach a photocell to his ear, and to use the changes in opacity with each pulse beat to drive a small counter; such a system works quite well providing the head is not moved sufficiently to cause slipping of the earpiece. Alternatively, the subject may be fitted with chest electrodes, and a cable passed to an electrocardiograph machine; this gives a very accurate figure for pulse rate, but involves the fitting of electrodes which may be disturbed by arm movement or by sweating. If the subject is moving freely within a prescribed area such as an ice-rink or a football pitch, then a small radiotelemeter may be worn. This amplifies the electrical signal from the heart and transmits it to a small radio receiver and electrocardiograph on the touch-line. If even greater freedom of movement is desired, then a small slow-speed tape-recorder can be worn; this type of device will record the electro-cardiogram for periods of up to twelve hours.
>
> The respiratory minute volume can be measured by either the Kofranyi-Michaelis meter or the Wolff IMP; in both cases, an observer must follow the subject and note the counter readings at suitable intervals; however, there seems no fundamental reason why such machines should not include either telemetry or tape recording of the counter movements. The main limitation of both devices is that they cannot handle a flow rate of more than 60 litre/min.

Other less direct indices of increased oxygen consumption such as the rise of deep body temperature or the associated secretion of catecholamines (noradrenaline and adrenaline) do not appear to offer any advantage over the measurement of ventilation and pulse rate.

Chronic Activity

Activity Questionnaires. For epidemiological purposes, it is often necessary to collect information on the activity of large groups of people over many months, and it is then tempting to use the subjects themselves as the source of the necessary labour. A retrospective questionnaire may be used, in which the subject is required to look back on perhaps the most recent year of his life, and to specify the intensity, duration and frequency of all active pursuits. Unfortunately, the quality of information obtained in this way is low, and in general the level of habitual activity is exaggerated by the subject. The accuracy can be improved if the subject is taken through the questionnaire in the form of an interview, but this can be a very tedious and time-consuming process. Often, the information obtained is not much better than could be derived from a simple three point scale as follows:

0 points—taking no regular activity to improve personal fitness
1 point —playing one active sport per week, or participating in jogging, or gymnastics
2 points—playing one active sport with regular training programme
3 points—playing more than one active sport with regular training

The simple scale works quite well if activity is stereotyped, as in the military services. In one survey, the author was able to account for 35 percent of the variation in physiological responses to exercise in terms of the simple points score, and it would be rash to conclude that more could have been achieved through using the very complex and sophisticated questionnaires available in the literature. Here we have an example of the general phenomenon that a simple and unequivocal test, well performed, gives as much or more information as complex tests that are either performed badly or have an inherent variability.

A prospective questionnaire, where the subject notes his activity as this occurs, is often more accurate than a retrospective questionnaire. Unfortunately, it may be necessary for the forms (Fig. 4) to be completed over several months, and many subjects then lose their initial enthusiasm for keeping a careful record despite frequent encouragement from the investigator. The mere act of keeping the record may also modify activity; in some individuals, the diary acts as a conscience, restricting time-wasting pursuits, while in others the extra recording necessitated by a change of activity is sufficient to keep the patient to a more restricted pattern. The accuracy of prospective records is

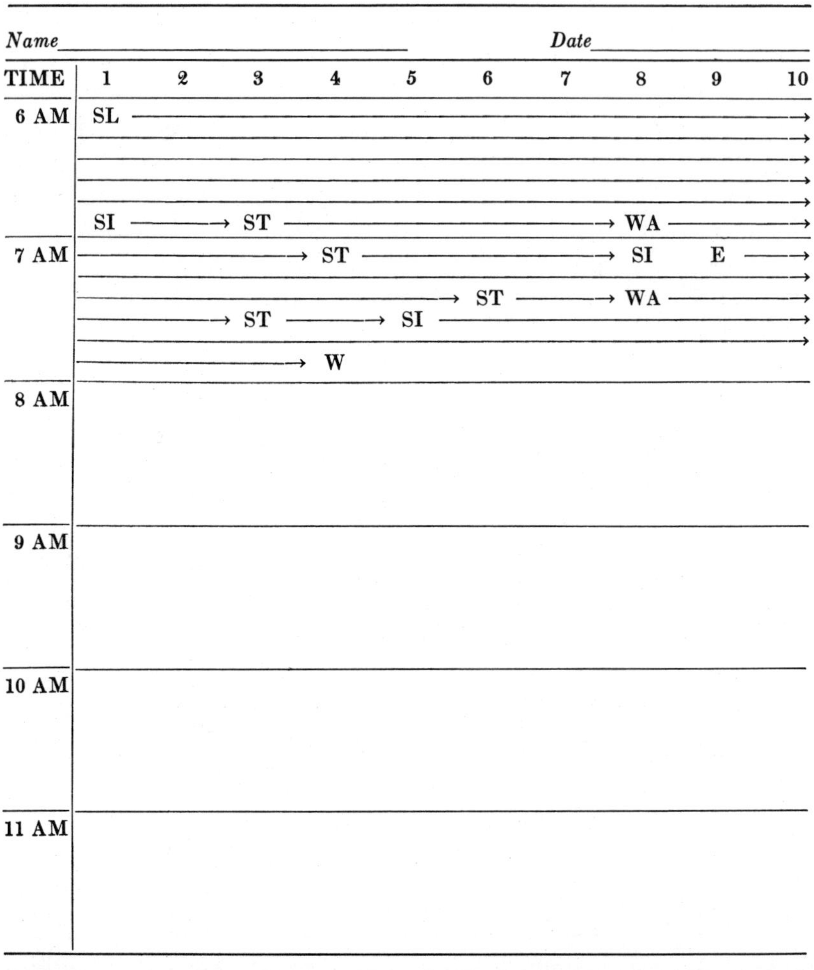

TIME	1	2	3	4	5	6	7	8	9	10

Name_____ Date_____

6 AM — SL —————————————————————————→

SI ———→ ST ————————————————→ WA ——→

7 AM ————————→ ST ———————————→ SI   E ——→

———————————————→ ST ———————→ WA ————→

————————→ ST ————→ SI ———————————————→

————————————→ W

8 AM

9 AM

10 AM

11 AM

Figure 4. A prospective diary record of habitual activity. The day is ruled into blocks of 10 × 6 minutes, and activities are indicated by a simple code (e.g. SL = sleep, SI = sitting, ST = standing, E = eating, WA = washing, WL = walking); a continuous line implies that activity has remained unchanged from that recorded for the preceding minute.

increased if they are kept by a trained observer, rather than by the subject himself; this approach is best suited to a factory or a barracks, where several individuals can be watched simultaneously. It becomes prohibitively expensive when the ratio of subjects to observers is one to one.

Sometimes it is useful to link the diary technique with "spot" measurements of the oxygen cost of listed activities; this approach has been particularly successful in calculating ration allowances for troops during manoeuvres of various types.

One final possibility for personal record keeping is an adaptation of the "points" system proposed by Lt. Col. Cooper in his best-selling paperback *Aerobics*. This system has the advantage that it is widely understood by the general public, and it permits the equation of a variety of different athletic activities. A suitable form for recording the weekly score is shown in Fig. 5.

DAY	Main Activities	Time Actually Active (min)	Points
Sunday	1. Jogging 1 mile	12 min	2
	2. Skiing	30 min	3
	3. —	—	—
Monday	1. Jogging 1 mile	12 min	2
	2. Walking 1½ miles	30 min	0
	3. —	—	—
Tuesday	1. Jogging 1 mile	12 min	2
	2. Squash	10 min	1½
	3. Walking 3 miles	60 min	1½
Wednesday	1. Squash	10 min	1½
	2. Walking 1 mile	20 min	0
	3. —	—	—
Thursday	1. Jogging 1 2/20 miles	12 min	3
	2. Skating	30 min	2
	3. Walking 3 miles	60 min	1½
Friday	1. Jogging 1 1/20 miles	12 min	3
	2. Squash	10 min	1½
	3. —	—	—
Saturday	1. Golf	9 holes	1½
	2. Walking 1 mile	20 min	0
	3. —	—	—
	Total Points for Week		*26*

Figure 5. Illustration of the use of Cooper's point system in a personal activity record.

Individual activities are awarded points according to the intensity and duration of effort, using the tables given in Cooper's book.*

* Some of the point values are open to question; however, this does not invalidate the usefulness of the underlying principle.

Instrumentation. One simple mechanical device for epidemiological measurements of chronic activity is a pedometer. This looks rather like a pocket watch and is hung from the belt or a side pocket. A ratchet controlling movement of the hands is released once for each swing of the leg. The speed of movement of the hands is adjusted according to pace length, so that the scale indicates the total mileage traversed. This device is most suited to sedentary workers whose principal source of energy expenditure is occasional walking. It does not give a reliable index of activity if much work is performed by the arms, or the ratchet is released by vibration of the body.

Tape recordings of the electrocardiogram can be used over an extended period; however, large scale trials await the development of a cheap tape recorder that will run at a constant speed even when subjected to vigorous vibration. The data reduction equipment that converts the ECG signal to a minute by minute pulse count is also complex and expensive at the present time.

If one is interested simply in the average pulse rate over a specified part of the working day, then it is possible to carry out the averaging of the ECG signal as the test proceeds. One device that will accomplish this is the Wolff electrochemical integrator (SAMI).* The signal from each pulse beat deposits a few molecules of silver on a gold electrode. After use, an electrical current is passed through the integrating cell to restore its initial chemical status; from the period of wear, and the current passed, the mean pulse count is deduced. The ECG amplifier and integrating cell is not much larger than a package of cigarettes, and it is readily slipped into the pocket of the subject; the main problem is to ensure that the sensing electrodes do not work loose, and the subject is provided with a small earphone so that he can "hear" any irregularity in the pulse signal fed to the apparatus. The SAMI pulse integrator has been used successfully by the inventor and his colleagues to demonstrate that the average heart rate of London bus drivers is appreciably lower than that of the "conductors" who collect the fares.

Assessment of Food Intake. There can be a surprisingly large discrepancy between the intake and the expenditure of energy if comparisons are made over the period of a day or two. However, it has been known since the classical studies of Voit (1831–1908) that the principle of the conservation of matter applies to man. Thus, if the study is extended over several weeks, and the body

---

* SAMI = Socially acceptable monitoring instrument.

weight remains constant, the average energy expenditure must equal the caloric value of ingested food, less small losses in urine, faeces, and (particularly alcohol) in exhaled gas. A careful record of food consumption can thus be used to assess the mean cost of protracted activity. Let us take the example of a miner, working at the pit face six hours per day for five days per week (Table I). From experiments where various food products have

TABLE I

TO ILLUSTRATE A CALCULATION OF THE ENERGY COST OF MINING FROM MEASUREMENTS OF FOOD CONSUMPTION

Food Intake	Weight gm	Energy Value, kcal
Protein	86	350
Fat	141	1230
Carbohydrate	414	1590
Alcohol	83	580
		3750
Losses in Excreta		150
Daily Expenditure		3600

Weekly Expenditure   25,200 kcal
Weekly Expenditure of Office Worker = 2300 × 7 = 16,100 kcal
Additional Energy Cost of Mining   = 9,100 kcal per 5 day week
                                                       = 1,820 kcal per 6 hr day
                                                       = 5.1 kcal per minute
Cost of Sitting at Office Desk   = 1.7 kcal per minute
Average Cost of Mining   = 6.8 kcal per minute

been burnt in a bomb calorimeter, it is known that the heat yields of protein, fat, carbohydrate, and alcohol are respectively 4.1, 9.3, 3.8, and 7.0 kcal/gm. The protein, fat, and carbohydrate content of the miner's diet is obtained from tables, and the corresponding energy value is calculated (3750 kcal/day); after allowing for loss of combustible material in the urine, faeces, and exhaled gas (about 150 kcal/day), the average intake and expenditure of energy must be 3600 kcal per day, or 25,200 kcal/week. This may be compared with the weekly energy expenditure of an office worker (16,000 kcal). Assuming that weekend and leisure pursuits are similar, the miner consumes 1820 kcal more energy than the office worker in six hours at the coal face—an excess expenditure of just over 5.1 kcal/min. The cost of sitting at an office desk is about 1.7 kcal/min, so the average rate of energy expenditure at the coal face must be 6.8 kcal/min.

It is interesting to note the large calorie yield of alcohol. In the example cited, the miner drank 3 pints of 6% beer per day—a conservative estimate for many mining communities! It is not surprising that sedentary workers who are fond of alcohol gain weight unless they make substantial reductions in the intake of conventional foodstuffs.

References

Shephard. R.J.: *Endurance Fitness.* Toronto. University of Toronto Press, 1969.

Shephard, R.J.: For exercise testing, please. A review of procedures available to the clinician. *Bull Physio—Pathol Resp (Nancy):* 6:425–474. 1970.

Andersen, L.A. *et al.: Fundamentals of Exercise Testing.* Geneva, WHO Monograph. 1971.

Shephard. R.J. (Rapporteur): Exercise tests in relation to cardiovascular function. *WHO Tech Rep, 388.*

Weiner, J.S., and Lourie, J.A.: *Human Biology—A Guide to Field Methods.* Oxford, Blackwell, 1969.

Mellerowicz, H.: *Ergometrie,* Munich, Urban & Schwarzenberg, 1962.

Durnin, J.V.G.A., and Passmore, R.: *Energy, Work, and Leisure.* London, Heinemann, 1967.

Cooper, K.H.: *The New Aerobics.* New York, Evans, 1970.

3

THE BASIS OF HUMAN PERFORMANCE

Before proceeding with our study of specific physiological and biochemical responses to physical activity, we will consider in more general terms the reactions of the body to this endogenous assault upon its environment. The ultimate disturbance of the milieu interieur depends not only upon the rate of the forward reaction, but also the nature and extent of any compensatory processes that may be invoked.

At a first inspection, the intensity of physical activity seems to be determined by the primary rate of the forward reaction—limiting factors include the local stores of biochemical fuels, the rate at which these stores can be supplemented from the blood stream, the rate at which combustion can occur, and the availability of oxygen to the active tissues. However, on closer examination, we find that activity is also dependent upon numerous feedback mechanisms. Some help the movement itself (for instance, the relaxation of antagonistic muscles). Others seek to restore the constancy of the internal environment (for instance, the increased activity of the cardiorespiratory system and the mobilization of liver glycogen). Others, again, inhibit the forward reaction; of these, inhibitory mechanisms originating in the cerebral cortex are perhaps the most important.

Factors Influencing the Forward Reaction

Brief Local Activity

Let us suppose that a specific group of muscles engage in a brief period of activity that does not require any substantial change in their length; a good example would be the performance of a simple handgrip test of muscular strength. The force that is developed depends largely upon the inherent strength of the muscles called into action. However, motivation, skill, and agility all help to determine whether the inherent potential of the muscle group is realized. *Motivation* is a complex phenomenon, and lies too much in the realm of the psychologist to discuss here; to a first approximation, we may regard an improvement of motivation as a removal of some of the normal inhibitory feedback from the higher centres of the brain. *Skill* is also a complex matter; it involves both constitutional aptitudes and the ability to learn new movement patterns. Information must be stored in the brain and relayed to the muscle fibres at an appropriate signal. *Agility* is strongly influenced by constitution and flexibility; the latter is maintained and developed by regular activity, appropriate warm-up procedures and adequate relaxation of antagonistic muscle groups.

If a muscle is allowed to shorten, a substantial part of the power developed by the contracting fibres is dissipated in overcoming internal viscous resistance. The external force is then markedly influenced by the *rate of shortening* of the muscle fibres, the temperature at which shortening occurs, and the extent of any imposed load.

Brief General Activity

Participation in a one hundred yard track and field event provides a good example of brief general activity. The rate of energy expenditure may be ten times that of a more protracted event such as a one mile race. The performance realised by the sprinter depends in part upon the static and dynamic strength of the active muscles, in part upon their energy stores, and in part upon the rate at which stored energy can be released. *Reaction time, skill,* and *motivation* also influence the outcome of the race, but the event is often completed without taking a single breath; the efficiency of the oxygen supply mechanisms thus makes no contribution to performance.

Sustained General Activity

The nature and extent of the body energy stores are such that activity cannot be sustained for much more than a minute in the absence of a steady oxygen supply. In more prolonged activity, such as a 5000 metre race, the rate of the forward reaction depends on the rate at which oxygen can be conducted from the atmosphere to the active tissues. A chain of transport mechanisms is involved, including the lungs, heart, circulation, extracellular and intracellular diffusion, and ultimately the transfer of electrons between a series of closely linked oxidation-reduction reactions.

The movement produced by a given energy expenditure depends upon the *mechanical efficiency* of the performer. This is influenced by such factors as inherent and acquired *skill*, the *posture* in which the activity is undertaken, and the proportion of the body musculature that can be brought to bear upon the task. *Strength* must be adequate to maintain posture and permit perfusion of the active muscles; on the other hand, an excessive development of muscle increases the body weight that must be propelled. If activity is pushed to the limit imposed by oxygen transport mechanisms, a number of unpleasant sensations must be overcome, and *motivation* then influences the rate of the forward reaction.

Very Prolonged Activity

If a population is observed closely, it is surprising how few industrial, recreational and domestic activities involve more than one hour of continuous work. However, there are occasional circumstances such as marathon running and long-distance cycling events where a more protracted effort is required.

The quantities of metabolic fuel stored within the active cells are inevitably finite, and are normally exhausted in sixty to ninety minutes. During sustained activity, local resources (glycogen and fat) must be supplemented by glucose and fatty acids derived from the blood stream. Once intracellular food stores are exhausted, performance becomes limited by the vascular supply of foodstuffs, and by possible adverse effects of a falling blood sugar level upon cerebral function.

Large quantities of *body fluid* are lost during prolonged work. *Exudation* into the tissues is increased, *sweat* production may amount to 1 to 2 litres per hour, and in some climates as much as 0.5 litres of water per hour may be lost in *exhaled gas*. In some circumstances, the forward reaction can thus be limited by the ability to replenish body fluids and associated mineral ions.

Inefficiencies in the conversion of chemical to mechanical energy lead to a progressive accumulation of *heat* within the body as work continues. The rise of body temperature is appreciable, even under temperate conditions, and in a warmer climate it can quite rapidly limit performance.

Habitual Activity

Little is known of the factors that cause some people to engage repeatedly in vigorous activity, while others remain content with a more sedentary existence. We suspect a large role is played by the influence of family and friends; possibly there are also "activity" centres within the brain that create a drive for energy expenditure.

Feedback Mechanisms Limiting Physical Activity

Brief Local Activity

If a muscle undergoes intense contraction without shortening, a series of feedback mechanisms are rapidly initiated. The rise of tension within individual fibres is sensed by local receptors. These tend to inhibit the contraction, but fortunately the body has evolved a mechanism for resetting the sensitivity of the control loop (the gamma reflex, p. 175). Activity can thus continue, while at the same time the muscle receptors inform the brain of the rate of rise of tension within the system.

One serious effect of the increasing intramuscular tension is an occlusion of the local blood supply. In the absence of a suitable feedback loop, this would inevitably limit the subsequent duration of muscular activity. Fortunately, the changing chemical environment within the muscle stimulates appropriate "chemoreceptors," and through a control loop that passes to the cardiac and circulatory centres of the medulla, a progressive increase of systemic blood pressure is induced. This improves, but does not fully restore circulation through the tensed muscles. A further feedback loop now comes into play. The rising systemic blood pressure stimulates fibres in the aorta and at the bifurcation of the common carotid arteries, and impulses tending to reduce systemic blood pressure are transmitted back to the medulla. Nevertheless, the local drive from the muscles remains dominant, and blood pressure continues to rise.

The time for which a muscular contraction can be held depends upon the balance that is struck between the local accumulation of metabolic by-products and their removal by the circulation. It is more problematical whether the cumulative change of chemical environment itself inhibits the forward reaction, or whether painful sensations associated with the build-up of waste products lead to a "voluntary" inhibition of activity mediated via the higher centres of the brain. Certainly, both the intensity and the duration of contraction can be enhanced by increasing the motivation of a subject.

If a muscle is allowed to perform external work by intermittent shortening against an external load, the duration of activity is extended. However, the forward reaction still ceases after a specific number of repetitions of a given task have been completed. Despite the intermittent nature of the contractions, blood flow may be inadequate to meet metabolic demands, and a failure of oxygen supply or a delay in restoration of the status quo may contribute to ultimate exhaustion. Nevertheless, the main limitation is motivational, and arises within the central nervous system.

Brief General Activity

Any system of feedback loops introduces an element of delay. The time involved in simple adjustments to exercise, such as the relaxation of antagonistic muscles, is a small fraction of a second, being determined by the speed of impulse transmission through connecting nerve fibres and intervening synapses.

Many of the cybernetic processes that regulate muscular activity operate much more slowly, and in events such as a fifty-yard dash there is thus little to inhibit forward movement except the inertia of the body and incomplete relaxation of the antagonistic muscles. Once motion is initiated, indeed, a conscious effort may be needed to check progress beyond the finishing line.

After some fifteen seconds of general activity, energy stores of phosphagen molecules (p. 398) and expendable oxygen stores (p. 152) are both exhausted. Over the next thirty seconds, further energy is derived largely from the incomplete breakdown of glycogen to lactate, a reaction that requires no oxygen but leads to an accummulation of acid waste products (p. 166). The local pH change provides negative feedback in two ways. It causes fatigue and pain within the active muscles, and also leads to a disproportionate breathlessness as the acid blood reaches the centres controlling respiration (p. 27). The "capacity" of the lactate system is exhausted in three quarters of a minute, and at this stage an unpleasant degree of breathlessness makes itself felt. There is thus a marked slowing of performance between a 440 yard run (45 seconds, average speed 20.1 mph) and an 880 yard run (one minute 45 seconds, average speed 17.2 mph).

Sustained General Activity

Sustained general activity initiates a chain of feedback mechanisms, the majority of which are designed to minimize chemical changes within the active tissues and the blood stream. The nervous pathways involved have yet to be specified in detail, but there is a surprisingly accurate matching of ventilation and blood flow to the increased peripheral demand; further, the output of the heart is selectively redistributed, meeting the needs of the active muscles and cutaneous circulation at the expense of the viscera and inactive tissues.

Performance of several minutes duration is normally limited by voluntary feedback. The individual so paces his efforts that demand equals oxygen supply, without trespassing upon the oxygen debt mechanisms used in shorter bursts of activity. Lactate accumulation, with attendant muscular fatigue, pain, and respiratory distress is deferred until the final half minute of an event and the subsequent recovery period. However, if an individual is to realize his full potential performance, the maximum oxygen intake must be developed as rapidly as possible and sustained throughout the subsequent course of the race. A consistent pace is helpful in minimizing wind resistance. If a competitor has the misfortune to be outpaced by his rivals, he tends to run too fast. Lactate then accumulates at an earlier point in the contest, and negative feedback results. If local fatigue, pain and breathlessness are ignored, the contestant may push himself to a second limit imposed by his oxygen transporting system. The heart cannot beat any faster, for if it attempted to do so its own oxygen supply would be compromised. The amount of blood pumped per beat has also reached the maximum possible value, and the output of the heart is still inadequate to meet the combined demands of skin, muscle, and brain. The blood supply to the brain falters. Coordination deteriorates, vision is impaired and consciousness is lost; central circulatory failure thus provides a potent method of arresting physical effort.

Very Prolonged Activity

A sensation of general weakness and fatigue is a common reason for the slowing and ultimate cessation of very prolonged physical activity.

The feedback mechanism involved may be the local accumulation of acid breakdown products of metabolism. Such compounds can build up steadily over the course of a working day, particularly if a task is performed in an unfavourable body position and rest periods are short or nonexistent.

A second potent factor is exhaustion of the glycogen stores; with maximum activity, this occurs in sixty to ninety minutes. Thereafter, exercise is dependent on the availability of oxygen and blood-borne metabolites. Short bursts of anaerobic work (as might be incurred when cycling up a steep hill) become virtually impossible. A number of "biochemical messengers" such as adrenaline and the pituitary growth hormone are released. These attempt to maintain blood levels of sugar and fatty acids by the breakdown of liver glycogen and depot fat respectively. At the same time, intramuscular concentrations of sugar and fat are supported by a more ready transport of these materials across the cell membrane. Liver glycogen stores are exhausted by one to two hours of maximum effort, and unless an athlete is provided with a sugary drink at this stage, there is a precipitate fall of blood glucose; this leads in turn to negative feedback from fatigue of the central nervous system.

In a hot climate, fluid loss may become a dominant factor. Initially, less blood is returned to the heart, and the output per beat thus drops. The blood flow to the viscera is further restricted in a desperate attempt to meet the combined needs of muscle and skin, but the possibility of compensation at the expense of the internal organs is small. Exercise may thus be terminated by central circulatory failure and loss of consciousness. Occasionally, a contestant may continue to stagger forwards by a supreme feat of willpower. Various dangerous positive feedback loops may then be activated, including failure of the sweat glands, with a rapid rise of body temperature, and failure of the kidneys and adrenal glands with diminishing regulation of both vascular tone and the composition of body fluids.

It is rare for a progressively rising body temperature to provide the necessary feedback to limit activity. However, an observer would do well to halt exercise when the body temperature passes 104°F, since there is then imminent danger of fatal hyperpyrexia.

Habitual Activity

Since little is known of factors provoking habitual activity, it is hardly surprising that we are equally ignorant as to the basis of satiety. Current "explanations" speak of changes in mood and arousal, induced by exercise, and possibly hormonal in origin. It is conceivable that a given individual becomes accustomed to a certain level of arousal, and persists with physical activity until this level is reached.

Relationship to Performance on the Track

Having considered the various factors that determine the maximum rate of energy release, and negative feedback loops that inhibit further performance, it is of interest to test how well physiological concepts match the actual performance of an athlete. Lloyd has carried out such an analysis for runners (Fig. 6). Ignoring

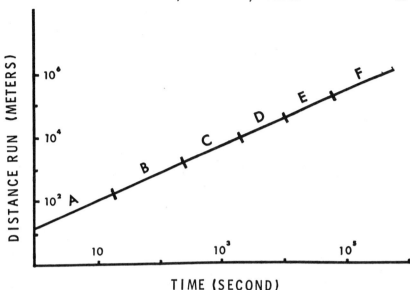

Figure 6. The relationship between distance run and record time. Data up to August 1965, collected by Lloyd. The time zones A-F are discussed in the text.

differences of body configuration between contestants in short, medium, and long distance events, and considering jointly all data from a fifty-yard dash to a marathon race, a suitable descriptive equation is as follows:

$$\text{Log } X = 1.11 + 0.9 \text{ Log } t$$

where X is the running distance in metres, and t is the record time for this distance, measured in seconds.

Many years ago, Hill argued that the energy of a runner (E) was derived from two sources—a store (S), and an "income" of R per unit time. According to this theory, the energy available for a race lasting t seconds would be given by a linear relationship of the type

$$E = S + Rt$$

The power P is equal to the rate of energy usage, so that

$$P = E/t = S/t + R$$

Furthermore, the running speed V is necessarily a function of power, so that

$$P = A + BV^n$$

where A, B, and n are constants. Thus we may write

$$S/t + R = A + BV^n$$

and if n can be made equal to unity, the last equation can be rewritten in the form

$$Vt = \frac{S}{B} + t(R - A)/B$$

In other words, the distance run $(X = Vt)$ becomes a linear function of t. At a first glance, this seems at variance with Lloyd's equation, with Fig. 6, and with our preceding discussion of the several critical factors that each limit power output for differing periods of time. However, in practice, a linear relationship can be attained if data is restricted to a brief range of times. One process is then dominant, and variations in speed and thus wind resistance are of secondary importance. Wind resistance varies as the third power of running speed (page 534); thus, if it accounts for 10 percent of the constant B at 11 mph, it will amount to 40 percent at 22 mph. Slopes applicable to different ranges of distance are shown in Fig. 7.

Line (a) describes the observed data quite well for events of 100–200 metre distance, but times for the 50 metre event are displaced to the right, presumably an expression of the effort involved in accelerating the body mass. The times under discussion (6–20 sec) coincide with the previously specified first phase of brief general activity. As the duration of an event is increased, the diminishing importance of inertia is offset by a progressive and probably an exponential exhaustion of oxygen and phosphagen stores.

Line (b) describes the data from 800 to 1600 metres, but the 400 metre point lies a little to the right; we are here dealing with the classical Hill equation—a combination of a steady oxygen intake and a fixed total oxygen debt—the normal basis of sustained general activity. The time required to cover 400 metres is a little greater than that predicted from the linear equation, since the maximum oxygen intake is not reached immediately; there is an "on-transient" lasting for a minute or more, depending upon the speed and efficiency of adaptation of the cardiorespiratory system to exercise. If we assume a fixed relationship between energy expenditure and the distance covered (0.065 kcal/m), we can estimate the maximum oxygen intake from the slope of line (b); the very reasonable value of 5.1 litre/min is obtained. The intercept of line (b) is 149 m, corresponding to 22.8 kcal, a very reasonable estimate of oxygen debt.

The slope of line (c), covering the range 1500 to 9000 metres (4 to 30 minutes of activity) is a little less than for line (b).

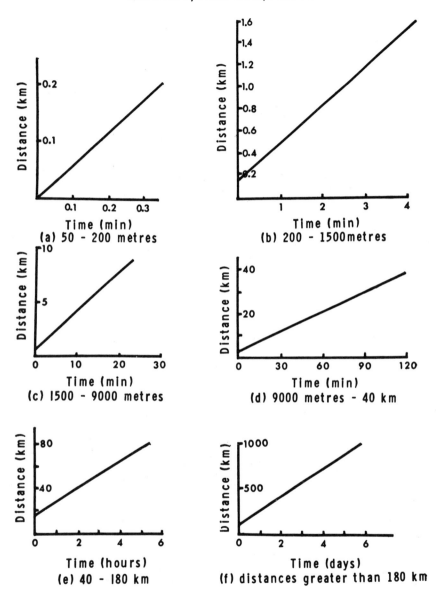

Figure 7. The relationship between time and distance run. Linear scales, based on data of Lloyd.

Expressing both slopes in terms of the equivalent oxygen intake, the respective values are 4.8 and 5.1 litre/min. The difference, about 6 percent, is most readily explained in terms of the diversion of an equivalent percentage of the cardiac output from the active muscles to the skin, in an attempt to minimize the rise of deep body temperature. It is also possible that the efficiency of effort has fallen somewhat due to a progressive increase of ventilation, an increase of systemic blood pressure (and thus cardiac work), a transition from carbohydrate to fat metabolism, and an accumulation of acid metabolites in the tissues. The zero intercept of line (c) amounts to 212 metres, equivalent to 32.8 kcal; it thus seems possible that secondary factors such as changes of metabolic fuel and a progressive heating of the body are beginning to distort the classical Hill relationship between distance, energy stores and oxygen supply.

A further break in the line occurs at about thirty minutes. The slope (d) now diminishes to 20.4 kcal/min, or (allowing for a high percentage of fat combustion) about 4.6 litre/min oxygen intake. The zero intercept increases to almost 1.3 km (74 kcal of energy). We are now reaching the phase of prolonged activity, where the rate of the forward reaction is influenced by the transport not only of oxygen but also of metabolic fuels and body heat. By analogy, the nature of the zero intercept changes to correspond with either a store of fuel or a heat sink.

Line (e) describes the data from two to five hours; the slope has now decreased to 14.1 kcal/min, or about 3.3 litre/min oxygen intake; we are looking very largely at the ability of the body to transport metabolic fuels, and oxygen supply mechanisms have become of lesser importance. The zero intercept of 13.4 km corresponds to 870 kcal. If we assume that 1 gm of glycogen yields 3.8 kcal of energy (p. 475), then this would imply an initial glycogen store of 230 gm. In fact, body glycogen stores amount to some 500 gm. (p. 479), but the figure of 230 gm. may be realistic for that fraction of the body musculature involved in distance running.

The final line (f) has a much shallower slope, because activity over such extended periods is necessarily varied in type (walking and jogging) with occasional pauses for massage, refreshment, and even sleep.

The measurement of distance and the timing of athletic events are both more precise than biochemical and physiological tests. It is thus interesting that laboratory concepts are substantiated by track performance. Nevertheless, we must turn to the procedures of exercise physiology and biochemistry in order to understand current human limitations and to suggest procedures whereby the performance of both the athlete and the worker may legitimately be enhanced.

Reference

Lloyd, B.: Presidential address, Section I (Physiology and Biochemistry), British Association. In *Advancement of Sciences*, 515–530 (1966).

4

THE CARDIOVASCULAR SYSTEM

The Dominant Role of the Circulation in Sustained Exercise

The dominant role of the circulation in sustained exercise is brought out by a simple calculation. Conductance, $\dot{U}$, is the reciprocal of resistance R; $\frac{1}{\dot{U}} = R$. Thus, if the conductance of oxygen, $\dot{U}_{O_2}$, is large, the resistance to its transport is small. Under normal conditions, the transport of oxygen from the atmosphere to the working tissues is limited by two conductances, arranged in series—alveolar ventilation (represented by the standard abbreviation*$\dot{V}_A$) and blood transport ($\lambda\dot{Q}$, the product of the solubility of oxygen in unit volume of blood, λ, and the cardiac output, $\dot{Q}$). The overall resistance, $1/\dot{U}$, is thus given by

$$\frac{1}{\dot{U}} = \frac{1}{\dot{V}_A} + \frac{1}{\lambda\dot{Q}}$$

Since the maximum value of $\dot{V}_A$ is about 80 litre/min, λ is close to unity, and the maximum value of $\dot{Q}$ is about 25 litre/min, the equation may be written:

$$\frac{1}{\dot{U}_{O_2}} = \frac{1}{80} + \frac{1}{1(25)}$$

In other words, the overall resistance to oxygen transport, $1/\dot{U}$, depends more on cardiac output than on alveolar ventilation. In the case of carbon dioxide, the solubility factor λ is larger (about 5), and the equation thus reads

$$\frac{1}{\dot{U}_{CO_2}} = \frac{1}{80} + \frac{1}{5(25)}$$

Elimination of carbon dioxide depends more on alveolar ventilation than on blood transport.

---

* See page 556 for a discussion of standard abbreviations.

Circulatory Priorities in Exercise

The basic functions of the circulation are to carry oxygen, metabolic fuels, vitamins, hormones and heat to individual cells, and to remove the end products of cellular metabolism (carbon dioxide, water, and excessive heat). In the resting state, this presents little problem. However, during intense exercise, the heart is fully stressed, and priorities must be reviewed if activity is to be sustained and local cellular damage avoided.

Individual tissues have differing oxygen needs. In some, the demand is relatively high (2–4 ml/100 gm/min); examples are the kidney, liver, brain, and the intestinal mucosa. In other tissues, oxygen usage is moderate (0.7–1.3 ml/100 gm/min, for example the spleen and lung) or low (0.3 ml/100 gm/min or less, for example fat, skin and bone). The demands of any given tissue vary with temperature. According to the "law" of Arrhenius, oxygen consumption ($\dot{V}_{O_2}$) is approximately doubled for every 10°C rise of temperature, according to the equation

$$\dot{V}_{O_2} = Ae^{-\mu/R_0 T}$$

where A, μ, and R_0 are constants, and T is the absolute temperature. We certainly cannot assume a body temperature of 37°C during sustained exercise. Even if the day is quite cool (say 20°C), the core temperature of a marathon runner can rise to 40–41°C. On the other hand, in colder weather the temperature of inactive peripheral tissues may fall quite markedly, perhaps to 20 or 25°C. When calculating circulatory demands, we must thus reckon with the fourfold variation in oxygen requirements induced by changes in tissue temperature.

Individual tissues also differ quite markedly in their susceptibility to oxygen lack. If a major artery of the arm is torn, a tourniquet can be applied for as much as twenty minutes without causing irreversible damage. On the other hand, if a branch of the coronary arterial tree is occluded either by spasm of the vessel wall or by lodgement of a blood clot, the tissue distal to the occlusion dies in five to ten minutes, giving the clinical picture of "coronary infarction." The brain is even more susceptible to loss of its normal blood supply. If the circulation is arrested (through cardiac standstill, or the irregular and ineffective pattern of ventricular activity known as fibrillation), then irreversible changes occur within four minutes. Subsequent attempts at resuscitation may be technically successful, but it is likely the patient will be permanently deprived of his higher mental faculties.

At rest, several body tissues are overperfused. The skin accounts for some 5 percent of oxygen consumption, yet it receives 10 percent of cardiac output; the kidneys, again, account for 10 percent of oxygen consumption, but receive 25 percent of the cardiac output. The explanation is that in these tissues the blood supply meets demands other than oxygen consumption—the elimination of heat in the skin, and of waste products in the kidney. During vigorous exercise, the blood flow to the kidneys and other visceral organs is progressively reduced. This change is particularly obvious if the environment is hot, and under such circumstances the flow may ultimately fall to less than a third of the normal resting value. At this stage, a considerable reduction of visceral function is seen; the ability of the kidney to excrete test substances such as para-amino hippurate is depressed, and the liver shows a parallel reduction in the clearance of bromsulphthalein from the circulation. In general, the effects of the visceral ischemia are reversible, but there is some cellular damage; enzymes from the renal and hepatic tissues are liberated into the blood stream, and the urine may contain red cells, casts, and protein (pp. 97, 233).

The blood flow to the skin is not reduced in moderate exercise—indeed, it usually increases, as more heat must be eliminated from the body. However, a rather sudden decrease occurs as the maximum oxygen intake is approached. The body makes a last desperate search for blood, and the face of the athlete assumes an ashen gray pallor. Certain drugs, such as amphetamines, produce cutaneous vasoconstriction at a lower intensity of exercise. Performance may be improved thereby, but the penalty is an impairment of heat elimination, and this penalty is reputed to have cost at least one life in an international contest (see further p. 323).

Exercise Cardiac Output and Heart Size

Heart Rate

The resting heart rate varies from less than 30 beats/min in a superb athlete to as much as 100 beats/min in a sedentary middle-aged executive awaiting his annual medical examination (p. 401). In general, readings are greater in women and in young children than in men; they are also increased by standing, smoking, and the recent ingestion of food. However, if these variables are controlled or eliminated, then there is a fairly close inverse relationship between cardiorespiratory fitness and pulse rate. Training increases the resting stroke volume without changing the cardiac output; thus there is an inevitable decrease of resting pulse rate.

When a young man performs maximum exercise at sea level, his heart rate is about 195 beats per minute. Transient values of up to 250 beats per minute have been recorded during a few seconds of very intense exercise, but it is unusual to find an adult who can maintain a rate of more than 200/min over several minutes. The factor limiting heart rate is unknown, but there is a regular decline of the maximum with age, so that in a 60-year-old man the peak value is no more than 155–160/min. In young women, the average maximum value is a little higher than in men of the same age (198/min); again, there is a progressive decline of this maximum with age. There have been suggestions that the maximum heart rate is a little lower in athletes than in sedentary subjects. However, this is difficult to document; most of the reports making this claim have not measured the pulse rate during an actual race, but rather have required the athlete to perform an unaccustomed mode of exercise in the laboratory.

A typical heart rate response to submaximum exercise is illustrated in Fig. 8. At the beginning of exercise, there is a rapid increase of pulse rate. If the work load is moderate, a plateau is reached in one to two min, but if the exercise is more severe, the rate continues to increase until the subject is exhausted. The factors regulating heart rate are discussed later in this Chapter, but we may note here that the initial rapid increase is partly a conditioned reflex, and partly

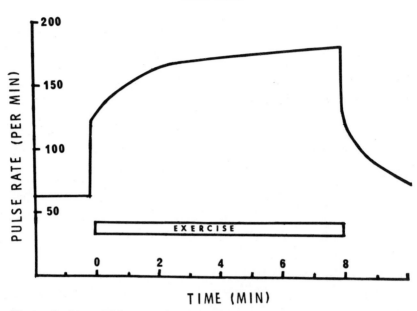

Figure 8. A typical heart rate response to a period of submaximal exercise.

a response to irradiation of impulses from the motor cortex. Further increments of pulse rate are a response to local vasodilation in the active muscles and stimulation of proprioceptors in the moving limbs. The final phase of slowly climbing pulse rate during exhausting work reflects several factors including a rising deep body temperature, the recruitment of less efficient muscles as fatigue sets in and a general increase of apprehension. Recovery after exercise also follows a complex curve—there is an initial rapid slowing, due to removal of cortical and proprioceptive stimulation, and a second slower phase when metabolites are being removed from the active tissues and body temperature is returning towards its normal resting value.

Over much of the working range, the plateau pulse rate is proportional to oxygen consumption (p. 26). However, higher rates are encountered for arm than for leg work, for static than for dynamic effort, and for exercise in a hot or emotionally charged rather than a "neutral" environment.

If exercise is discontinuous, the completeness of recovery depends upon both the intensity of work and the length of the intervening rest periods. With relatively light effort, many repetitions may be undertaken, and there is a complete recovery between each bout, but if the exercise is more severe, a cumulative displacement of the recovery pulse rate is seen. For the purpose of interval training, this cumulative stress is allowed to develop until it is adjudged that the necessary training stimulus has been applied (p. 449). In industry, rest pauses should be of sufficient length that recovery is fairly complete. The necessary time is longer in a hot than in a cool environment, suggesting that a major factor in delayed recovery is an elevation of the deep body temperature.

Stroke Volume

The stroke volume of the resting subject depends upon body posture. When lying down, it may be 120 ml per beat, but when standing or sitting it is only about 80 ml. The reason for this difference is that blood pools in the veins of the leg when a person is standing erect. Most types of exercise improve the venous return from the lower half of the body. Thus, if a man is exercising his legs in an upright or a seated position, his stroke volume increases progressively from 80 to about 120 ml as the oxygen consumption increases to perhaps 50 percent of his maximum oxygen intake. On the other hand, if a standing subject performs exercise with his arms, blood tends to remain pooled in the lower half of the body, and the stroke volume is much poorer. If the subject is recumbent, the legs are at or above heart level, and there is little tendency for blood to pool in the lower half of the body even before exercise is commenced. Thus, under these circumstances, the resting stroke volume is quite large, and it does not increase with exercise.

The stroke volume is increased by cardiorespiratory training. Thus, while a sedentary young man may have a maximum cardiac output of 24 litre/min (200 x 120 ml), an athlete may have a maximum output as high as 30–36 litre/min (200 x 150–180 ml). One factor contributing to the larger stroke volume of the athlete is an increase of blood volume. It follows that any factor leading to a decrease of blood volume (excessive sweating, prolonged hyperventilation in dry mountain air, prolonged physical effort) is associated with a reduction of stroke volume.

End-diastolic Volume

The heart is not completely emptied with each beat. At rest, some 70 to 80 ml of blood remain within the left ventricle. Thus, the exercising heart may increase its output either by filling more fully during diastole, or by emptying more completely during systole. Both mechanisms are probably operative.

The relationship between diastolic filling and stroke volume was first explored by Starling, at the beginning of the present century. He used an isolated dog "heart-lung" preparation. This enabled him to vary the degree of diastolic filling and to measure the resultant stroke volume rather precisely. He was able to produce beautiful curves showing that as diastolic filling increased, there was a progressive increase of stroke volume until a certain limit was reached (Fig. 9). Beyond this point, further filling led to the dangerous situation of a progressively decreasing stroke volume.

Unfortunately, Starling's preparation was dissected free of all nerve supply; furthermore, it did not receive the normal complement of circulating catecholamines such as adrenaline and noradrenaline. Some authors have thus found difficulty in reproducing Starling's results in exercising man. The explanation seems that when exercise is performed, a combination of increased activity of the sympathetic nerves, decreased activity of the parasympathetic system, and an outpouring of catecholamines moves the operating characteristic of the heart leftwards to a new Starling curve; a larger stroke volume is produced for a given filling, and at least initially the heart is emptied more completely at each beat. Part of the "reservoir" provided by the end-systolic volume is thus driven into the active part of the circulation.

It is not unknown for patients with valvular disease of the heart to pass the "hump" of the Starling curve. While they remain on the ascending limb, a worsening of their valvular

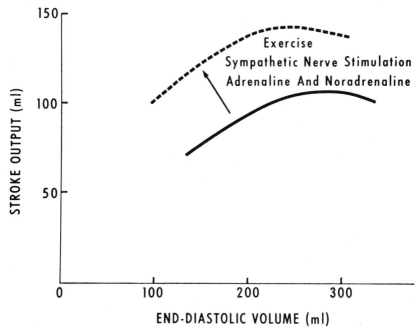

Figure 9. The relationship between end-diastolic volume and stroke output of the ventricle ("Starling's law of the heart"). Note the effects of exercise, sympathetic nerve stimulation, and administration of adrenaline and noradrenaline upon this relationship.

leakage or the demands of mild exercise are met by an increase of stroke volume—the heart failure is said to be "compensated." However, exercise of unaccustomed severity or a further deterioration of the diseased valve may bring them to a position where a further increase of diastolic volume leads to a diminution of stroke volume. Heart failure is now said to be "decompensated," and urgent treatment is required. The blood volume must be reduced (by diuretics and a low salt diet), and the operating characteristics of the heart must be moved to a more favourable Starling curve (by the use of drugs such as digitalis). It is unlikely that healthy people either can or will exercise to the point of decompensation. Certainly, subjective complaints and loss of the erect posture normally prevent this from occurring.

The Starling mechanism was originally thought responsible for the increased cardiac output of exercise. Muscular activity increased the return of blood from the leg veins, thereby increasing the diastolic volume and thus the stroke output. Unfortunately for this hypothesis, the diastolic volume is not necessarily increased in exercise, and it is now realised that the body has more important mechanisms for the increase of cardiac output during work. The main role of the Starling mechanism is probably to equalize the output of the two sides of the heart. Let us suppose that in maximum exercise, the output of the right ventricle increased from 5 litre/min to 25 litre/min, while that of the left ventricle increased from 5 litre/min to 24 litre/min; in a mere five minutes, the entire blood volume would be waterlogging the lungs. Fortunately, the Starling mechanism permits a much more precise balancing of output between the two circulations, and such problems are avoided.

Heart Size

The approximate heart volume is calculated quite readily from posteroanterior and lateral chest radiographs (Fig. 10);

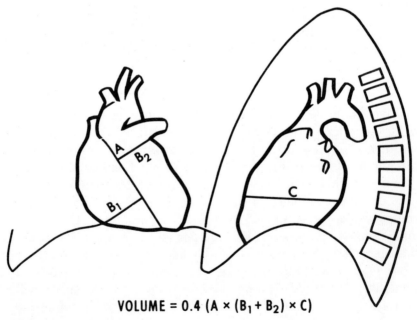

$$\text{VOLUME} = 0.4 \, (A \times (B_1 + B_2) \times C)$$

Figure 10. Calculation of the cardiac volume from postero-anterior and lateral chest radiographs.

the volume (ml) is 0.4 (A x B x C), where A, B, and C are measurements of the three principal dimensions in centimetres.

There is a general relationship between physical activity and heart size; thus the heart volume of a sedentary young man is about 11 ml/kg of body weight, while that of an athlete may be as much as 14 ml/kg. The heart is particularly well-developed in endurance athletes, such as long distance cyclists. It is generally assumed that hypertrophy of the cardiac muscle has occurred in response to the repeated demands of exercise. Careful studies to separate inheritance of a large heart from a true training response have yet to be carried out in man, but we know that a similar hypertrophy of the heart muscle can occur when it has to work against an abnormal valvular narrowing (as in pulmonary valvular or infundibular stenosis).

Radiographic measurements unfortunately do not distinguish clearly between a well-developed, hypertrophied muscle, and an enlarged but thin, dilated and failing heart. Clues can sometimes be drawn from other features of the radiograph, such as congestion of the lung fields, but often the question must be resolved by relating heart volume to working capacity or maximum oxygen intake.

Techniques of Measuring Cardiac Output

Direct Fick Method. The ideal way of measuring cardiac output ($\dot{Q}$) in man is to apply the direct Fick principle to samples of blood obtained at cardiac catheterization:

$$\dot{Q} = \frac{\dot{V}_{O_2}}{(C_{a,O_2} - C\bar{v},_{O_2})}$$

where V_{O_2} is the oxygen consumption (measured under steady state conditions), C_{a,O_2} is the oxygen content of arterial blood, and $C\bar{v},_{O_2}$ is the oxygen content of a specimen of mixed venous blood drawn from the pulmonary artery. Unfortunately, the risks of cardiac catheterization do not justify its application except for diagnostic purposes; even in the absence of cardiac disease, there is a 2 to 3% incidence of serious complications (mainly abnormalities of heart rhythm).

The Dye Method. A second popular clinical procedure is based on the injection of a dye that is rapidly removed from the circulation;

indocyanine green is commonly used. There have been attempts to monitor blood-stream concentrations of this dye using an earpiece, but they have not achieved great success. Accurate estimation of cardiac output apparently requires intracardiac injection of the dye with subsequent collection of blood samples by arterial puncture. Some have argued that such procedures can be applied to normal subjects, but in addition to the hazards of catheterization arterial puncture carries an appreciable risk of thrombosis with a possible need for subsequent amputation. A medically qualified investigator may choose to offer himself as a subject, but it is difficult to suggest that uninformed patients accept such risks for scientific purposes.

The CO_2 Rebreathing Method. The choice of procedure for the applied physiologist thus lies between CO_2 rebreathing and the inhalation of a foreign gas. The CO_2 rebreathing method applies the Fick procedure to the exchange of carbon dioxide:

$$\dot{Q} = \frac{\dot{V}_{CO_2}}{(Ca,\ co_2 - C\bar{v},\ co_2)}$$

The steady-state output of carbon dioxide is measured by the standard open-circuit method. "Arterialized" capillary blood is obtained from a small stab wound of the finger tip or the ear lobe and its CO_2 content determined; providing the finger is adequately heated, the arterioles become widely dilated, and the CO_2 tension of the blood speciman thus obtained corresponds closely with that of the arterial blood. Alternatively, the arterial CO_2 tension can be estimated from a continuous record of alveolar CO_2 levels (Fig. 11). When the subject is at rest, the CO_2 tension in the final portion of the expirate (the "end-tidal" sample) coincides rather closely with

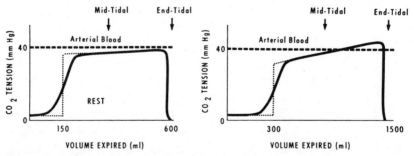

Figure 11. The tension of carbon dioxide over the course of a complete expiration. Note that at rest, the end-tidal sample approximates closely to the composition of arterial blood, but that in exercise, the arterial blood value lies midway between midtidal and end-tidal readings.

the arterial value; during vigorous exercise, variations of CO_2 tension over the course of the breathing cycle are larger, and commonly the best approximation to the arterial tension is given by an average of mid-tidal and end-tidal readings. The mixed venous CO_2 reading is obtained by rebreathing from a bag containing 5% to 10% CO_2 in oxygen. If the "correct" mixture is chosen, the continuously recorded CO_2 tension shows a few oscillations as the gas in the bag mixes with that within the lungs, and then a plateau is reached (Fig. 12); at

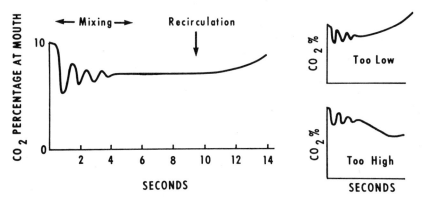

Figure 12. Estimation of mixed venous CO_2 tension by the rebreathing method. If the "correct" initial mixture is chosen, there is a plateau of some six seconds duration prior to the onset of recirculation. If the initial mixture contains too little CO_2 the plateau is replaced by an upward slope, while if the concentration is too high, there is a downward slope.

this stage, the alveolar gas tension equals that in the mixed venous blood, and CO_2 is neither excreted nor absorbed. The plateau is temporary in nature, and if rebreathing is continued for more than twelve or fifteen seconds, the record shows a secondary upward curve. Rebreathing dams back CO_2 within the body, and blood with an increased CO_2 content quickly starts to appear at the lungs; "recirculation" is said to have occurred. The time available to define the plateau is much shorter in vigorous exercise than at rest, sometimes being as brief as seven to ten seconds.

The Foreign Gas Method. The foreign gas method applies the Fick equation to the uptake of a very soluble gas such as acetylene or nitrous oxide. Again, there is a brief period of rebreathing from a small bag. The first four breaths are used to mix the bag contents with the alveolar air, and the investigator examines changes over the next three to six breaths. The increase of nitrogen concentration reflects any decrement in volume of the lung/bag system, and decreases in oxygen and acetylene concentrations are used to calculate the cardiac output according to the equation

$$\dot{Q} = \left(\frac{\dot{V}_{O_2}}{Ca, C_2H_2}\right) \frac{\Delta C_2H_2}{\Delta O_2} \qquad \dot{Q} = \left(\frac{\dot{V}_{O_2}}{Ca, C_2H_2}\right) \frac{\Delta C_2H_2}{\Delta O_2}$$

Ca, C_2H_2 is the arterial concentration of acetylene, assumed equal to the average of concentrations found in the bag at the fourth and seventh breaths, multiplied by a factor describing the solubility of acetylene in arterial blood. ΔC_2H_2 is the change in acetylene concentration from the fourth to the seventh breath, the latter figure being corrected for any decrement in the volume of the lung/bag system. ΔO_2 is the change in oxygen concentration, calculated in a similar manner. When the method was introduced by Grollman, in 1929, the gas samples were analysed chemically. Carbon dioxide and oxygen were first absorbed, and then the acetylene was burnt to CO_2 and water vapour. The method was cumbersome, and in an attempt to gain accuracy, high concentrations of acetylene (up to 20%) were used; these were subjectively unpleasant, tended to be anaesthetic, and had the unfortunate habit of occasionally exploding in the patient's lungs. The figures that Grollman obtained for the resting cardiac output are now recognised to have been rather low. This was partly because he used an erroneous solubility coefficient for acetylene, and partly because rebreathing was continued for too long, so that the composition of the final gas sample was influenced by recirculation. The development of gas chromatograph techniques has greatly speeded up the necessary analyses, and has made possible the use of lower (1%), nonexplosive and subjectively more pleasant acetylene concentrations. Nitrous oxide can be used in the same type of rebreathing system, gas concentrations being determined by either infrared or chromatographic analysis.

Some authors have used an open-circuit semisteady state method with foreign gases such as nitrous oxide. The gas mixture is inhaled for a rather long period, and the procedure becomes open to one objection of the original Grollman method, namely that recirculation causes erroneously low cardiac output values.

Relative Merits of Foreign Gas and CO_2 Methods. The main objection to the CO_2 rebreathing method is that in the resting state the difference of CO_2 tension between arterial and mixed venous blood specimens is small (about 6 mm Hg). Since it is difficult to determine CO_2 tensions to nearer than 1–2 mm Hg, the arteriovenous difference tends to be overshadowed by measurement errors. Fortunately, in maximum exercise, the arteriovenous tension differences rises to 30–40 mm Hg, and it can then be determined with much greater relative precision. The foreign gas method works quite well in normal healthy men, but the analyses are more time-consuming than for the CO_2 rebreathing method. Neither the foreign gas nor the CO_2 rebreathing procedure work well in a patient with chronic chest disease, because the permissible period of rebreathing is too short to develop an equilibrium between the poorly ventilated regions of the lung and the rebreathing bag.

Heart Sounds and Murmurs

Heart sounds and murmurs are the province of the clinician rather than the applied physiologist. However, "murmurs" can arise in a perfectly normal heart and if misinterpreted they may cause unnecessary invalidism. A brief comment on their genesis thus seems appropriate. Normally, the blood moves with a "laminar," or streamline flow pattern. This implies a regular gradient of flow rate from the rapidily moving central part of the blood stream to a stationary film bordering the vessel walls. A flow pattern of this type makes no sound that can be detected by a stethoscope; the sole cardiovascular noise thus consists of two heart sounds (I, "Lubb," and II, "Dupp"). The "Lubb" sound is initiated by vibration of the atrioventricular valves and the "Dupp" sound arises from a similar vibration of the aortic and pulmonary valves. Laminar flow implies that one film of blood is slipping smoothly over another. As the speed of flow is increased, there ultimately comes a "critical velocity," V_c, where this orderly shearing process breaks down, and an irregular "turbulent" pattern of flow develops. The critical velocity can be calculated according to the equation:

$$V_c = \frac{R\eta}{\delta r}$$

where R is a constant, the "Reynolds number," about 1000 to 2000 for a straight and smooth-walled tube, η is the viscosity of the blood, δ is its density, and r is the radius of the blood vessel.

If the blood flow is increased sufficiently, whether by exercise or by anxiety, the critical velocity may be reached. Turbulence and a murmur then develop.* It is heard first in the early part of systole, over the aortic region. Let us suppose the cause is anxiety. If the patient is told he has a murmur, his anxiety may be even greater at a subsequent examination. The cardiac output is further increased, turbulence becomes more extensive, and the murmur is heard over a larger area of the chest for a longer fraction of the cardiac cycle. A vicious circle of restricted activity, anxiety, and increasing murmur may thus be created. Anaemia is another source of an "innocent" murmur; the tendency to turbulence is here brought about partly by a decrease of blood viscosity, and partly by an increase of cardiac output in an attempt to compensate for the decreased oxygen carrying capacity of the blood.

Pathological murmurs are localized areas of turbulence. The cause may be a narrowed, roughened or leaky heart valve or an abnormal communication between the pulmonary and systemic circulations (for example atrial and ventral septal defects, and persistent ductus arteriosus). The abnormal pattern of blood flow and the roughening of the vessel wall have the effect of lowering the Reynolds number. Pathological murmurs may be localized to the region of the abnormality but are often propagated over a quite a wide area of the chest. They are usually louder than an "innocent" murmur, they may extend into diastole, and they do not readily disappear with rest.

If a pathological murmur is present, the work of the heart is generally increased by the associated abnormality, and any exercise programme should be arranged in close consultation with the patient's cardiologist. However, it is increasingly recognized that many "cardiac" patients benefit from an exercise regime tailored to their condition and the demands of their daily life.

* Clinical readers may object that "innocent" murmurs are supposed to disappear with exercise or a change of posture. Murmurs that respond in this way probably arise from small ventricular septal defects. If the pressure in the pulmonary circulation is raised, the shunting of blood diminishes until the murmur is no longer audible.

The Blood Supply to the Heart Muscle

The heart muscle receives a substantial blood flow even at rest—about 80 ml/100gm of tissue per minute, or in a 400gm heart, 320 ml/min, some 5 percent of the resting cardiac output. In exercise, this flow may increase fivefold. A number of unusual features of the coronary circulation deserve specific comment.

Oxygen Extraction

Coronary blood drains largely to the coronary sinus, and blood samples collected from this site have an exceedingly low oxygen content (1–2 ml/100 ml, compared with the normal resting "mixed venous" oxygen content of some 15 ml/100 ml). Arterial blood has an oxygen content of about 19 ml/100 ml. Thus the heart muscle succeeds in extracting 17 or 18 ml of oxygen from each 100 ml of blood, whereas other tissues extract no more than 4 ml per 100 ml. The economical usage of coronary blood flow presents a problem during exercise. In the general circulation, the arteriovenous oxygen difference increases progressively with work load, reaching a limiting value of 13–14 ml/100 ml in sedentary subjects, and 15–16 ml/100 ml in athletes; however, in the coronary circulation, any increase of oxygen needs can be met only by an increased blood flow.

Absence of Oxygen Debt

A second mechanism whereby the skeletal muscles can accomodate an increased metabolic demand is through the accumulation of an oxygen debt. This is not possible in heart muscle. If the circulation is interrupted, metabolism can be sustained only by the small reserves of oxygen stored in the red cell and muscle pigments (haemoglobin and myoglobin). Perhaps because the heart muscle is entirely dependent on oxidative metabolism, the cellular structure shows an unusually large number of mitochondria.

External Compression of Vessels

Because the coronary vessels are imbedded in the heart wall, they are subject to external pressure with each contraction of the ventricles. The left ventricular systolic pressure is normally five or six times as great as that in the right ventricle; in consequence flow through the left coronary artery is completely stopped for much of systole (Fig. 13), whereas flow through the right coronary artery shows relatively minor fluctuations over the cardiac cycle.

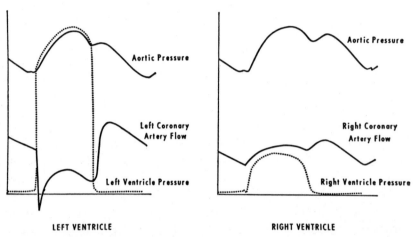

Figure 13. The perfusion pressure and flow in the left and the right coronary arteries over the course of the cardiac cycle. (Schematic, based on data presented by Gregg, 1962.)

During exercise, the left ventricular systolic pressure increases, but the right ventricular systolic pressure shows little change, The pressure available for perfusion of the right coronary artery is thus effectively increased. However, the left ventricle is less fortunate. Its workload is increased by the rise of left ventricular systolic pressure and the coronary vessels are also subject to greater compression. If the diastolic pressure is raised, there may be some increase in the pressure perfusing the left coronary artery. However, flow is restricted to the diastolic phase of the cardiac cycle, and this is progressively shortened as the intensity of exercise is increased. For these reasons, it is usually the left ventricle which develops signs of oxygen lack during vigorous exercise.

Regulation of Blood Flow

Since the heart muscle cannot develop an oxygen debt and oxygen extraction from the blood in the coronary circulation cannot be increased beyond the normal resting value, a mechanism for the rapid and accurate adjustment of blood flow to the increased metabolic demands of exercise is essential.

> A large sympathetic and parasympathetic nerve supply to the heart has been described, and some coronary vasodilatation can be induced by a stimulation of the stellate ganglion. However, there is no good evidence that the autonomic nerves play any important role in the normal response to exercise. Occasionally, they may be responsible for a reflex vascular spasm. A good example of this is an attack of cardiac (anginal) pain induced by a walk on a frosty morning. Exercise induces mouth breathing, and the cold dry air stimulates vagal receptors in the air-passages, thus initiating a spasm of both the bronchi and the coronary arteries.

The main basis for the increased coronary blood flow of exercise is probably a local accumulation of metabolites and CO_2, coupled with a reduced oxygen tension. Noradrenaline has a direct dilator effect on the coronary vessels; adrenaline also has some direct dilator action, with a stronger indirect dilator effect through (a) stimulation of metabolism in the vessel wall and (b) an increase of diastolic pressure in the systemic circulation. Both compounds are liberated into the circulation during exercise, and could thus contribute to the increase of coronary flow.

> If an attack of angina occurs, this is commonly treated by adminstration of an organic nitrite such as amyl nitrite or the longer acting glyceryl trinitrate. At one time, such compounds were thought to produce a beneficial effect by dilating the coronary vessels. However, it is now accepted that they act in part by reducing the systemic blood pressure and thus the work of the heart, and in part by easing external compression of the coronary arteries.

The Collateral Circulation

Substantial anastomoses occur between the main coronary vessels, particularly at the apex of the heart. These anastomoses are important in reducing the area subject to infarction if blockage of a major coronary artery should occur. Proponents of the view that exercise reduces the liability to "coronary" attacks have suggested that physical activity encourages development of collateral channels; it is postulated that the "anoxic" stimulus dilates potential anastomotic pathways (p. 518). Unfortunately, attempts to demonstrate either enlargement of the existing coronary tree or the development of new collateral vessels as a specific result of enforced activity have been rather disappointing.

Exercise and Sudden Death

There is some evidence (p. 509) that exercise may increase the immediate liability to death from cardiac arrest or ventricular fibrillation. Several explanations of this phenomenon may be advanced. Firstly, narrowing of the vascular supply may moke a patch of heart muscle relatively anoxic, and thus more irritable—a potential focus for abnormal rhythms including ventricular fibrillation. Secondly, a more general oxygen-lack (ischemia) may develop in the heart muscle because hardening of the coronary vessels prevents a normal dilatation in response to the increased oxygen demands of exercise. Ischemia may be sufficient to cause death of myocardial tissue (infarction) and thus cardiac arrest. Thirdly, a frank occlusion of a coronary vessel may be induced by exercise. One suggested explanation notes the drop in pressure as the blood flows past a fatty plaque on the vessel wall. With exercise, there is an increase of flow and thus of pressure drop across the plaque. Haemorrhage tends to occur into the plaque from the up-stream side and this progressively occludes the coronary vessel. Alternatively, the increased flow of exercise may dislodge a thrombus from the vessel wall, and this can then block a smaller artery.

The Work of the Heart

Some General Principles

The energy of the circulation is degraded to heat as frictional (viscous) and turbulent work are performed within the blood vessels. In order to maintain the energy content of the system and thus the blood flow, work must be performed by the heart. As in any mechanical pump, the work performed per stroke (W) is given by the product of pressure (P_v) and volume change ∂V integrated over the ejection phase of the cardiac cycle:

$$W = \int_{V_d}^{V_s} P_V \, \partial V$$

To a first approximation, this integral equals the product of the mean ventricular ejection pressure $\bar{P}_v$ and the stroke volume Q_s:

$$W = \bar{P}_V \cdot Q_s$$

A typical pressure-volume diagram for the left ventricle is shown in Fig. 14. Normally, both ventricles contain some 160 ml of blood at the end of diastole, and only 80 ml is expelled as the heart contracts; the remainder constitutes a reserve that tends to be drawn upon during exercise.

The Work Performed

In the resting state, the left ventricle performs approximately 0.1 kg-m of useful work per beat (the mean pressure is about 100

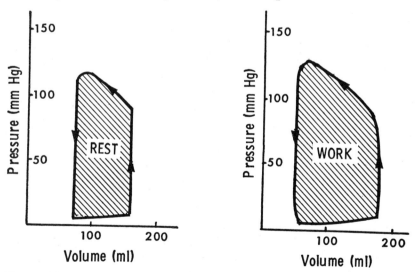

Figure 14. Pressure/volume diagrams for left ventricle. The work performed with each heart beat is indicated by the area of the pressure/volume diagram.

mmHg, or 0.13 kg/cm², and a typical stroke volume is 80 cm³).
Thus if the heart is beating 70 times per minute, the useful workload totals some 7 kg-m/min. The mean pressure in the right ventricle is about a fifth as great as in the left, so that the useful work
performed by this chamber is about 1.4 kg-m/min. Although the
workload of the heart is small, the efficiency is also low, since a
great deal of mechanically "useless" work is performed against the
tension in the heart wall (T). The "useless" work can be calculated
from the expression

$$W = \alpha \int_o^t T \,\partial t$$

where α is a constant to convert the integral of tension over the contraction period to the same units of work as the pressure-volume
product. Thus the mechanical efficiency E is given by

$$E = \frac{\int_{V_d}^{V_s} P_v \,\partial V}{\int_{V_d}^{V_s} P_v \,\partial V + \alpha \int_o^t T \,\partial t}$$

At rest, E is about 3 percent, but in exercise it may increase to
10 to 15 percent. The main determinant of cardiac work is the tension T, and this in turn is related to the ventricular pressure according to the law of Laplace:

$$P_v = T \left[\frac{1}{R_1} + \frac{1}{R_2} \right]$$

R_1 and R_2 are the radii of the ventricle in two dimensions.

It can be appreciated from the foregoing, that an increase of
blood pressure due to anxiety can produce both a substantial
increase in the workload of the heart, and also a lowering of
mechanical efficiency. On the other hand, moderate rhythmic
activity gives rise to a substantial increase of useful cardiac
work, with little increase of mean ventricular pressure; the
efficiency of the exercising heart thus rises markedly, while the
total work load only increases slightly. For this reason, it is
often better for the postcoronary patient to take exercise than
to sit at home in a state of ever-increasing anxiety. Work involving substantial muscular tension (isometric exercise, or the
lifting of heavy weights) provides an important exception to

this rule. Such activity gives a large increment of mean blood pressure, and thus a large increase in the total cardiac workload.

For a given cardiac output, a rapid heart rate is less efficient than a slower rhythm. This is to be anticipated from the foregoing theory. The duration of the individual contraction is similar whether a large or a small volume of blood is expelled from the heart; thus an increase of heart rate increases the total tension work per minute.

Clinicians sometimes use the so-called "tension-time index" as a measure of the cardiac workload. Despite its impressive name, this is no more than the product of heart rate and systolic blood pressure. The true figure for the total work performed by the heart per minute is given by

$$\left(\int_{V_d}^{V_s} P_v \, \partial V + \alpha \int_o^t T \, \partial t \right) f_h$$

where f_h is the heart rate. Since T is closely related to P_v, the tension-time index would reflect the work performed if the stroke volume and the duration of the contraction phase were both constant. During exercise, the second is more likely to be constant than the first; fortunately for the tension-time index, it is the larger component of the total cardiac work load.

The Oxygen Cost of Cardiac Work

Let us suppose that in vigorous exercise the useful work performed rises from 7 kg-m/min to 42 kg-m/min, and that the efficiency increases from 3 percent to 10 percent. The heart of the exercising patient is then performing a total of 420 kg-m of work per minute, or nearly 1 kcal. This requires an oxygen consumption of about 0.2 litre/min.

Direct measurements of oxygen consumption in the dog heart support these calculations. At rest, oxygen usage is about 10 ml per 100gm of tissue and in maximum exercise this rises to 60 ml/100gm. Since the human heart weighs about 350gm, on a proportionate basis it would have a maximum oxygen usage of 0.21 litre/min.

Given a maximum cardiac output of 25 litre/min, the oxygen cost of pumping blood is 8 ml of oxygen per litre of cardiac output. This is a substantial charge upon the total oxygen intake, although it is very much less than the equivalent oxygen transport (120 ml of oxygen per litre of cardiac output).* There thus seems little danger that the point will be reached where the oxygen cost ·of pumping blood exceeds the extra oxygen introduced into the body thereby.

The Electrocardiogram and Exercise

Preliminary Inspection of the Electrocardiogram

Most clinicians like to examine a 12-lead electrocardiogram prior to exercise; this includes the three standard limb leads (I, right arm to left arm; II, right arm to left leg; III, left arm to left leg) and nine "unipolar" leads in which the potential is measured relative to Wilson's central terminal (leads I, II, and III, each joined to a common terminal through a 5000 ohm resistor).

It has been argued that electrical changes in the heart during a cardiac cycle can be represented by the movement of a small dipole (a conductor with a positive charge at one end, and a negative charge at the other) in a three dimensional space. It might seem that the entire information content of the electrocardiogram could be obtained if potentials were recorded in three planes at right angles ("orthogonal") to each other. However, in practice, additional information is obtained as an exploring electrode is moved over the chest wall; the voltages thus recorded reflect the characteristics of the immediately underlying myocardium. An abnormality may thus be detected in some chest leads, and not in others.

The potentials to be recorded are very small, and the amplitude of all ECG waves is markedly dependent on the impedances interposed between the heart and the recorder, particularly at the points of contact between the skin and the recording electrodes. No particular significance can thus be attached to a low voltage signal. Some authors have claimed an association between a large, upright T wave and a large stroke volume, however, this may reflect in part the fact that fit individuals have less subcutaneous fat. Certainly, the association between the two variables is not very close, and there are easier ways to assess the cardiac stroke volume. Detailed interpretation of the electrocardiogram is the responsibility of a cardiologist, but it may be helpful to note other features that he can

---

* If the maximum oxygen intake is 3 litre/min, and the cardiac output is 25 litre/min, then 120 ml of oxygen are transported per litre of blood flow.

deduce from a study of the electrical record. The electrical axis of the heart is influenced by the position of the heart in the chest and by ventricular hypertrophy. Left axis deviation (with a large R wave in Lead I, and an S wave in Lead II) is seen with the horizontally placed heart of an obese subject (Fig. 15), while right axis deviation (with an S wave in Lead I and a large R wave in Lead III) is seen in a thin individual with a vertically placed heart. Hypertrophy of the left ventricle usually produces left axis deviation, but the voltage of the various waves is much greater than with a a simple rotation of the heart (for instance, the S wave in Lead V_1 is > 1.5mV, and the R wave in Leads V_4, V_5 or V_6 is > 2.5mV). Similarly, hypertrophy of the right ventricle produces right axis deviation, with tall R waves in Leads V_1 and V_2, and conspicuous S waves in Leads V_5 and V_6. Left ventricular hypertrophy (Fig. 15) may be a result of athletic training, in which case it is associated with a slow resting pulse rate, or it may reflect an abnormality such as narrowing of the aortic valve (aortic stenosis). Right ventricular hypertrophy is almost always pathological, reflecting pulmonary stenosis or hypertension.

The rate of conduction of the electrical impulse through the myocardium is influenced by the ionic composition of the plasma. This is reflected in the PR interval. The normal range is 0.16–0.22 seconds. An increase in the concentration of potassium ions (such as in fresh water drowning) lengthens the PR interval, while an increase of sodium ions (as in salt water drowning) has the reverse effect (see p. 296).

What are some of the danger signs in a preexercise electrocardiogram? It is important to exclude imminent or recent myocardial infarction. This is suspected if there is a prominent Q wave and elevation of the ST segment when the exploring electrode is placed immediately over the affected area of myocardium. If the infarct is on the posterior surface of the heart, the ST segment may be depressed rather than elevated. In doubtful cases, it is helpful to show a progression of change when electrocardiograms are repeated over the course of several days. Acute myocarditis is a second important contraindication to exercise; this also may lead to depression of the ST segment and inversion of the T wave. Exercise should not be undertaken if there is a probability of recent pulmonary embolism. A large embolus leads to tachycardia and ECG evidence of right heart

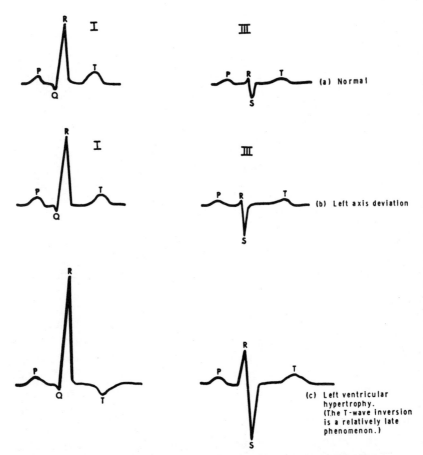

Figure 15. The influence of left-axis deviation and left ventricular hypertrophy upon the appearance of Leads I and III of the electrocardiogram.

strain (including inverted T waves over the right side of the chest), but smaller emboli may give no abnormal ECG appearances. Gross abnormalities of rhythm are also of concern, particularly bursts of rapid ventricular rhythm (ventricular tachycardia) with independent P waves.

Caution must be observed when exercising patients with atrial flutter or fibrillation. In atrial flutter, an irritable focus gives a rapid succession of P waves (up to 250–300/min), and only the third or fourth impulses are transmitted to the ventricle; in atrial fibrillation, there are irregular and rapid "f" waves, and the ventricular contractions are slow and irregular in timing. Other indications for caution include the Wolff-Parkinson-White syndrome, marked atrioventricular block, and left bundle-branch block. The Wolff-Parkinson-White syndrome arises from premature excitation of one of the two ventricles and is due to an abnormality of conduction in the region of the a-v node. The ECG shows a shortened P-R interval and a widened QRS complex. Heart block at the a-v node is shown by a lengthening of the P-R interval, with failure of transmission of a proportion of impulses to the ventricle; it usually indicates some underlying abnormality of the myocardium, and there is a danger of progressing to a Stokes-Adams attack, with complete ventricular asystole. An a-v block must be distinguished from a sinu-atrial block; the latter is a normal expression of increased vagal tone, and is not uncommon in an athletic individual. With a-v block, one or more beats may be "dropped" completely and sometimes there is a QRS complex without a preceeding P wave ("ventricular escape"). Bundle-branch block is indicated by a broadening of the QRS complex, and is a cause for concern mainly because it indicates underlying heart disease; left bundle branch block is usually pathological, but some degree of right bundle branch block is a common finding in athletes.

Mention should also be made of a number of innocent sources of apparently irregular heart rate. Sinus arrhythmia is a normal finding that is more common in athletic than in sedentary individuals; the heart rate quickens during inspiration and slows during expiration. The ECG has a normal form, and the rhythm becomes more regular as exercise is commenced. The underlying mechanism is probably the Bainbridge reflex (p. 91). Ectopic beats may arise from an irritable focus in the atrium, the a-v node, or the ventricle; in the last case, the P wave is absent and the QRS complex has a broadened and abnormal form. The cause of ectopic beats may be excessive smoking or anxiety; if this is their basis, they become less frequent as exercise is commenced.

The Response to Exercise

The ST Segment. As the intensity of exercise is increased, the oxygen consumed by the heart muscle outstrips the oxygen supplied by the coronary vessels. Hypoxia is usually more severe in the left than the right ventricle, and this leads to a progressive change in the ST segment of the electrocardiogram—first a depression of the S-ST junction (Fig. 16) and then a

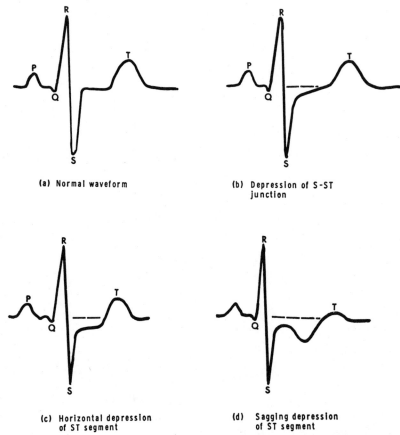

(a) Normal waveform

(b) Depression of S-ST junction

(c) Horizontal depression of ST segment

(d) Sagging depression of ST segment

Figure 16. The effect of progressive oxygen lack on the electrocardiogram.

horizontal or downward sloping depression of the entire ST segment (Fig. 16). The underlying physiological mechanism is a functional impairment of the "sodium pump" (p. 175), with delayed repolarisation of the cell membranes within the ventricular muscle.

If the coronary vasculature is healthy, oxygen lack does not progress beyond a slight junctional depression even in maximum exercise. However, if the coronary vessels are narrowed by atheroma, junctional depression appears at a rather light work load and substantial depression of the entire ST segment develops with more severe effort. This provides the basis of a number of exercise tests. The *Master test* has been widely used by clinicians for some thirty years. The patient is required to climb backwards and forwards over a double nine-inch step for 1½ minutes (Single Master test) or three minutes (Double Master test). The rate of climbing is varied somewhat with age and weight, but generally the terminal pulse rate is about 120 beats/min. An abnormal response is reported if the ST segment of the recovery electrocardiogram is depressed by more than 1 mm (0.1 mV); a patient showing such a response has an above average risk of premature death from coronary heart disease. There are two main criticisms of the Master test (a) the level of effort required of the average patient is rather mild, and (b) the test imposes a greater stress on elderly than on young patients (since the maximum pulse rate declines with age, p. 51). Some laboratories carry out *maximum exercise tests* on all patients submitted for electrocardiographic examination, but this seems unnecessarily risky. A reasonable compromise is record the electrocardiogram when patients are exercising at a fixed percentage (75%) of their maximum aerobic power. It is not necessary to measure the oxygen consumption directly for this purpose. The required intensity of stress can be defined adequately for clinical purposes by using an *age-related target pulse rate*; 160 at age twenty to thirty, 150 at thirty to forty, 140 at forty to fifty, and 130 at fifty to sixty. The threshold for the reporting of an abnormal ST depression is held at 0.1 mV when carrying out the more vigorous forms of exercise test. Hence, the proportion of any given population diagnosed as having impaired coronary flow is larger with a target pulse test than with a traditional Master two-step test.

Marked depression of the S-ST junction has some pathological significance. The tracing is regarded as abnormal if the ST segment is upward sloping yet remains 0.1 mV or more below the iso-electric (zero) potential at the origin of the T wave.

Accurate measurements of ST displacement are difficult during vigorous exercise. The main problem is a wandering baseline, a reflection of varying electrode impedance, and it can be overcome by analogue and/or digital computing techniques. An analogue computer is used to superimpose an arbitrary number of ECG tracings (for instance, 16 or 32 successive beats); the averaged signal is then presented either as a visual display or as a series of perhaps 1024 (2^{10}) discreet voltage readings. Although this type of data reduction overcomes the problem of baseline drift, a single abnormal beat (such as a ventricular extrasystole) can cause a grossly inaccurate averaged signal. A digital computer can be programmed to give a similar but more sophisticated solution of the same problem. The 1024 measurements are made on each of forty-eight successive heart beats. The computer programme then selects sixteen of the forty-eight beats that have a mutually similar wave-form, and calculates an averaged tracing from these sixteen beats.

ST depression is a nonspecific sign. It indicates a disturbance of the ionic balance across cell membranes, irrespective of the cause of this disturbance. It is thus important to exclude chemical malfunctioning of the "sodium pump" (due to drugs such as digitalis), and altered plasma electrolyte concentrations (due to the use of diuretics or hyperventilation) before concluding that the coronary vessels are narrowed.

Other changes in the electrocardiogram. The extrasystoles of the anxious patient commonly become less frequent with effort. However, an abnormality of rhythm that appears for the first time during exercise, whether a form of heart block or a series of extrasystoles, is usually an expression of local oxygen lack. The irritability of the myocardium is increased not only by local hypoxia but also by an increase in the concentration of circulating catecholamines (adrenaline and noradrenaline). Abnormalities of rhythm are not particularly helpful in diagnosing the coronary prone patient. Nevertheless, they are an indication to halt an exercise test, and if ignored, there is a risk that ventricular tachycardia and even ventricular fibrillation may develop. Both ST depression and disturbances of rhythm are often worse in the period immediately following exercise, and thus if there is any doubt about the patient's condition it is wise to stop a test. Various factors contribute to the worsening of myocardial status in the immediate postexercise period; these include a fall in the mean systemic blood pressure and a continuing decrease in the oxygen content of arterial blood.

Ventricular Fibrillation

Ventricular fibrillation is an irregular writhing contraction of the ventricles that is ineffective in expelling blood from the heart. Unless treated, it is rapidly fatal. The cause is usually a local irritation of the myocardium. A variety of factors such as electric shock, drowning, anticholinesterase poisoning, and myocardial infarction can all trigger an attack, and the combination of myocardial ischaemia and catecholamine secretion may induce an attack during vigorous exercise—particularly if there is associated anxiety. The treatment is to apply one or more "shocks" to the chest wall, using an external defibrillator. The intense voltage leads to a complete depolarisation of the myocardium, and it is hoped that when repolarisation occurs a normal rhythm will recommence.

The first designs of defibrillator used up to 250 volts of alternating current, applied directly to the heart muscle through an emergency incision in the chest wall. Unfortunately, many people were not prepared to take the drastic measure of opening the chest when treating a casualty. Accordingly, external defibrillators were devised. It was then necessary to increase the potential to some 750 volts, and there was a danger that the rescuer himself might be sent into fibrillation by careless handling of the equipment. Partly for this reason, and partly because of difficulty in timing brief shocks reliably, the preferred technique is to use a direct current defibrillator. A small condenser (about 2.5 μF) is charged to a very high voltage (5000 volts); the charge Q is given by

$$Q = VF$$

Where V is the potential, and F is the capacity. If the absolute values are as quoted, the charge is $(25 \times 10^{-6}) \times 5000 = 0.125$ Coulombs. The stored energy is equal to $\frac{1}{2}$ QV, or 312.5 watt-sec. In practice, the applied shock is increased progressively from 100 to 350 watt-sec, depending on the age of the individual, the thickness of the skin and underlying fat, and the response to an initial shock.

It is difficult to obtain reliable statistics on the success of ventricular defibrillation. In some institutions, all patients "brought in dead" have been given this treatment, in order to familiarise staff with the procedure. Often, there has been some doubt of the diagnosis. Nevertheless, it seems likely that a properly used defibrillator will save the lives of a substantial number of patients who would otherwise die, and any physician carrying out vigorous exercise tests on middle-aged adults would be wise to have such equipment available. If the precaution is observed of monitoring the electrocardiogram during testing, episodes of ventricular fibrillation will be less likely, and in the event that an arrhythmia does develop, a clear diagnosis can be made immediately. The success of the defibrillating procedure is markedly influenced by attendant hypoxia; in a well-oxgenated heart it is by no means easy to induce persistent fibrillation by a direct electric shock, but once the coronary blood flow has stopped, it becomes quite difficult to restore a normal rhythm.

Cardiac Arrest

Ventricular contractions may cease as a sequel to a developing heart block, as a secondary response to the various stimuli inducing ventricular fibrillation, or as a result of the increase in plasma sodium ion concentration accompanying salt-water drowning. The heart may also fail to restart following an otherwise successful defibrillation. If the ECG is being monitored, there will be a complete absence of electrical activity. If an electrocardiogram is not available, there will be no pulse palpable in the carotid artery, and no heart sounds audible over the myocardium. Owing to the rapidity of irreversible brain damage (p. 50), treatment must be started immediately, even in the absence of a physician.*

Sometimes the heart can be restarted by a vigorous blow on the chest, but if this fails, cardiac massage must be undertaken. The patient is placed on a rigid surface, since much of the energy of a potential rescuer can be dissipated by the springs in a bed or mattress. Vigorous pressure is applied over the sternum some sixty times per minute. The ribs and underlying viscera are protected by interposing the free hand of the rescuer. If ventilation has ceased, a second person must apply mouth to mouth or some other form of artificial respiration (p. 155). There is little question that in the dog a very effective arterial pressure can be developed by external compression of the chest. In man, the thorax is more rigid, and the pressures achieved are quite marginal for survival. "Systolic" pressures of 100 mmHg have been recorded, but the pulse wave has a spiky form, with a very low diastolic reading. Further, there is commonly an increased venous pressure reducing the gradient available for perfusion of the vital organs. Nevertheless, there have been many instances where this form of resuscitation has been successful.

Some authors still recommend that if the condition of the patient does not improve within a minute, the thorax should be opened by a broad incision through the fourth or fifth interspace, and internal massage should be commenced. However, such a procedure is restricted to licensed physicians.

If resuscitation is successful, the patient must be watched very carefully over the next forty-eight hours. The heart remains ab-

---

* Permissible forms of treatment vary in different provinces and states (see p. 543). The current policy of the Ontario College of Physicians and Surgeons is that "suitably trained registered nurses" may carry out external cardiac massage.

normally irritable, but the likelihood of a recurrence of arrest or fibrillation can be reduced by administration of procaine amide. The brain may respond to the anoxic episode by subsequent swelling ("cerebral oedema"). Various measures are adopted to minimize the likelihood of permanent brain damage at this stage. They include reduction of the circulating blood volume, and deliberately induced hypothermia.

The teaching of cardiac massage now forms an important part of emergency training, and a number of the "manikins" devised for instruction in artificial respiration (p. 160) indicate whether a first aid worker is developing an adequate blood pressure by external compression of the chest.

Energy in the Cardiovascular System

Forms of Energy

The energy of the cardiovascular system exists in three forms—pressure, potential energy, and kinetic energy.

Pressure energy P is self-explanatory. Potential energy is stored in a fluid if it is above some arbitrary reference level; in the case of the circulation, the reference level is that of the heart. The quantity of energy involved depends on the density of the fluid (δ), the gravitational acceleration (g), and the height (H) above the reference level. Kinetic energy is present in a fluid by virtue of its motion; it depends on density (δ) and the velocity of flow (v). Thus the total energy content E of blood flowing through a given vessel is

$$E = P + \delta gH + \tfrac{1}{2}\delta v^2$$

In the resting state, there is little kinetic energy at most points in the circulation, so that the equation simplifies to

$$E = P + \delta gH$$

During exercise, kinetic energy accounts for an increasing proportion of the total energy, particularly in the great veins and the pulmonary circulation, where the pressure energy remains low.

Some energy is degraded to heat during the course of the circulation, and this loss is restored to the arterial side of the circulation by cardiac activity. In addition, a continuous interchange of the three forms of energy occurs as the blood passes through the vascular system.

Effect of Posture

A change of posture converts pressure energy into potential energy and vice-versa. Thus in the erect position, the circulation to the head and neck is at a low pressure; indeed, in the neck veins, the pressure is negative relative to the heart, and the vessels collapse. The extent of body tilting necessary to induce venous collapse is used as a rough clinical measure of central venous pressure. In the dorsum of the foot, the potential energy is negative, but there is a substantial hydrostatic pressure of 80–90 mmHg. The arteries are relatively indistensible, and any increase of intravascular pressure has a small and rather uniform effect on their blood content (Fig. 17); in contrast, the venous system is very readily distensible, and a small increase of intravascular pressure is enough to distend the leg veins to near their full capacity. The blood thus pooled re-

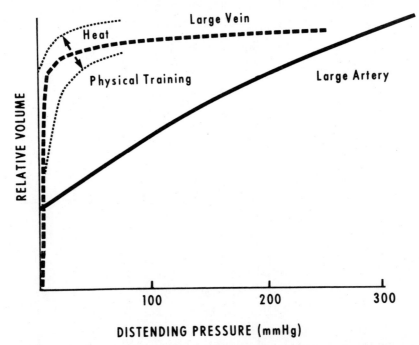

Figure 17. A comparison of pressure/volume curves for a large systemic artery and a large systemic vein. Note the influence of heat and of physical training upon the venous pressure/volume curve.

duces the venous return and (through operation of the Starling mechanism and other reflexes, p. 55) reduces the stroke output of the heart. The blood pressure tends to fall and impulses from the pressure receptors of the aortic arch and carotid sinus diminish. Then compensatory mechanisms come into play—the heart rate accelerates, and the sympathetic discharge to the leg veins is increased, thereby decreasing their capacity at a given distending pressure.

The rate and extent of adaptations to a sudden change of posture are used in some older tests of "fitness" (p. 402). Certainly, there is good evidence that whereas a sedentary person responds to the upright position with an immediate decrease of blood pressure, an individual in a good state of cardiorespiratory training may show a small increase of blood pressure. The individuals most prone to a fall of arterial pressure on standing have avoided the stress of gravity for some time: examples include cases of prolonged bed rest, astronauts engaged in space exploration, and possibly athletes involved in prolonged swimming contests. It seems that if normal gravitational forces are not experienced periodically, the veins fail to constrict on standing. Manifestations of this loss of adaptation include tiredness, dizziness on standing rapidly, and frank "faints"; all reflect an inadequate blood supply to the brain. There may be an associated autonomic reaction, usually described as a *vaso-vagal attack*—the skin then becomes pale, moist and clammy, the subject feels nausea and the pulse rate which has been rapid suddenly slows. At the same time, the arteries supplying the muscles dilate widely. The victim "bleeds into his muscles," the blood pressure falls dramatically and loss of consciousness is rapid. If the individual concerned is allowed to lie down, the hydrostatic load distending the veins is removed, blood floods back to the heart increasing the stroke volume, and recovery is rapid. However, there have been incidents of misguided enthusiasm, particularly on the parade-ground, where fainting guardsmen have been held erect by their colleagues with serious if not fatal deprivation of blood supply to the brain.

The capacity of the veins at any given distending pressure is increased by a rise of body temperature. Under such circumstances, the total blood volume is also reduced by sweating and exudation of fluid. A faint is thus most likely to occur in hot weather. A further problem faced by the unfortunate guardsman is lack of movement. Exercise normally diminishes venous pooling; the contraction of the leg muscles forcibly pumps blood back towards the heart, and this process is helped by the subatmospheric pressures generated within the chest (the "thoracic pump"). However, venous return remains difficult if arm work is performed in an upright position. Under such conditions, the blood content of the leg veins may actually increase (hence the small cardiac stroke volume when arm work is performed). Immediately following any type of vigorous exercise, the system is particularly vulnerable to a failure of venous return. The body is hot, and the arterioles are widely patent, permitting rapid filling of the veins. If it is necessary for a subject to remain standing after exercise, he should cease his efforts gradually (warm down); among other useful functions, this keeps the muscle and the thoracic pumps operating at an adequate level.

Effect of Gravitational Acceleration

There is a dramatic increase of venous pooling if a subject encounters increased gravitational acceleration. Sudden exposure to 3 to 6g for 20 to 30 seconds was a common experience among fighter pilots during and immediately following World War II. The acceleration was normally in a footward direction, leading to ischaemia of the brain; twenty seconds exposure to 3.5 to 4g was sufficient to cause some impairment of vision (a "grey out"), and 4 to 6g for a similar period caused loss of consciousness. Tolerance of gravitational stress was worsened by poor physical condition, fatigue, a hot environment and overindulgence in alcohol. Concomitant exercise increased g tolerance. A more practical remedy for the fighter pilot was to fit an "anti-g" suit; this applied a counter-pressure to the lower half of the body whenever the aircraft banked and the aerobatic capacity of the pilots was greatly extended thereby. As accelerations were further increased, a new physiological problem appeared; a large part of the total pulmonary blood flow was directed to the lower third of the lungs, and at the same time an increase in the effective density of the pleural fluid led to collapse of the air spaces in this region. In consequence, venous blood was shunted through the collapsed segments of lung and into the arterial circulation without oxygenation.

Occasionally, increased gravitational forces were developed in the headward direction; if severe, these led to a "red-out" (unconsciousness preceded by congestion of the eye). There was a risk of cerebral damage if headward accelerations exceeded 3g.

Much greater accelerations are now encountered in rocket launching, and the astronaut minimizes the physiological effect by lying in the prone position. Much greater decelerations may be encountered in collisions of either vehicles or competing sportsmen; however, the duration of the deceleration is short, and the stresses are imposed on bones and ligaments rather than on the cardiovascular system.

Kinetic Energy

We have noted that in the resting circulation, very little energy is in the kinetic form. The exception to this generalisation is the blood in the large veins and atria. The filling of the ventricles depends on energy stored in the atrial blood, and the diastolic pressure may actually be higher in the ventricles than in the atria. Since kinetic energy is proportional to the square of velocity, the situation changes markedly during exercise—a six fold increase of flow gives a thirty-six fold increase of kinetic energy, and in maximum effort a quarter or more of the total energy within the pulmonary artery may be in the kinetic form. This is important when measuring arterial pressures—unless a pressure gauge or catheter with a lateral tapping is used, the kinetic energy is added to or subtracted from the observed pressure, and a change of flow and thus of kinetic energy may be interpreted as a change of pressure.

Pressures in the Systemic Circulation

The Arterial Pulse Wave

A simple *polygraph* was devised by Mackenzie (1853–1925) to record the radial pulse at the wrist. He distinguished several types of irregularity—the "youthful" type, corresponding to our "sinus arrhythmia," the "adult" type, corresponding to ventricular extrasystoles, and the "dangerous" type, corresponding to auricular fibrillation.

The Cameron *"heartometer,"* popular in many physical education laboratories, is basically an indirect method of recording the brachial pulse wave; an arm cuff inflated to 10 mmHg above diastolic pressure is coupled to a mechanical pressure recorder. A system of coloured lights gives a crude index of systolic and diastolic blood pressures. Some workers have attached great significance to the "heartometer" oscillations, calculating not only their amplitude and duration, but also first and second differentials of the tracings. There is certainly a relationship between the amplitude of the primary pulse wave and cardio-respiratory fitness (p. 401); this reflects the fact that pulse pressure varies with $\dfrac{\text{stroke volume}}{\text{arterial distensibility}}$

However, a large pulse pressure can reflect not only the large stroke volume of a fit subject but also the rigid arteries of an older person. Sometimes these possibilities can be distinguished by inspection of the pulse record. In general, both systolic and diastolic pressures are higher if the arterial wall is rigid, and the rise and fall of pressure are also more rapid under these conditions. The "heartometer" tracing is also influenced by the nature of the overlying tissue, particularly the texture of the skin, the amount of subcutaneous fat, and any tension in the arm muscles. In view of the very indirect nature of the recording, complex mathematical treatment of "heartometer" data seems neither necessary nor desirable.

> The rate of transmission of the pressure wave from the heart to the peripheral arteries is inversely related to the square root of the distensibility of the great vessels. Thus the pulse wave travels only about half as fast (5 m/sec) in a young person with elastic arteries as in an older person with some vascular hardening (10 m/sec). The rate of travel depends also on the mean systemic blood pressure. As this is increased, the arteries are put under stretch; their effective elasticity then declines, and the pulse wave travels more rapidly.

The Venous Pulse Wave

A very light mechanical or electrical tambour can be placed over one of the large veins to obtain indirect recordings of the venous pressure. The central venous tracing usually shows three oscillations corresponding to atrial contraction (a wave), the pressure wave transmitted from the underlying artery (c wave), and the rise of venous pressure as the atria refill (v wave). Because the Starling curve is shifted to the left in exercise, an increased stroke volume can be developed with remarkably little rise of venous pressure. However, if a patient exercises to the point where the heart is failing, there is then a considerable elevation of venous pressure, the great veins are distended, and the a and v waves are transmitted much more forcibly to the recording tambour.

The Measure of Systemic Blood Pressure

The standard clinical method of measuring systemic arterial pressure has been used for some seventy years. It dates from the design of the mercury sphygmomanometer by Riva-Rocci (1896), and the description of the sounds made by blood as it pulsed under the arm cuff (Korotkov, 1905). It is difficult to appraise the accuracy of the clinical technique, since it is a problem to record pressures simultaneously from the same limb by direct and indirect methods. However, there is general agreement that under resting conditions the pressure at which sounds can first be heard corresponds fairly closely with the systolic pressure recorded from a catheter in the brachial artery (Fig. 18). There is often a more substantial discrepancy between the directly recorded diastolic pressure and the stethoscopic estimate, whether the observer records the point when the sounds lose their tapping quality "(fourth phase") or when they are no longer audible ("fifth phase").

The accuracy of indirect measurements can be improved by careful training of the observers. Practical measures include listening to standard tape recordings of the Korotkov sounds, instruction in the dangers of digit preference (some people will consistently record a pressure ending in a zero or a five), choice of a correct cuff width (use of too large a cuff leads to overestimation of pressures) and adoption of a standard rate of cuff deflation (2 mmHg per second). Unfortunately, the error of indirectly measured pressures is greater during exercise. Difficulty arises partly because it is difficult to listen to the Korotkov sounds on a moving subject, and partly because the appearance and disappearance of the sounds is less clear-

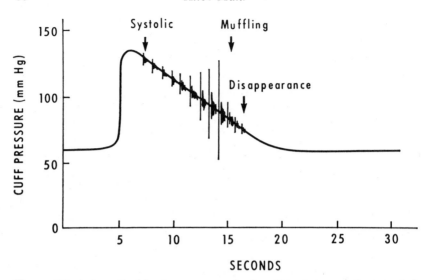

Figure 18. Automatic blood pressure recorder. Korotkov sounds recorded from the brachial artery are superimposed upon a pressure record from the syphygmomanometer cuff. The systolic pressure is indicated by the first appearance of the Korotkov sounds, the diastolic readings by their muffling and (if desired) their disappearance. The cuff is automatically inflated to 150 mmHg twice in every minute.

cut in exercise. Fortunately, the diastolic pressure changes little in the usual types of rhythmic exercise. For some purposes, it may thus be sufficient to measure the systolic pressure during activity, and to assume that the diastolic reading does not change from its resting value. Some authors believe that the indirect figure for systolic pressure is grossly inaccurate during exercise. In one study, readings were 8–15 mmHg less than catheter estimates during exercise, and exceeded the catheter figures by 16–38 mmHg during recovery. Considerable care must thus be used when interpreting exercise data.

Direct intravascular recording of arterial pressures is not usual in applied physiology. Unless direct benefit accrues to the patient, the risks of arterial puncture are not justified. However, there are a number of automatic devices that make repetitive indirect measurements of the systemic blood pressure. One was devised by the author while working at Porton (1958). This incorporates a small pump that inflates a sphygmomanometer cuff to just above systolic pressure once every thirty seconds; over the next fifteen seconds, the pressure drops to 60 mmHg, and the cuff is then completely deflated for fifteen seconds; if greater accuracy is required, the cycle length can be increased to sixty seconds. The pressure within the cuff is monitored continuously by an electrical transducer. A microphone is strapped over the brachial artery, and this detects the Korotkov sounds, which are superimposed on the pressure record (Fig. 18). The points of appearance, muffling, and disappearance of the sounds are noted as in standard clinical practice. The main difficulty when using the technique for an extended period is that activity tends to displace the microphone from the optimum recording site.

The Interpretation of Resting Blood Pressure

Since exercise induces a rise of systemic blood pressure, it is wise to exclude from very vigorous activity those individuals with a pathologically high resting blood pressure. However, the precise point at which an abnormally high resting blood pressure (hypertension) should be diagnosed is a matter of dispute. The blood pressure is greatly increased by anxiety, and much thus depends on the degree of relaxation that is achieved. Pressures also rise over the course of the day, and the systolic pressure is increased following a heavy meal; finally, both systolic and diastolic pressures increase by 10 to 15 mmHg over the span of adult life. The clinician usually attaches more significance to an increase of diastolic than of systolic pressure. A diastolic reading of 90 mmHg is viewed with suspicion, and a reading of 100 mmHg or more is indicative of hypertension.

The Influence of Activity on Systemic Blood Pressure

The immediate effect of rhythmic physical activity is a progressive increase of systolic pressure, varying in extent with the intensity and duration of effort; on the other hand, most authors find little or no increase of diastolic pressure during rhythmic work (Fig. 19). Isometric exercise (p. 162) gives a large and rapid increase of both systolic and diastolic pressures, even if the contracting muscles form a rather small fraction of the total muscle bulk. The rise of pressure is first seen when the active muscles are contracting at more than 15 percent of their maximum force, and it reaches a peak when the contraction is some 70 percent of maximum effort. There is a close parallel between the reduction of muscle blood flow by the isometric

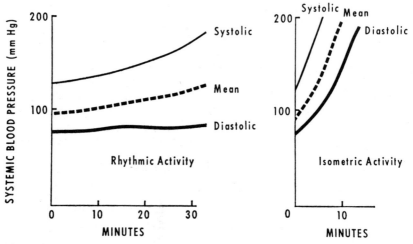

Figure 19. A comparison of the increments in systemic blood pressure induced by rhythmic and isometric muscular contractions.

effort and the corresponding rise in mean systemic blood pressure. The hypertension seems mainly an attempt by the body to compensate for compression of the intramuscular vessels. The local stimulus is not precisely identified, but it is known that the nerve pathway involves the sensory fibres of the dorsal column of the spinal cord. The response is thus absent in syringomyelia, a disease that damages this part of the spinal cord. A second factor that may contribute to the rise of blood pressure is a tendency to make a forced expiratory effort against a closed glottis (the Valsalva manoeuvre). This action leads to an increase of intrathoracic pressure and thus of peripheral systemic pressure, (see pressure breathing, p. 155). It is a common occurrence during weight-lifting feats, but is less likely to be involved in the hypertension that accompanies more modest hand grip efforts.

The difference of blood pressure response to rhythmic and isometric exercise has important application to the design of rehabilitation programmes. Rhythmic exercise places little strain upon the heart unless it is so prolonged that there is a large increase of systolic pressure and thus of tension work. On the other hand, even a few minutes of sustained isometric

contractions, weight lifting, or the supporting of body weight
from the arms can give a disastrous rise of blood pressure and
thus of cardiac work. Most authors believe the rise of blood
pressure carries a risk of bursting an aneurysm or some other
weak point in the walls of the great vessels; however, if a
Valsalva manoeurve is performed, this provides some protection to the intrathoracic vessels through a simultaneous increase
of extramural pressures.

The long-term effects of exercise upon the resting systemic
blood pressure are still the subject of dispute. Some workers
have found a small (5–10 mmHg) reduction of pressure in
those attending a regular exercise class, but it is difficult to
dissociate this apparent improvement from the greater familiarity of the subjects with the laboratory and the observer as the
experiment proceeds.

Mechanisms of Regulation in the Systemic Circulation

Cybernetics

The regulation of the circulation is effected by one of the many
cybernetic control mechanisms in the body. The primary variable
that is controlled is the central blood pressure; specialized sensors
detect deviations from control settings in the aorta and at the
bifurcation of the common carotid arteries, thus protecting the
blood supply to the brain except in unusual circumstances. There
is a typical cybernetic loop—an input from the sensors via the
carotid sinus nerves, regulating centres (the cardiac and vasomotor centres in the medulla), and a negative feedback via
the autonomic nerves supplying the heart and blood vessels.
However, information from many other sources (Fig. 20) may
alter the "setting" of the medullary centres, and in some cases
both the output of the heart and the local reactions of the
blood vessels may override the general control mechanisms.

Sensory Input

Impulses from the higher centres of the brain can have a
marked influence on the "setting" of the cardioregulatory and

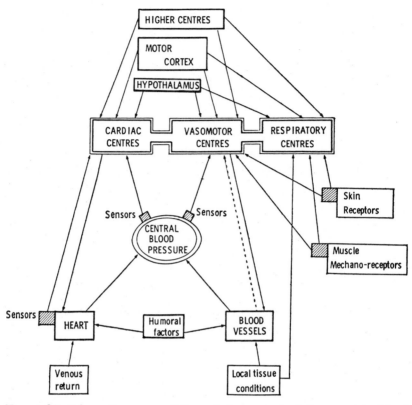

Figure 20. Schematic representation of the control of the systemic blood pressure.

vasomotor centres. Anger, anxiety, and other emotional responses can increase both heart rate and blood pressure, thereby throwing a heavier load upon the heart than vigorous exercise (p. 66). In the athlete, conditioned reflexes from the cerebral cortex may initiate similar changes immediately prior to a race.

Information may also irradiate from the motor cortex to the cardiac and vasomotor centres. When voluntary activity is initiated, there is a tremendous increase in the neural discharge from the motor regions of the brain; the majority of impulses travel via the pyramidal fibres to the anterior horn cells of the spinal cord, where they are relayed to the contracting muscles.

However, a small proportion of the neural signals reach the cardioregulatory centres of the medulla oblongata, thereby contributing to the early increase of heart rate in the first few seconds of exercise.

Centres regulating body temperature are found in the hypothalamus. If body temperature rises as a result of exercise or exposure to a warm environment, impulses irradiate from the hypothalamus to the cardioregulatory and vasomotor centres, inducing tachycardia, vasodilatation and an increase in the blood flow to the skin.

The medullary centres concerned with the circulation may also receive impulses from the centres controlling respiration. Thus, on exposure to a low pressure of oxygen, the respiratory centres are stimulated by impulses from the carotid bodies, and irradiation of this information to the vasomotor centre gives a marked rise of blood pressure.

Finally, information is transmitted to the medullary centres from a wide range of peripheral receptors. The most important are the nerve endings of the prime sensors in the carotid sinus and the aortic wall. These receptors send depressor impulses to the cardioregulatory centre when the systemic blood pressure rises; they are more receptive to the rate of pressure change than to the mean pressure level, and thus their rate of discharge for any given mean pressure is greater when the pulse pressure is increased. A second group of receptors important in the context of exercise are located in the muscles and joints; these are stimulated by either active or passive limb movements, and account for a substantial part of the increase of heart rate during exercise. Receptors have also been described in the great veins, the atria, the ventricles, and the pulmonary arteries. These intra vascular receptors are occasionally stimulated by exposure to industrial irritants such as organic nitriles, but their normal functional significance is less certain. If the great veins are deliberately distended, the receptors within their walls usually initiate an increase of heart rate (the "Bainbridge Reflex"). However, this reflex is unlikely to be involved in the tachycardia of exercise, since the cardiac output of a normally active person is increased without an increase of venous filling pressure.

Cardiac Regulation

The heart rate is normally slowed by impulses passing down the vagus nerve, and is speeded through increased activity of the sympathetic nerves. Similar effects can be induced experimentally by the injection of massive doses of the substances (acetyl-choline and noradrenaline) that normally transmit nerve signals from the endings of the vagal and sympathetic fibres to the cardiac pacemaker in the sinuatrial node. However, both transmitter substances are broken down rapidly in the body, through the action of appropriate enzymes (choline-esterase and amine-oxidase, respectively). It it thus unlikely that either compound can accumulate under physiological conditions. However, acetyl-choline may reach a pharmacologically active concentration if the choline-esterase is inhibited. This occurs during poisoning with certain organo-phosphorus compounds used as insecticides and chemical warfare agents ("nerve gas"). If poisoning is severe, the rate of sinus rhythm is greatly slowed, and "heart block" may also develop at the atrioventricular node (p. 73).

Trained athletes have a slow resting heart rate (30–60 beats per minute) relative to untrained men (70–80 beats per minute). The resting cardiac output is rather similar in the two groups, but the athlete has a larger stroke volume than the nonathlete. Much of the literature from Eastern Europe extols the virtues of what is called "vagotonia"; the rate of vagal discharge is probably greater in a trained individual than in one who is untrained, but other mechanisms undoubtedly contribute to the slow heart rate of the athlete, and "vagotonia" scarcely merits the mystic significance with which it is sometimes endowed.

The exercise response (p. 52) normally involves an increase of the sympathetic and a decrease of the vagal discharge. However, recent experiments on dogs have shown that some increase of cardiac output is still possible in completely denervated hearts, presumably through the operation of Starling's law (p. 55).

Muscle Blood Flow

Measurement of Peripheral Blood Flow. Venous occlusion plethys-mography is the standard technique for measurement of blood flow to skin and muscle. The method works best on the upper limb. The classical design of plethysmograph consists of a rigid metal or perspex cylinder, with a tightly fitting rubber sleeve at either end. The arm is slipped through the sleeves, and the cylinder is filled with water at a "neutral" temperature (33–34°C). Any change in the dimensions of the enclosed limb segment is transmitted by the water to a suitable recording device. The veins are first emptied by raising the limb above heart level. Venous return is then blocked by in-flating a blood pressure cuff to 50–60 mmHg, and the blood flow is deduced from the initial rate of swelling of the enclosed segment.

In some applications, both hand and forearm are enclosed by the plethysmograph. However, it is more usual to measure flow to the hand and the forearm separately. The hand is largely representative of skin blood flow, while the proximal part of the forearm reflects mainly muscle blood flow. For the forearm measurements, the return of blood from the hand is obstructed by a second cuff, distal to the plethysmograph and inflated to above arterial pressure.

The water-filled plethysmograph is at best heavy and cumber-some. It severely restricts movement of the limb, and commonly discharges its water content at an inopportune moment. It is thus increasingly replaced by a series of two or more mercury-in-rubber strain gauges. Fine silastic capillary tubes are filled with mercury; their electrical resistance then varies with the extent to which they are stretched, and if they are fitted around a limb, they can be used in the same manner as a classical plethysmograph. The strain gauges have several important advantages. In particular, they are light, and can be worn during vigorous exercise without impeding normal heat loss. Unfortunately, the quality of records obtained during physical activity is poor, since muscle contractions themselves change limb dimensions. It is thus quite common to examine flow immediately following physical activity; as we shall see below, the postexercise measurement is distorted by restriction of flow during movement.

Methods that can be used during exercise are remarkably few. The rate of heat loss from an electrically warmed intramuscular probe gives a qualitative index of muscle flow. However, the re-sponses observed vary considerably with displacements of the exploring needle towards or away from major arteries. The rate of removal of radioactive material (such as $Na^{24}Cl$) indicates the average blood flow through the nutritive capillaries of a muscle (blood flowing through arteriovenous anastomoses does not contribute to the clearance of radioactive compounds). Counting must extend over a minute or more to obtain a reasonably accurate reading and measurements are distorted if the relationship between the limb and the counter is altered (as may happen during physical activity). The ideal method of measuring blood flow to an active limb has yet to be devised.

Regulation of Muscle Blood Flow. The nerve fibres supplying the intramuscular blood vessels are derived entirely from the sympathetic system; however, they are of two distinct types— adrenergic fibres, which release noradrenaline and cause vasoconstriction, and cholinergic fibres, which release acetyl-choline and cause active vasodilatation. The adrenergic fibres normally exert a substantial constrictor tone, and a decreased adrenergic discharge plays a larger role in increasing flow than does an increased activity of the cholinergic fibres. As would be expected from the foregoing discussion, both adrenaline and noradrenaline have a direct constricting effect upon the muscle blood vessels; however, they also have a slower indirect dilating effect. In the case of adrenaline, a stimulation of metabolism within the vessel wall is thought to be responsible for the late vasodilatation; the mechanism for noradrenaline involves the sympathetic nerve fibres in some manner that has yet to be elucidated.

The immediate effect of exercise is an increased adrenergic discharge, and thus there is a tendency for muscle blood flow to be reduced throughout the body. This can be regarded as a necessary precaution, to prevent overperfusion of inactive muscle groups. It is difficult to demonstrate any specific modulation of this neural activity in fibres supplying the vasculature of active muscles, and it must be presumed that the constrictor effect of the nerve impulses is countermanded by local vasodilator metabolites. A number of likely candidates (oxygen lack, a decrease in pH, accumulation of lactate, histamine, and bradykinin) have now been excluded, but several possibilities such as the extracellular accumulation of potassium ions or adenosine triphosphate remain to be explored.

Despite vasodilation, muscle flow may be impaired by physical activity (see also section 9.2). During rhythmic work, flow is increased several fold, but it is still impeded somewhat by contractions, and is much greater in the intervals of relaxation (Fig. 21). Isometric contractions start to restrict blood flow when the force developed is 15 percent of a maximum contraction, and if the force is more than 70 percent to 80 percent of maximum the vessels are completely occluded. This point can be demonstrated experimentally by fitting a cuff around the upper arm and inflating it to above arterial pressure; if muscle contractions are at more than 70 percent of maximum force, the time to fatigue is uninfluenced by inflation of the cuff (Fig. 43)

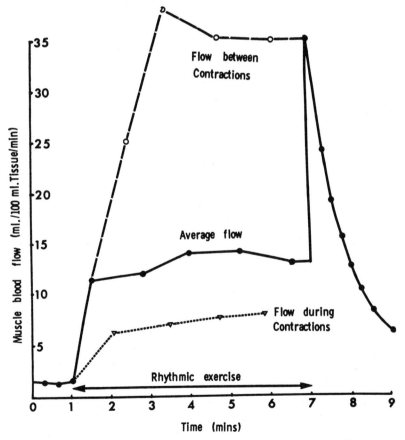

Figure 21. The influence of rhythmic exercise on muscle blood flow. (Based on a study of Barcroft and Dornhorst, *J Physiol, 109*:402, 1949).

Skin Blood Flow

The skin blood flow increases quite rapidly in a hot environment. The main mechanism is a reduction in the normal vasoconstrictor tone, mediated via sympathetic nerve fibres distributed in the sheaths of the blood vessels. There is also some local dilatation of the vessels in response to warmth, even when the sympathetic nerves have been surgically removed. However, the cholinergic dilator fibres seen in muscle are absent from the skin. This can be demonstrated by experiments on the heated hand; the local blood flow is not diminished either by injecting atropine (which would block the transmission of cholinergic impulses) or by infiltrating the somatic nerves with local anaesthetic. A further mechanism of vasodilatation in a hot environment may be a local response of the subcutaneous vessels to bradykinin, an active compound released during activity of the thermal sweat glands.

Much of the increased flow to the extremities by-passes the normal capillary circulation; blood passes directly from the small arterioles to the venules through a series of arteriovenous anastomoses. Heat loss is thus occurring primarily from superficial veins. Blood flowing via this pathway by-passes the tissues, and oxygen extraction is therefore minimal. The extent of such "nonmetabolic" flow largely determines the maximum arteriovenous oxygen differences reached in exhausting exercise. A well-trained subject loses a larger proportion of his total heat production by sweating, and less by pumping blood through the arteriovenous anastomoses. Mainly for this reason, he develops an overall arteriovenous oxygen difference of 16–17 ml/100 ml of blood, compared with 13–14 ml/100 ml in an untrained subject.

The decrease of blood flow to the extremities in the cold reflects a shutting down of the arteriovenous anastomoses. The reduction in blood flow is particularly marked if physical activity involving intense vibration is performed in the cold; spasm then affects not only the arteriovenous anastomoses, but also the capillaries supplying the metabolic needs of the digits. Some individuals are particularly susceptible, and a distinct syndrome (Raynaud's disease) is recognised by clinicians. The usual descriptions refer to men operating pneumatic drills, but the condition is also quite common in forestry workers operating chain saws. The critical frequency of vibration is high (~100 cycles per second), and attempts to eliminate such frequencies from mechanical equipment have not been particularly successful. Not all workers are affected; there seems an undue sensitivity to both vibration and cold in those who are susceptible. Extensive surgery, such as removal of the sympathetic nerve supply to the limb, has sometimes given one or two years of relief; however, the severity of the disease process does not generally warrant such drastic intervention, and the operation itself tends to cause an increased sensitivity of the vessels to catecholamines, thereby reducing the likelihood of an ultimate cure.

Visceral Flow

We have noted previously (p. 49) that a number of the visceral organs such as the kidneys receive more than their fair share of the total cardiac output at rest, and that visceral flow is drastically reduced when exercise is performed in the heat. Such changes reflect mainly an altered balance of sympathetic and parapathetic nerve discharge. However, the catecholamines also have a direct constricting effect on the visceral vessels, and to the extent that blood levels of catecholamines are increased by physical activity (p. 244), these hormones may also contribute to the redistribution of blood flow. The maximum possible redistribution is perhaps 2–3 litre/min, no more than 10 percent of the total exercise requirement of 20–30 litre/min.

Some Problems of Circulatory Regulation

Collapse. Collapse at the end of an exhausting race is by no means uncommon, particularly in a hot environment. The immediate symptoms are due to a failure of the blood supply to the brain. Intense dilatation of the arteries and veins within the limbs is supplemented by a decrease of blood volume due to sweating; the blood pressure can no longer be maintained, and premonitory local symptoms such as mental confusion, or blacking out of part of the visual field are followed—often quite rapidly—by loss of consciousness.

No harm results if the patient falls to the ground, activity is stopped, fluids are provided, and the body is cooled by tepid sponging. However, more serious consequences may supervene if a contestant is urged to his feet and continues to struggle towards the finishing line. Failure of the sweat glands, a progressive rise of body temperature, renal failure, and exhaustion of the adrenal glands may all occur, sometimes with fatal consequences.

Deaths from heat collapse and its complications are a recognized hazard of United States football games, particularly if the contestants wear nylon clothing that is impervious to sweat (see also p. 302). A more general increase of "cardiovascular" deaths occurs in the steamy cities of the southern United States during hot spells. A third group particularly prone to heat problems are workers in deep underground mines.

Pressure Breathing. The term "pressure breathing" is something of a misnomer, since respiration would be impossible in the absence of pressure; what is usually implied is a pressure higher than normal ("positive pressure breathing") or lower than normal ("negative pressure breathing"). The pressure may be intermittent (as in various mechanical respirators) or continuous ("positive" pressure, as developed by a weight lifter performing a Valsalva manoeuvre, or supplied to an aviator operating at altitudes in excess of 40,000 feet; "negative" pressure as encountered by a snorkel diver with a surface line). Intermittent "positive" intraalveolar pressure can restrict the pulmonary circulation; normally, alveolar pressure exceeds pulmonary arterial pressure towards the apex of the lung, but if the alveolar pressure is increased, perfusion becomes impossible in a much larger proportion of the lung, with consequent "wastage" of much of the induced ventilation. A respiratory pump with a phase of "negative" intraalveolar pressure assists venous return to the chest, and leads to more uniform perfusion of the lung; however, in practice, these advantages are outweighed by the onset of collapse in the more dependent and better perfused parts of the lung. Theoretically, the "negative" pressure also increases the formation of oedema fluid within the lung, but this disadvantage is hard to demonstrate experimentally.

The earliest aviation pressure breathing equipment simply increased the intrathoracic pressure. This led to distension of the chest, with stimulation of airway stretch receptors, and a very uncomfortable pattern of shallow panting breathing. The next development was to wear an air-filled suit that applied counterpressure to the chest and abdomen. This made respiration much more comfortable, but presented a major problem to the circulation; if the suit pressure was, say, 100 mmHg, venous return from the limbs ceased until the veins had filled to this new, higher pressure. Assuming the body withstood the immediate crisis without collapse, there was a progressive loss of fluid into the limb tissues, and this further reduction of effective blood volume—plus the attendant swelling and discomfort of the tissues—commonly led to a vasovagal attack in one to five minutes. The obvious remedy was to enclose the entire aviator in a "full-pressure suit"; the main reason for reluctance to accept the obvious was that the inflated suit acted as a rigid splint, preventing necessary movement of the limbs.

The snorkel diver has the entire body surface exposed to a higher pressure than alveolar gas. He is thus engaged in continuous "negative" pressure respiration. As with intermittent negative pressure, there is a risk of causing collapse of parts of the lung, and breathing is carried out with a relatively small alveolar gas volume. If the airway is closed and the external pressure is further increased, then the chest may be compressed to its minimum dimensions (residual volume), yet leaving the air pressure within the lungs substantially less than that in the pulmonary capillaries. Haemorrhage into the lung tissues is then likely (the "thoracic squeeze" syndrome p. 277).

Shock. Shock is a term so abused by many writers that it currently has little meaning. It was a frequent diagnosis in both world wars, particularly in casualties that had suffered severe haemorrhage, and it is best defined as a loss of blood volume to which the body cannot readily adjust. Let us suppose that an experimental animal such as a cat is bled repeatedly. At first, the removal of 10–20 ml of blood gives only a transient fall of blood pressure. However, if the bleeding is repeated at short intervals, adjustment becomes slower and incomplete in character. For a time, recovery is still possible if the animal is tended carefully, but ultimately the blood pressure is reduced to a critical mean value (between 40 and 50 mmHg) where further removal of blood leads to an irreversible deterioration of condition.

It seems likely that the irreversible changes reflect an in-adequate blood supply and thus oxygen lack in certain vital organs—possibly the brain, kidneys, liver, and intestines. The large intestine has an enormous bacterial population, and death of this region leads to a massive circulatory infusion of microorganisms ("septicaemia"). Under field conditions, such infection is supplemented by local con-tamination of injuries and the situation may later be complicated by exhaustion of defence mechanisms such as the adrenal glands.

The "shocked" patient has a cold, pale and sweaty skin, since there is an intense constriction of the subcutaneous blood vessels in an attempt to maintain the systemic pressure. At one time, it was common practice to "treat" the cold skin by heavy blankets and even radiant heat cradles. This inevitably led to a dilatation of the superficial vessels, a further fall of blood pressure, and rapid death. The essential item of treatment is a rapid restoration of circulating fluid—preferably by an appropriately matched blood transfusion. If this is not immediately available, a physician can give an infusion of plasma or a glucose/dextran polymer mixture. Drinks such as tea are of doubtful benefit in serious cases; in the absence of blood protein or a high molec-ular weight polymer, the fluid is rapidly excreted, and in the event that surgical treatment of the injury is required, the drink may be vomited during induction of anaesthesia. However, prevention of haemorrhage, elevation of the legs, and bandaging of the limbs are useful first-aid measures.

Exercise and the Pulmonary Circulation

The pulmonary circulation has a number of special features that merit separate discussion. Pressures in the pulmonary artery are normally quite low (about 18 mmHg systolic and 7 mmHg diastolic). Further, the entire system is very disten-sible; a threefold increase of blood flow can be accomodated without a significant rise of presure, and even in maximum exercise a healthy young person probably does not exceed pressures of 25/10 mmHg.

The pulmonary arteries, and to a greater extent the pulmonary veins function as a variable reservoir for the left ventricle. At rest, some 500 ml of blood is "stored" in the lungs, and in ex-ercise there may be three times this quantity. Little of this store is in contact with alveolar gas. The blood content of the pulmonary capillaries is no more than 100 ml at rest, rising to perhaps 200 ml in vigorous exercise. The cross-section of the pulmonary capillary bed undergoes a threefold expansion in vigorous exercise, and since the maximum cardiac output may reach six times the resting value, the speed of flow through the capillaries is increased by exercise. A typical red cell spends 0.75 sec in the pulmonary capillaries of a resting man, but only 0.35 sec during exercise. When a man is standing upright, the pulmonary arterial pressure is close to zero in the upper third of the lung. Under these circumstances, the alveolar gas pressure may exceed pulmonary arterial pressure, thereby interrupting blood flow through the upper part of the lung. Since exercise raises pulmonary arterial pressure, perfusion of the upper parts of the lung may be improved by vigorous work; unfortunately, this advantage is sometimes offset by a parallel increase of alveolar gas pressures.

Normally, there is little tendency for fluid to escape from the pulmonary capillaries. However, the balance can be upset if "negative" pressure breathing is carried out when capillary permeability has been increased by prolonged oxygen lack or chemical poisoning. Oxygen lack also raises pressures in the pulmonary circulation, a factor that may contribute to the development of high altitude oedema (p. 258).

Exercise and the Microcirculation

The role of the arteriovenous anastomoses in by-passing the capillary microcirculation has already been mentioned (p. 97). We shall discuss here the behavior of the capillaries proper, with particular reference to physical activity.

The large increase of muscle blood flow during—and immediately following—vigorous exercise is matched by a large increase in the number of patent capillaries within the active muscles. August Krogh (1874–1949), a famous Danish physiologist, made many of the classical studies on capillary behaviour, and he reported a twenty-fold increase of capillary density (from 5/mm² at rest to >100/mm² during exercise). Krogh faced many technical difficul-

ties in making his estimates, and the subsequent introduction of
rapid freezing techniques has greatly improved the precision of
morphometric work by minimising tissue distortion. Current authors
set the capillary density at about $200/mm^2$ for rest and $600/mm^2$
for exercise.

The increased count expands the effective surface area of the
muscle capillaries and thus increases the tissue diffusing capacity (p. 140). It also shortens the average distance between
the capillaries and the metabolically active sites within the
muscle cells, thereby enabling tissue diffusion to proceed with
a smaller terminal gradient of oxygen pressure.

Some fluid normally "leaks" from the blood into the tissues
at the arterial end of the capillaries. The hydrostatic pressure
in this region may be 30 mmHg, compared with 8 mmHg or
less in the tissues. There is thus a net hydrostatic pressure of
22 mmHg, tending to produce exudation. This is opposed by
osmotic forces. The plasma colloid osmotic pressure is some
25 mmHg, compared with 10 mmHg for the extracellular fluid.
Hence, there is a net osmotic pressure of 15 mmHg opposing
the 22 mmHg hydrostatic pressure, and a resultant pressure of
7 mmHg driving fluid from the capillaries into the tissues. At
the venous end of the capillaries, the hydrostatic pressure is at
least 15 mmHg less, while the osmotic forces are largely unchanged. Thus there is a net pressure of about 8 mmHg favor-
ing resorption at the venous end of the capillary, and fluid does
not accumulate in the tissues. However, the balance is a delicate one, and is upset by either an increase of hydrostatic
pressure within the capillaries (exercise, prolonged standing,
heart failure, pressure breathing) or a reduction of the effective
plasma osmotic pressure (starvation and changes of capillary
permeability, p. 239).

In exercise, the pressure within the capillaries may rise by
at least 10 mmHg. The initial loss of fluid from the circulation
has been set at 0.4 ml/min per 100 ml of muscle, or if 20 kg
of muscle are active, 80 ml/min. If this rate of loss continued
throughout sustained activity, it would represent a serious drain
upon a total blood volume of 5 litres. Fortunately, the exudation of fluid increases both tissue hydrostatic pressure and

plasma colloid pressure, so that the process is rapidly self limiting. However, the red-cell count is increased by 5 to 10% immediately after vigorous exercise; such haemoconcentration is helpful in the transport of both oxygen and hydrogen ions by the blood, but it also increases viscosity thereby increasing the cardiac workload. Although exudation of fluid tends to be self-limiting, other mechanisms help to conserve blood volume during exercise. Urine formation virtually ceases, and the tone of the venous reservoirs is increased.

The permeability of the capillary wall, and thus the effective osmotic pressure gradient can be upset by large changes of intravascular oxygen and carbon dioxide tensions. However, changes of the required order are unlikely unless the circulation is completely interrupted for a substantial period of time.

References

Burton, A.C.: *Physiology and Biophysics of the Circulation.* Chicago, Year Book Medical Publishers, 1965.

Fishman, A.P., and Richards, D.W.: *Circulation of the Blood: Men and Ideas.* New York, Oxford University Press, 1964.

Carlsten, A., and Grimby, G.: *The Circulatory Response to Muscular Exercise in Man.* Springfield, Thomas, 1966.

Guyton, A.: *Circulatory Physiology: Cardiac Output and its Regulation.* Philadelphia, Saunders, 1963.

Hamilton, W.F.: *Handbook of Physiology.* Section 2: Circulation. Baltimore, Williams & Wilkins, 1963–1965, vol. 1, 2, 3.

Shepherd, J.T.: *Physiology of the Circulation in Human Limbs in Health and Disease.* Philadelphia, Saunders, 1963.

Roskamm, H., Reindell, H., and König, K.: *Körperliche Aktivität und Herz-und Kreislauferkrankungen.* Munich, Barth, 1966.

Rose, G.A., and Blackburn, H.: *Cardiovascular Survey Methods.* Geneva, WHO, 1968.

Wood, P.: *Diseases of the Heart and Circulation.* London, Eyre & Spottis-woode, 1968.

Dimond, E.G.: *The Exercise Electrocardiogram in Office Practice.* Springfield, Thomas, 1961.

Shephard, R.J. (Rapporteur): *Exercise Tests in Relation to Cardiovascular Function.* Geneva, WHO, 1968.

Chapman, C.B.: Physiology of muscular exercise. *Amer Heart Ass Monog 15.* New York AHA, 1967.

Wade, O.L., and Bishop, J.M.: *Cardiac Output and Regional Blood Flow.* Oxford, Blackwell, 1962.

West, J.B.: *Ventilation/Blood Flow and Gas Exchange.* Oxford, Blackwell, 1965.

de Reuck, A.V.S., and O'Connor, M.: *Problems of Pulmonary Circulation.* London, Churchill, 1961.

Aviado, D.M.: *The Lung Circulation.* Oxford, Pergamon, 1965.

Physiology Society Symposium: Physiological basis of circulatory shock. *Fed Proc: 29,* 1832, 1970.

Reeve, E.B., and Guyton, A.C.: *Physical Bases of Circulatory Transport. Regulation and Exchange.* Philadelphia, Saunders, 1967.

Nunn, J.F.: *Applied Respiratory Physiology With Special Reference to Anaesthesia.* London, Butterworths, 1969.

Gillies, J.A.: *A Textbook of Aviation Physiology.* Oxford, Pergamon, 1965.

Harrison, T.R., and Reeves, T.J.: Cardiac resuscitation and electrical treatment of arrhythmias. In: *Principles and Problems of Ischemic Heart Disease.* Chicago, Year Book Medical Publishers, 1968.

Greene, D.G.: Drowning. In Fenn, W.O., and Rahn, H. (Eds.): *Handbook of Physiology.* Section 3, Respiration. Baltimore, Williams & Wilkins, 1965, vol. 2.

Altman, P.L., and Dittmer, D.S.: *Respiration and Circulation.* Bethesda, Md., Federation of American Societies for Experimental Biology, 1971.

5

THE RESPIRATORY SYSTEM

The Ventilatory Conductances and Their Role in Sustained Exercise

Classical physiology has conceived respiration as proceeding through a series of closely linked stages—"external" ventilation (the exchange of gas between the atmosphere and the alveolar spaces), pulmonary diffusion (the exchange of gas between the alveoli and pulmonary capillary blood), blood transport, tissue diffusion (the exchange of gases between peripheral capillaries and the tissues), and finally tissue respiration. It was necessary to discuss the blood transport term when dealing with the cardiovascular system (p. 48); in this connection, we noted that the several stages of gas exchange could be represented by a chain of conductances, each offering a finite impedance to the movement of gas from the atmosphere to the working tissues. Oxygen intake was mainly dependent on blood transport, while carbon dioxide elimination depended on both alveolar ventilation and blood transport.

Let us now examine the stages other than blood transport. Air flows into and out of the chest in response to forces developed by the respiratory muscles and the elasticity of the thoracic cage and lung tissues; these forces overcome viscous and turbulent air flow resistance, viscous resistance to tissue displacement, and the inertia of both the air molecules and heavy viscera such as the liver. The external ventilation is normally measured at the mouth. Unfortunately, not all of the recorded volume is effective from the viewpoint of gas exchange (Fig. 22). Part is spent in ventilating the conducting airways (the anatomical dead space). A further part is "wasted" in ventilation of lung regions that are either poorly perfused or have an inadequate diffusing capacity (the so-called "alveolar dead space"). Only the ventilation of appropriately perfused alveoli contributes to the overall gas exchange. A variable part

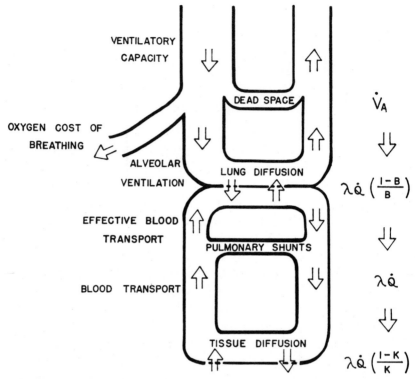

Figure 22. The conductances concerned in respiratory exchange, and the corresponding partial pressures of oxygen. For the meaning of the symbols, see page 556.

Diagram reproduced by permission of Ontario Medical Review.

of the total oxygen intake is consumed by the respiratory muscles. This is obviously not available for the performance of external work. Thus, when assessing the suitability of a given pattern of breathing during exercise, we must consider not only the alveolar ventilation that is achieved, but also the possible disadvantage to other active tissues of an increase in the work of breathing.

The impedance to gas transfer at any stage in the respiratory chain is given by the reciprocal of the corresponding conductance (p. 48). Thus, the impedance to movement of oxygen between the atmosphere and the alveolar spaces is proportional to the reciprocal of alveolar ventilation $\left(\dfrac{1}{\dot{V}_A}\right)$. Reference to an electrical analogy suggests a second simple measure of impedance. Suppose that a number of conductors are arranged in series; then the proportion of the total voltage drop that occurs across any one conductor depends simply on the proportion of the total impedance offered by this conductor. Let us now equate voltage with oxygen partial pressure. There is a finite drop of oxygen pressure, from some 150 mmHg in inspired gas (P_{I,O_2}) to almost zero pressure in the active tissues (P_{t,O_2}). This pressure distributes itself between the several conductances of the oxygen transport chain in proportion to the contribution each makes to the overall impedance. The relevant gradients for alveolar ventilation and blood transport are readily seen; these are, respectively, from inspired to alveolar gas ($P_{I,O_2}-P_{A,O_2}$), and from arterial to mixed venous blood ($P_{a,O_2}-P_{\bar{v},O_2}$). We are considering the conductances as arranged in series, and this apparently implies that the gradient for pulmonary diffusion is from alveolar gas to arterial blood ($P_{A,O_2}-P_{a,O_2}$), while that for tissue diffusion is from mixed venous to tissue gas ($P_{\bar{v},O_2}-P_{t,O_2}$).

The last two gradients are at variance with traditional views on gas diffusion. The diffusing capacity of the lungs ($\dot{D}_L$) is normally expressed as the rate of gas transfer per unit of pressure gradient between alveolar gas and a hypothetical "mean capillary" blood specimen. The hypothetical "mean capillary" pressure (Fig. 23) is so calculated that exactly half of the observed oxygen uptake has occurred by the time that blood traversing the pulmonary capillary vessels reaches this pressure ($P_{\overline{pc},O_2}$). The diffusing capacity for oxygen is then calculated according to the equation

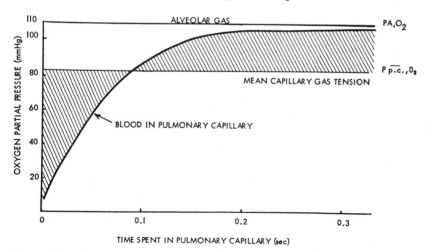

Figure 23. The concept of a mean pulmonary capillary oxygen tension that will permit the observed oxygen exchange. The line is drawn in such a manner that the two shaded areas are of equal size.

$$\dot{D}_L = \frac{\dot{V}_{O_2}}{(P_{A,O_2} - P_{\overline{pc},O_2})}$$

The reason why the gradient in our model is $(P_{A,O_2} - P_{a,O_2})$, rather than $(P_{A,O_2} - P_{\overline{pc},O_2})$ is that we are really studying not diffusion alone, but rather the interaction between blood transport and diffusion. The corresponding impedance is a complex quantity $\left(\dfrac{B}{1-B}\right)\dfrac{1}{\lambda\dot{Q}}$, where B is an exponent based on the ratio of pulmonary diffusing capacity to blood transport $(B = e^{\frac{-\dot{D}_L}{\lambda\dot{Q}}})$

Similarly, in the tissues, we are studying the interaction between blood transport and tissue diffusion. The relevant impedance is again a complex quantity $\left(\dfrac{K}{1-K}\right)\dfrac{1}{\lambda\dot{Q}}$ where K is an exponent based on the ratio of tissue diffusing capacity to blood transport $(K = e^{\frac{-\dot{D}_t}{\lambda\dot{Q}}})$.

As in any chain of conductances, the overall impedance $\dfrac{1}{\dot{U}}$ is given by the sum of the individual components:

$$\frac{1}{\dot{U}} = \frac{1}{\dot{V}_A} + \left(\frac{B}{1-B}\right)\frac{1}{\lambda\dot{Q}} + \frac{1}{\lambda\dot{Q}} + \left(\frac{K}{1-K}\right)\frac{1}{\lambda\dot{Q}}$$

Fortunately, the more complex second and fourth terms are not very important during maximum exercise at sea level. For most purposes, the equation describing gas transport thus simplifies to the form we have already discussed in the section on the cardiovascular system:

$$\frac{1}{\dot{U}} = \frac{1}{\dot{V}_A} + \frac{1}{\lambda\dot{Q}}$$

However, there is some evidence that the term describing the interaction between pulmonary diffusion and blood transport can be important if the alveolar oxygen pressure falls. This is the case when vigorous work is performed at moderately high altitudes and when underwater swimming is sustained by breath-holding rather than by the use of breathing equipment.

External Ventilation

The Respiratory Minute Volume

The normal resting respiratory minute volume is about 4 litre/min BTPS per square metre of body surface area. Thus, a ventilation of 7.2 litre/min BTPS would be anticipated in a young man with a body surface area of 1.80 m². The breathing frequency depends on the state of training of the individual. Athletes generally breathe more slowly than sedentary individuals. A rate of fourteen breaths per minute would be typical of a sedentary young man; with a ventilation of 7.2 litre/min, this would imply a tidal volume of 500 ml BTPS.

When exercise is undertaken, there is a triphasic increase of ventilation. The triphasic response has a similar basis to that described for the increase of pulse rate (p. 52 and Fig. 8). There is an initial rapid increase of ventilation in response to conditioned reflexes and an irradiation of impulses from the motor cortex. The second phase is largely a response to the stimulation of muscle and joint proprioceptors. With moderate effort, a plateau of ventilation is reached in one to two minutes, but with more severe work, a third phase of slowly increasing ventilation is seen. Many factors contribute to the third phase, including the accumulation of acid metabolites, and a rise of deep body temperature.

The ventilatory response to a given work load is usually reported in terms of "steady-state" data; a "steady-state" is assumed when the body has been allowed four or five minutes to adapt to the new level of metabolism. A typical response curve is sketched in Fig. 24. At moderate work loads, there is a linear relationship between the respiratory minute volume and the oxygen cost of a given type of work, but as the intensity of effort is increased, a disproportionate hyperventilation develops. This parallels and probably reflects the accumulation of acid metabolites in the blood. The threshold of disproportionate hyperventilation varies from 50 percent to 80 percent of aerobic power, depending on the state of training of the individual, the type of exercise that is performed and the strength of the muscle groups involved.

During maximum exercise, an average young man reaches a ventilation of 90–120 litre/min BTPS; rather higher values are encountered in athletes. The rate of breathing increases with effort, but values of more than thirty-five to forty breaths per minute are unusual. Thus, the tidal volume increases to a maximum of 2500–3000 ml BTPS. As in the resting state, the

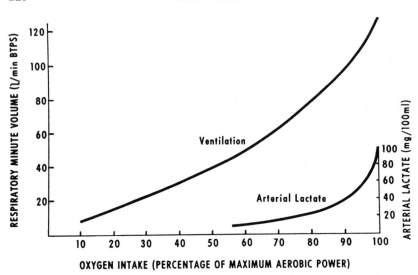

Figure 24. "Steady-state" ventilatory response to various work-loads, expressed as a percentage of aerobic power. Note that the ventilation is greater for a given level of arm work than for a corresponding rate of leg work (compare Fig. 3).

exercising athlete has a slower and deeper pattern of breathing than a sedentary individual. The efficiency of respiration is sometimes examined in terms of the "ventilatory equivalent" (Veq); this is simply the number of litres of ventilation (BTPS) required to supply each 100 ml STPD of oxygen that is consumed. If the resting oxygen consumption is 250 ml/min STPD, then the corresponding Veq is given by 7.2/2.50 = 2.87. The Veq remains at or near the resting level in moderate work, but it increases in exhausting exercise. If a young man has a maximum oxygen intake of 3000 ml/min STPD and a maximum exercise ventilation of 120 litre/min BTPS, then the ventilatory equivalent at this level of effort is 120/30 = 4.00. The athlete has a low ventilatory equivalent, both at rest and during vigorous exercise. High values are encountered in children, but once the adult Veq is reached, there is little subsequent change with ageing. In general, old people show a normal ventilatory response to moderate work loads, but become exhausted at a lower intensity of effort than those who are younger.

Exercise Ventilation and Lung Function Tests

Vital Capacity and Its Subdivisions. At one time, the vital capacity (the maximum volume that can be exhaled following a maximum inspiration) was hailed as a simple test of physical fitness. Indeed, Dreyer (1920) published a book that consisted largely of a series of tables of expected vital capacities, and he entitled this work *The Assessment of Physical Fitness.* Certainly, the measurement is influenced by muscular strength, and athletes who participate in sports that lead to development of the chest muscles (for instance, rowers and kayak paddlers) often have a large vital capacity in relation to their height; however, the general association between vital capacity and fitness is not particularly close.

The resting tidal volume of 500 ml represents no more than 10 percent of the vital capacity in an average young man; however, in maximum exercise tidal volumes of 3000 ml may account for as much as 60 percent of the vital capacity. The exercise-induced increase of tidal volume takes place mainly at the expense of the inspiratory reserve (Fig. 25). As during performance of a maximum voluntary ventilation test (p. 113), a subject who is working maximally breathes over the range 30 percent to 90 percent of vital capacity. There are several practical reasons for avoiding the final 30 percent of expiration; the maximum force that can be developed by the expiratory muscles is declining (p. 132), the airways are becoming progressively narrowed, and the compliance of the lungs (the change of volume for a unit change of pressure) is decreasing due to a progressive collapse of alveolar units in the basal regions of the lung. The final 5 percent to 10 percent of inspiration is also avoided because the inspiratory muscles can develop only a limited force when the chest reaches this degree of expansion (p. 132).

The vital capacity decreases by 20 percent to 25 percent over the span of adult life. It is also 20 percent to 25 percent smaller in the female than in the male. If elderly or female subjects try to reach the same intensities of work as a young man, they must either breathe faster or operate over the less

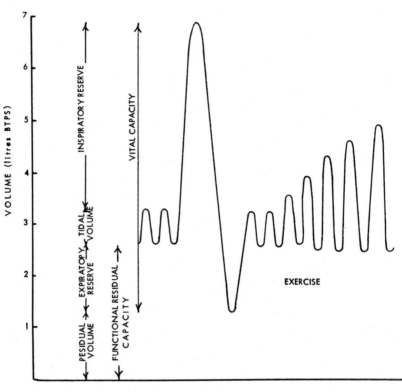

Figure 25. Static lung volumes. Note that on passing from rest to exercise, the tidal volume increases mainly at the expense of the inspiratory reserve, and the expiratory reserve remains relatively unchanged.

favourable part of their vital capacity. Partly for this reason, effort is more commonly limited by breathlessness as a subject becomes older.

If account is taken of age, sex and height, a multiple regression equation (p. 13) can predict an individual's vital capacity with a standard deviation of about 10 percent; possible equations for this purpose are as follows:

$$\text{Standing VC (men)} = 56.3\,H - 17.4\,(A) - 4210$$
$$\text{Standing VC (women)} = 54.5\,H - 10.5\,(A) - 5120$$

where H is the standing height in centimetres and A is the age in years. The vital capacity is technically a simple measurement, and for this reason the precision of the prediction equations is better than for many lung function tests. Nevertheless, the standard deviation of 10 percent implies that one person in forty has a vital capacity that is less than 80 percent of the predicted normal value. Disease must thus produce a gross destruction of lung tissue or rigidity of the thoracic cage before this can be detected by an isolated measurement of vital capacity. One way of making the test more sensitive is to repeat measurements annually. A sudden increase in the normal rate of ageing may give a useful warning of the onset of disease.

The Maximum Voluntary Ventilation

The maximum voluntary ventilation (MVV) may be defined as the maximum volume of air that a subject can respire in fifteen seconds. The test was originally developed by Hermannsen (1933) as the "Atemgrenzwert," and it provides a useful dynamic measure of ventilatory power. However, the results obtained are influenced markedly by the dynamic properties of the recording apparatus, the motivation of the subject and the breathing frequency he adopts. Many early investigators used a water-filled spirometer to measure the respired volume. Unfortunately, the water columns in the spirometer oscillated at certain breathing frequencies, and erroneously large volumes were recorded. Thus the impression was formed that the optimum frequency for the MVV test was forty to seventy breaths per minute. More recent studies have used low resistance equipment that does not resonate, and the largest volumes have then been recorded at rates of ninety to one hundred and ten breaths per minute.

The MVV of healthy young men is 160–200 litre/min BTPS. In athletes, values as high as 250 litre/min are not uncommon. In the elderly and in female subjects values are 20 percent to 25 percent smaller than in an average young man. The MVV is normally measured while the subject is at rest, and under such conditions it is difficult to sustain maximum effort. Within fifteen minutes, ventilation falls to some 50 percent of the fifteen second value, even if hypocapnia is avoided by supplying the subjects with carbon dioxide. If a similar decrease of MVV occurred during exercise, it could seriously limit prolonged effort. However, recent studies have shown that the MVV is initially larger and is better sustained if subjects engage in vigorous effort. Several factors may contribute to this increase of ventilatory performance including (a) secretion of catecholamines, leading to a decrease of airway resistance, (b) an increased sensory input to the respiratory centre, and (c) a "warm-up" of the chest muscles due to the general rise of body temperature (p. 190).

Although a subject can develop perhaps 80 percent of his resting MVV throughout fifteen minutes of vigorous activity, it is not necessarily advantageous to do so. The added hyperventilation leads to a considerable increase in the oxygen cost of breathing (p. 133), without a commensurate gain of oxygen intake. Thus the margin between the ventilation commonly observed in maximum exercise (90–120 litre/min BTPS) and the maximum practical ventilation may not be as large as measurements of MVV would suggest.

The sensation of shortness of breath commonly occurs when ventilation exceeds 50 percent of the MVV and on this basis some authors have calculated a "dyspnoea index":

$$\text{Dyspnoea Index} = \frac{\text{observed exercise ventilation}}{\text{MVV}} \times 100$$

Everyone is agreed that subjects are aware of increased breathing during exercise, but there is some discussion whether such "breathlessness" should be distinguished from the unpleasant sensation of laboured breathing ("dyspnoea") encountered by certain types of patients. Those who feel breathlessness is pleasant are in general physiologists who have studied only moderate levels of exercise. Discussion with athletes and inspection of the sculptures of Tait MacKenzie are enough to convince the present author that the breathlessness of maximum effort can be acutely unpleasant even for a normal person. On the other hand, it may not have the same neurological basis as a patient's dyspnoea. One explanation of dyspnoea has invoked the γ loop mechanism (p. 171); the body is thought to perceive disproportion between fibre length and tension in the respiratory muscles. Disproportion may arise from stiffening of the lung (pulmonary oedema), stiffening of the rib cage (various bone and joint diseases), or narrowing of the airway (bronchospasm or the use of high resistance respiratory equipment). It may also develop in normal maximum effort, secondary to an expiratory collapse of the airway (p. 118). Chemical stimuli make no direct contribution to the sensation, although accumulation of lactate may be associated with dyspnoea because it induces more intense respiratory effort.

The development of *"second wind"* is associated with a transition from dyspnoea to the more normal breathlessness of effort. There is little agreement as to why subjective comfort should increase. Some authors have suggested the primary explanation is an improvement of muscular efficiency, particularly a more rapid relaxation of antagonistic muscles, after "warmup" has occurred. A second factor may be a decrease in the blood levels of anaerobic metabolites. Although lactate accumulates in the first minute of exercise, when the circulation has not adapted to the increased metabolic demands of the active muscles (Fig. 42), if the intensity of effort is less than 60 percent to 70 percent of maximum aerobic power, much of this lactate is metabolized as the exercise continues. One objection to the second explanation is a poor correlation between the course of cardiovascular adjustments and the time when second wind develops. However, this may merely reflect a slow diffusion of lactate into the circulation, since even with maximum effort the arterial lactate concentration does not reach a maximum until two to four minutes after exercise has ceased.

Another unpleasant sensation associated with prolonged and vigorous effort is a *"stitch."* This is a sharp and rather severe pain felt laterally over the lower part of the chest wall. Some authors have attributed it to a spasm of the diaphragmatic muscles, while others have postulated that ischaemia of the diaphragm is responsible.

Forced Expiratory Volume. The MVV is an exhausting test for an elderly or a sick person, and if there is some point of structural weakness in the lung (for instance, a partly calcified tuberculous cavity), this may be disrupted by the forcible breathing. Thus clinicians commonly study the time course of a single forced expiration, initiated from full inspiration. The MVV expiration extends from 90 percent to perhaps 30 percent of vital capacity, so that for much of their course the FEV and MVV curves overlie one another. Some clinicians calculate an "indirect MVV," multiplying the volume expired in the first second ($FEV_{1.0}$) by a constant (usually 40). The procedure is based on out-dated views concerning the optimum breathing rate for the MVV test. We may note also the general point of philosophy that the information content of an $FEV_{1.0}$ reading is not increased by such multiplication—indeed, if the observer is bad at mathematics, the answer may actually deteriorate! Current practice is thus to interpret the $FEV_{1.0}$ either as a number in its own right, or as a percentage of the total forced vital capacity. A young and healthy adult can expel 81 percent to 85 percent of his vital capacity in one second. The percentage diminishes to about 70 percent of the forced vital capacity at the age of sixty. It is also reduced by exposure to irritant vapours (such as high concentrations of air pollutants), finely suspended particles (such as tobacco and industrial dusts), and cold air. The $FEV_{1.0}$ is normally recorded by a water-filled spirometer, and the record then shows a small initial lag due to inertia of the spirometer bell (Fig. 26); this lag should be ignored in calculating the $FEV_{1.0}$.

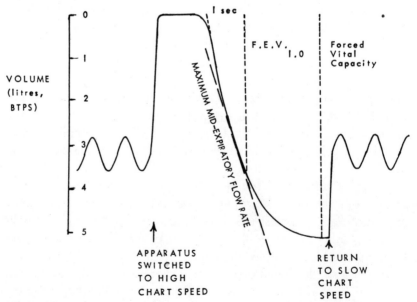

Figure 26. A typical forced expiratory volume curve, recorded by a water-filled spirometer. Note the initial lag due to inertia of the spirometer bell.

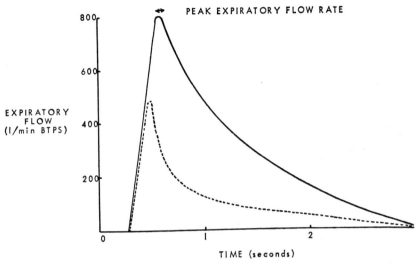

Figure 27. Forced expiratory flow curves: (solid line) young adult of above average fitness; (dashed line) older subject with early collapse of airways.

The true form of the forced expiratory flow curve is revealed by recording the pressure drop across a screen flowmeter (pneumotachograph). The flow rate rises very rapidly to a peak of about 600 litre/min, and then shows an "exponential" fall (Fig. 27). The initial peak flow depends very much on the maximum force that can be exerted by the chest muscles, while the subsequent decline of flow rate depends largely on collapse of the air passages (Fig. 28). At the commencement of expiration, the pressure within the smaller airways exceeds the pleural pressure, and the "equal pressure point" is not reached until the expirate is traversing the major airways; in this region the walls are supported by cartilaginous plates, and collapse is unlikely to occur. However, the balance of forces changes as expiration proceeds. When perhaps 60 percent of the vital capacity has been expelled, the elastic recoil of the lungs is much smaller (Fig. 28b). The airways also are narrower and in consequence the "equal pressure point" is reached in the finer airways where collapse can readily occur. Attempts at more forcible expiration are now fruitless; further collapse may occur but the expiratory gas flow cannot be increased. A number of factors exaggerate the inherent tendency to airway collapse, including (a) weakening of the cartilaginous plates, (b) a decrease in the elastic recoil of the lungs and (c) a spasm of the finer airways. Factors (a) and (b) are both natural responses to ageing, exaggerated by smoking and emphysema; factor (c) favours collapse by increasing

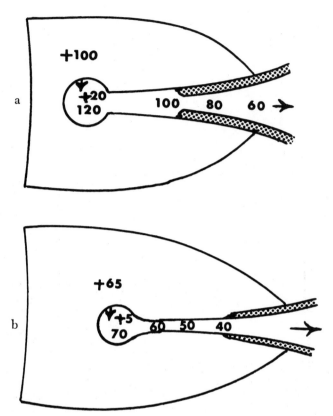

Figure 28. Illustration of the basis of airway collapse during a forced expiration. (*a*) *Commencement of expiration.* The pleural pressure of 100 mmHg is attributed to forces developed by the expiratory muscles and the "elastic recoil" of the thoracic cage. The intraalveolar pressure is boosted to 120 mmHg by the elastic recoil of the lungs. The pressure within the airway does not drop to intrapleural pressure until the major airways are reached. Here, cartilaginous plates prevent airway collapse. (*b*) *60% of vital capacity expelled.* The pleural pressure is now 65 mmHg. The elastic recoil of the lungs has decreased to 5 mmHg, so that the intraalveolar pressure is only 70 mmHg. Further, the finer parts of the conducting airway are now narrower, and the pressure thus drops more quickly on passing along the airway. The "equal pressure point" is thus reached in the finer branches of the airway that lack stout walls, and collapse tends to occur. Attempts at more vigorous expiration are fruitless, merely increasing the tendency to collapse.

the pressure drop from the alveolar spaces to the major bronchi. In a young person, "equal pressure collapse" does not develop until some 60 percent of the vital capacity has been expelled; thus, this phenomenon is only marginally involved in the respiratory pattern of maximum effort (ventilation from 90% to 30% of vital capacity). However, in an older person or an emphysematous patient, the equal pressure point is reached when only 30 percent or 40 percent of vital capacity has been exhaled, and. airway collapse may then seriously restrict exercise ventilation.

It would seem logical to examine the tendency to airway collapse by measuring flow during the latter part of expiration. This is done by fitting a tangent to the middle portion of the FVC curve (Fig. 26). The reading thus obtained is known as the *maximum midexpiratory flow rate* (MMEF).

Although portable bellows spirometers are available, the measurement of $FEV_{1.0}$ and MMEF is a little cumbersome for large scale field studies. One alternative is to measure the *peak expiratory flow rate*. A simple vane anemometer is used. This records the maximum flow that can be sustained for 10 milliseconds. From the pattern of the expiratory flow curve (Fig. 27), it might be thought that this reading would reflect muscular strength rather than airway resistance. However, in practice there is an appreciable deterioration of peak flow due to smoking and other causes of airway narrowing, and the peak flow meter is a useful epidemiological tool.

Residual Volume. The residual volume is the gas volume that cannot be expelled from the chest by a forcible expiration (Fig. 25). It can be measured quite simply. One approach is to note the dilution that occurs when a subject rebreathes from a spirometer circuit containing a known initial percentage of helium. An alternative method records the changes in both mouth and box pressures when a subject enclosed in a rigid box makes a forcible expiratory effort against a closed shutter. In general, the "body-box" readings are larger than those obtained by helium dilution since (a) equilibration of helium with poorly ventilated regions of the lung may be incomplete and (b) the body-box method takes account of both air "trapped" beyond points of airway collapse, and gas in the stomach and intestines.

The residual volume is about 22 percent of total lung capacity in children and young adults, but increases to as much as 40 percent of the total lung capacity by the age of sixty. Account must be taken of the residual gas volume when determining the percentage of body fat by underwater weighing (p. 486). The residual volume must also be known to calculate (a) the *functional residual capacity* (Fig. 25), (b) the total volume of gas within the lungs (alveolar volume), and (c) the dangers of "thoracic squeeze" (p. 276) and lung rupture (p. 291).

The alveolar gas volume influences the rate of change of gas tensions within the lung during breath holding, and the extent of oscillations in tension that occur over the course of the breathing cycle. The mean alveolar volume also influences the work of breathing, since the elastic forces developed by the chest and lungs are a nonlinear function of volume (Fig. 29).

Alveolar Ventilation

We have noted already that a part of the external ventilation is "wasted" in the dead space. The extent of this inefficiency can be seen if we calculate the ratio of dead space to tidal volume, using the classical Bohr equation:

$$\frac{V_D}{V_T} = \frac{P_{A,CO_2} - P_{E,CO_2}}{P_{A,CO_2} - P_{I,CO_2}}$$

The partial pressures of carbon dioxide in inspired gas (P_{I,CO_2}) and expired gas (P_{E,CO_2}) are readily determined. The corresponding alveolar pressure (P_{A,CO_2}) may present a little more difficulty, since it must be averaged over both a multitude of alveolar units, and also over a typical breathing cycle. Equilibration of carbon dioxide across the lung membrane is fairly complete, and under most conditions the best measure of the average alveolar carbon dioxide tension is provided by specimens of arterial or "arterialized" capillary blood. At rest, there is close agreement between arterial and "end-tidal"[*] gas pressures, the small discrepancy reflecting temporal and spatial mismatching of ventilation and perfusion—the so-called "alveolar" component of dead space. During vigorous exercise, the end-tidal sample may have a higher CO_2 pressure than arterial blood; this is due in part to larger oscillations of gas com-

---

[*] The "end-tidal" sample is the final portion of a normal expirate. It may be collected as such, using a suitable sampling device, or the corresponding readings may be noted from a continuous record of expired gas concentrations.

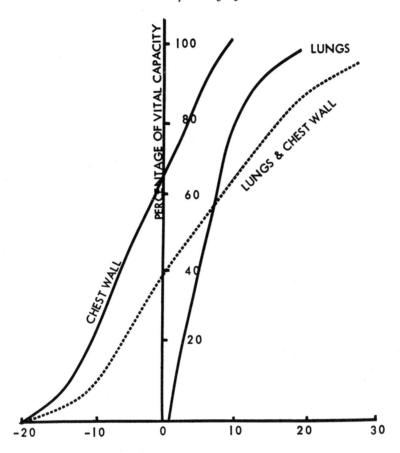

Figure 29. The influence of lung volume on the compliance of the chest wall and of the lungs (the compliance at any volume is given by the ratio $\Delta V/\Delta P$).

position over the breathing cycle and in part to a more uniform distribution of ventilation and perfusion.

The V_D/V_T ratio of the resting subject is about 0.3. The dead space of 150–180 ml is largely "anatomical," an expression of the volume of the conducting airways; the "alveolar" component contributes 30 ml or less to this total.

During exercise, two main factors increase the anatomical dead space—an expansion of the airways, and a reduction of mixing time. An increase of mean alveolar volume leads to a physical expansion of the conducting airways. This expansion is approximately proportional to their contribution to the total lung volume. Let us consider an airway that comprises an inelastic element (mouth, throat, and larynx) of volume 40 ml, and an elastic element (trachea, bronchi, and bronchioles) of volume 110 ml. If the total initial lung volume is 3000 ml, and a breath of 1000 ml is inhaled, then the conducting airway expands by $110 \times \dfrac{1000}{3000}$ ml $= 37$ ml.

A more important problem is created by the shortening of gas mixing time. Exchange between alveolar gas and newly inhaled air is dependent on the retrograde diffusion of mixed gas from the lungs through the smaller to the larger air passages. A post-inspiratory pause of two to three seconds is necessary if this diffusional exchange is to be reasonably complete. When the respiratory rate is increased to thirty-five to forty breaths per minute, such time is plainly not available. Computer calculations, based on the passage of gas into a theoretical model of the bronchial tree suggest that during maximum effort the dead space should increase to 500 or 600 ml. In practice, volumes of 300–400 ml are more usual, and it would seem that diffusional mixing is supplemented by axial gas flow[*] and a physical massaging of the airways by the lungs and heart.

If the alveolar component of dead space is included by the use of arterial blood samples, the calculated exercise V_D/V_T ratio lies in the range 0.20–0.25. The lowest ratio (and thus the most efficient ventilation) is obtained at or near the normal breathing frequency (35–40/min).

Detailed knowledge of possible changes in alveolar dead space during exercise is lacking. At rest, the studies of West and his colleagues suggest that the upper part of the lung is grossly overventilated ($\dot{V}_A/\dot{Q}$ ratio 3.3), while the lower part of the lung is somewhat overperfused ($\dot{V}_A/\dot{Q}$ ratio 0.6). Limited studies in moderate exercise indicate similar $\dot{V}_A/\dot{Q}$ ratios for the

---

[*] With "axial" or laminar flow, air passes through the centre of a bronchiole, leaving a film of alveolar gas lining its wall.

upper and lower parts of the lung. No data are yet available for vigorous effort. One reason for the paucity of information is that measurements are technically difficult during exercise. The subject must inhale a single breath of a radioactive gas such as $C^{15}O_2$, and hold himself stationary while the absorption of this material from the lungs is followed by a battery of scintillation counters (Fig. 30). Because of the difficulties in direct experiment, it is of interest to consider the question on a theoretical basis.

Milic-Emili has shown that the regional distribution of venti-

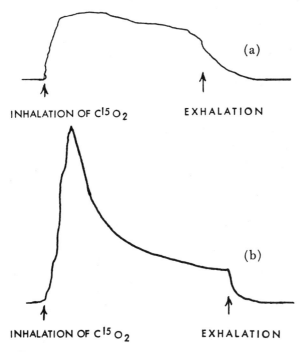

INHALATION OF $C^{15}O_2$ EXHALATION

Figure 30. Illustration of the method of assessing ventilation/perfusion relationships. The breath is held following inhalation of radioactive carbon dioxide ($C^{15}O_2$). Scintillation counts are recorded at selected levels on the chest surface. The graphs illustrate the behaviour of (a) the upper part of the lung and (b) the lower part of the lung. (a). *Scintillation counts from upper part of lung.* Small initial rise indicates poor ventilation. Slow subsequent fall indicates perfusion. (b). *Scintillation counts from lower part of lung.* Large initial rise indicates good ventilation. Rapid subsequent fall indicates good perfusion.

lation depends upon the initial lung volume. At low lung volumes, air is distributed preferentially to the upper regions of the lung, and these rapidly approach maximum expansion (Fig. 31); at this stage, the gravitational gradient of pleural pressure is enough to maintain collapse in the more dependent regions of the lung. At larger initial lung volumes, air is distributed preferentially to the lower parts of the lungs. In maximum exercise, ventilation extends over a large part of the vital capacity range, and in consequence a relatively uniform distribution of ventilation may be anticipated.

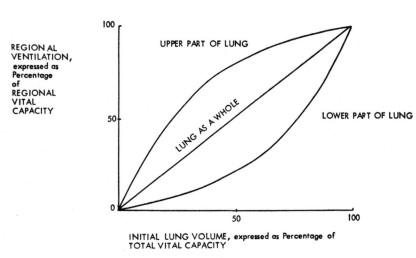

Figure 31. Illustration of the influence of initial lung volume on regional ventilation of the lung. The upper part of the lung fills early, and the lower part of the lung late in the course of a vital capacity inspiration. (Based on experiments of Milic-Emili).

West has carried out extensive studies of the regional distribution of pulmonary blood flow and he distinguishes three lung zones. These arise from the gravitational gradient of pulmonary arterial and venous pressures. In the upper zone, the alveolar pressure exceeds both arterial and venous pressures, and no perfusion can occur. In the middle zone, the arterial pressure exceeds alveolar pressure, but this in turn exceeds venous pressure; blood flow thus fluctuates with variations of alveolar pressure. In the lower zone, both arterial and venous pressures exceed alveolar pressure, and perfusion is independent of respiration. During vigorous exercise, the pulmonary arterial pressure rises, and even when standing it exceeds alveolar pressure except at the apex of the lungs; perfusion is then almost independent of alveolar pressure, and a relatively uniform perfusion of the lungs may be anticipated.

The present author's observations suggest that in near maximum effort the alveolar dead space is normally small and relatively independent of the posture in which exercise is performed. However, if the subject deliberately increases his tidal volume by voluntary hyperventilation, there is a sharp worsening of ventilation/perfusion relationships, and this creates a substantial alveolar dead space.

The Work of Breathing

General Concepts

Work is performed in moving air in and out of the chest. Ignoring for the moment the complication of turbulent air flow, we may represent the pressure P that must be developed in terms of the simple equation

$$P = K_1V + K_2\dot{V} + K_3\ddot{V}$$

where V is the change in chest volume, $\dot{V}$ the rate of change of volume (velocity), $\ddot{V}$ the rate of change of velocity (acceleration), and K_1, K_2, and K_3 are constants. The first term (K_1V) refers to the pressure developed against the elasticity of the rib cage, lungs, and lining film of "alveolar surfactant." Much of the energy stored in the expanded chest can be utilized during expiration, provided that the second and third terms of the equation are sufficiently large. This seems true during vigorous exercise, although it is not the case during normal quiet breathing. The second term ($K_2\dot{V}$) relates to work performed against airflow resistance and the viscosity of the moving tissues; it is by far the largest of the three terms during vigorous effort. The third term ($K_3\ddot{V}$) refers to work performed in accelerating both gas molecules and heavy viscera including the liver and chest wall.

Elasticity

The elasticity of the chest wall and lungs is normally expressed in terms of compliance. Compliance is the reciprocal of elasticity. Over the middle range of lung volumes, the compliance of the lungs (C_L) is about 200 ml/cmH$_2$O, and the compliance of the chest wall (C_C) is of a similar order. The overall compliance of the chest and lungs (C_{C+L}) is given by the equation:

$$\frac{1}{C_{C+L}} = \frac{1}{C_C} + \frac{1}{C_L}$$

and is thus about 100 ml/cmH$_2$O.

Compliance curves are somewhat sigmoid in shape (Fig. 29). It is thus important to specify the lung volume at which measurements are made when considering whether an individual has a normal lung and chest compliance. The shape of the compliance curves has relevance to artificial respiration. In order to produce a given tidal volume, a much larger pressure must be exerted during forcible deflation of the chest (back-pressure method) than during forcible inflation (arm lift, bellows and mouth to mouth techniques).

Congestion of the lungs may lead to a considerable reduction of lung compliance; a substantial positive pressure is then needed to produce even a small expansion of the lungs. Rescuers who are being trained in mouth to mouth resuscitation should use manikins that can simulate not only the normal lung compliance, but also the reduced compliance of a typical casualty. A reduction of compliance may create problems when ventilation is sustained by mechanical means. If a respirator provides air to the patient until a certain cut-off pressure is reached, the typical pressure setting (20–30 mmHg) may be developed before the victim has received an adequate tidal volume. Bellows resuscitators are fitted with a "relief" valve in order to avoid damage to the lungs. This again operates at a pressure of 20–30 mmHg, and if the compliance is low, a vigorous compression of the bellows causes most of its contents to escape via the relief valve.

Much has been written regarding the influence upon ventilation of regional differences in resistance and compliance. The authors concerned have assumed that the lungs and airways are a "damped" system, and that the rate of filling of any given lung unit is proportional to the product of its resistance and compliance, the so-called "time constant." On the basis of this theory, one would anticipate that as the breathing rate was increased, ventilation would be progressively restricted to those lung units with a short time constant; also, the apparent compliance of the lungs would decrease with an increase of breathing frequency. Frequency-dependent compliance is a well-recognised phenomenon in old men with emphysematous lungs; on the other hand, young and healthy subjects can increase their breathing frequency to one hundred breaths per minute without materially altering their lung compliance from values determined under "static" conditions. This does not necessarily imply all lung units have equal time constants. One possible explanation of why the breathing rate has no influence upon the compliance of a young person is that the system is normally underdamped rather than overdamped. The present author has studied pressure changes following a sudden interruption of airflow at the mouth (Fig. 32). Old and emphysematous subjects show a slow "ex-

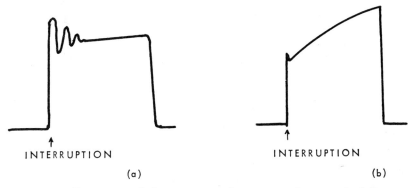

INTERRUPTION   INTERRUPTION

(a)   (b)

Figure 32. Illustration of the pressure changes at the mouth following the sudden interruption of expiratory air flow. (a) Healthy young subject (response is underdamped, and overshoots the equilibrium value). Old and emphysematous subject (response is overdamped, with a slow, "exponential" approach to the equilibrium value).

ponential" rise towards the final equilibrium pressure, as would be anticipated from the "time constant" theory; however, young and healthy subjects overshoot the equilibrium pressure, and the record then oscillates about the final mean value. Obviously, if the system is underdamped, we cannot expect simple time-constant theories to apply to our data.

Resistance

Airflow Resistance. The resistance to airflow includes both laminar and turbulent components. To a first approximation, the pressure drop associated with laminar air flow is proportional to flow rate and gas viscosity, while the pressure drop for turbulent air flow is proportional to gas density and the square of the flow rate. This information can be summarised in the form of the equation

$$P = K_1 (F) + K_2 (F^2)$$

where P is the resistive pressure drop, F is the rate of airflow, and K_1 and K_2 are constants proportional to viscosity and density respectively. Flow is normally laminar in the smallest airways, but generalized turbulence develops in the nose, throat, and trachea, and more localized areas of turbulence are found at points of branching in the major bronchi. The combination of laminar and turbulent flow leads to a non-linear overall pressure/flow curve of the type

$$P = KF^n$$

where n is an exponent of about 1.66. Resistance is essentially the ratio of pressure to flow; since the overall function is nonlinear, the calculated resistance depends on flow rate. Physiologists arbitrarily report resistance at a flow of 0.5 litre/sec. When measured in this way, the resistance from the mouth to the alveoli is about 2 cmH_2O pressure per litre per second flow, while the resistance from the external nares to the pharynx is of a similar order.

If any substantial ventilation is required, subjects inevitably prefer to breathe through the low resistance pathway (the mouth). This is particularly unfortunate if vigorous exercise is being performed out of doors on a cold, dry day. The normal "air-conditioning" mechanism of the nose is by-passed, and the trachea is subjected to a steady stream of cold dry air. This thickens the tracheal mucus, slows the movement of the tracheal ciliae, and may stimulate tracheal nerve endings inducing both bronchospasm and anginal pain.

As the ventilatory volume increases, generalized turbulence spreads progressively from the trachea into the bronchi. However, calculations of the Reynolds number (p. 61) suggest that turbulence rarely extends beyond the seventh order of bronchial branching except when work is performed at very great depths. The reason for more extensive turbulence in the diver is that the critical velocity is inversely proportional to ·gas density. The use of low density gas mixtures (such as 80% helium, 20% oxygen) is helpful to the diver for two reasons—the extent of turbulence is diminished, and there is also a decrease of the turbulent resistance coefficient K_2 at any given rate of airflow. Unfortunately, helium has a somewhat greater viscosity than nitrogen, so that the laminar flow resistance coefficient K_1 is increased by about 10 percent.

During rest and light work, a substantial increase of airway resistance can occur before the subject complains of any difficulty in breathing. This question has been studied quite extensively in the cotton spinning industry. Workers in cotton plants develop the condition of byssinosis, a reaction to particles of cotton dust that includes a progressive increase of airway resistance over the working week. Perhaps because disability is of gradual onset, no symptoms are reported until the resistance is at least four times the normal resting value (8 cmH_2O/litre/sec). "Tightness of the chest" is then noted. A similar picture is reported by the asthmatic, and by men exposed to large doses of organophosphorus insecticide. The physiological basis of the "tightness" is less certain—perhaps the γ loop mechanisms are signalling that the tension in the respiratory muscles is inappropriate to their length; perhaps also the mean chest volume increases as a partial adaptation to the spasm of the airways.

In vigorous effort, the tolerance to increased resistance is much poorer. Military respirators ("gas masks") are required to have a total resistance of less than 10 cmH_2O at an inspiratory flow of 85 litre/min. If this standard is not met, the subject complains of intense dyspnoea, and physical effort is limited by difficulty in breathing (p. 133, 153). Some workers have suggested that inspiratory resistance is more unpleasant than an expiratory load, but the present author was not impressed with this distinction when he studied the question on service volunteers. All breathing resistance is unpleasant when a man is working hard, and in consequence apparatus used for respiratory measurements should have a very low flow resistance (p. 414).

Laboratory measurements of airway resistance are commonly made by enclosing the subject in the body box used also for determinations of residual volume. The apparatus is cumbersome, but individual measurements are relatively easy once the equipment is installed. The main disadvantages are (a) the need to adopt a rapid and unnaturally shallow pattern of breathing, and (b) the difficulty in performing exercise while enclosed within the box.

Field measurements of resistance can be used to demonstrate the immediate effects of smoking on the airways. They may also be helpful in an epidemiological study. Thus, if bronchospasm is developing in one area of a factory or one part of a city this may provide a clue as to the nature or source of the irritant material. The simplest field apparatus is a peak flow meter (p. 117); other possibilities include a portable bellows spirometer, and an interrupter valve. The last device interrupts airflow at the mouth for a period of perhaps 50 milliseconds. A rapid equilibration of pressure occurs between the alveoli and the mouth (Fig. 32), and the final pressure reading is sufficiently close to the initial alveolar value to permit the calculation of airway resistance.

A substantial part of the total airway resistance arises in the first three or four orders of the bronchial tree. The resistance of this region is increased by reflex stimulation of nerve endings within the trachea; common stimuli include cold air, dust, nerve gas, insecticides, and the inhalation of vomit by an unconscious patient. On the other hand, with allergic reactions (for instance, the response to moulds and irritants, asthma, and the "anaphylactic shock" induced by poison ivy and jellyfish stings) the increase of airway resistance occurs mainly in the finest air passages. A peripheral type of spasm is particularly likely if the irritant material is conveyed to the lungs via the pulmonary circulation. Because the initial airflow resistance of the finer air passages is small, there may be little increase in overall airway resistance. However, the affected parts of the lung show a very slow rate of mixing with foreign test gases such as helium.

Exercise is often accompanied by a small decrease of airway resistance, but in sensitive individuals there may be a subsequent increase (exercise-induced asthma). The "bronchodilation" is generally attributed to the release of catecholamines (noradrenaline and adrenaline); these produce their effect partly by constricting vessels lining the airway, and partly by initiating an active dilatation of the bronchial muscles. A further factor reducing airflow resistance is an increase of mean alveolar volume during exercise. This automatically leads to some expansion of the airway. The manner in which exercise can cause asthma has yet to be fully explained; possible contributing factors are the inhalation of cold, dry air, and the aspiration of mucus.

Tissue Resistance. The tissue resistance is usually estimated as the difference between the total resistance to forced inflation of the chest and the airway resistance, and like most "difference" measurements it is difficult to calculate with certainty. Part of the tissue resistance is attributable to incomplete relaxation of antagonistic muscles and this component diminishes with either a local or a general "warm up" of the tissues (p. 190). Ageing increases the rigidity of the thoracic cage and thus tissue resistance.

Inertia

The inertial work involved in acceleration of gas molecules and heavy abdominal viscera is normally but a small part of the total cost of breathing. However, it can have important consequences, as much of the acceleration of gas occurs in the narrower air passages, distal to the "equal pressure point" (p. 118). Since the viscous resistance to airflow is low in this region, the forces involved in acceleration may determine whether airway collapse occurs during expiration. Inertia is also important to the damping of oscillations within the airway. As we have noted above, the normal bronchial tree is underdamped, and in consequence a distressing "chatter" may develop in the valves of any breathing equipment that is worn. The damping ratio (h) in a simple breathing circuit is given by the formula

$$h = \frac{R}{2} \sqrt{\frac{C}{L}}$$

where R is the resistance, C is the compliance, and L is the inertance. The behaviour of the human airway is rather more complex. Nevertheless, it is generally true that damping can be improved by a reduction of inertance (breathing a low density gas mixture such as helium), or (less desirably) by an increase of R or C. Conversely, the situation is worsened if the density is increased, as may occur during diving.

The Pressure-volume Diagram

The total work performed per breathing cycle is indicated by the pressure-volume integral. It is thus possible to plot a maximum pressure-volume diagram for the chest (Fig. 33), and in this way to demonstrate the maximum work that can be performed by the respiratory muscles. The diagram is commonly drawn under "static" conditions, by having a subject draw varying fractions of the vital capacity into his lungs and then make a maximum inspiratory or expiratory effort against a closed valve. The volumes thus recorded must be corrected for the 5 percent to 15 percent change in pressure of the sys-

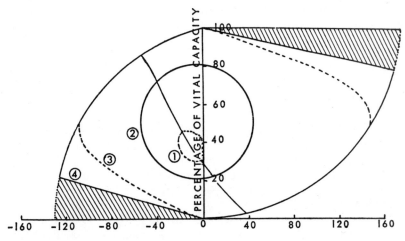

INPIRATORY PRESSURE (mmHg)   EXPIRATORY PRESSURE (mmHg)

Figure 33. Pressure-volume diagrams for the chest. (1) Normal quiet breathing; (2) maximum exercise; (3) maximum voluntary ventilation; (4) maximum "static" pressure-volume diagram. The shaded areas indicate the correction applied for gas compression and expansion during the development of the recorded pressures.

tem produced by the respiratory efforts; for this reason, it is not possible to determine the maximum inspiratory pressure at 0 percent of vital capacity, or the maximum expiratory pressure at 100 percent of vital capacity. During quiet breathing, only a very small fraction of the maximum pressure-volume diagram is utilized. The size of the pressure-volume loop increases with exercise, but even during maximum effort it rarely occupies more than a quarter of the static diagram. During a maximum voluntary ventilation, the dynamic diagram is still somewhat smaller than the static, partly because the volume of the system changes before the muscles are able to develop their maximum tension, and partly because of limitations imposed by the inherent force-velocity relationships of the respiratory muscles (p. 182).

The Oxygen Cost of Breathing

The oxygen cost of the breathing process could theoretically be calculated from the work performed (the area of the pressure-volume diagram for the lungs and chest). The difficulty with this approach is that the figures suggested for the mechanical efficiency of breathing range very widely from 1 percent to 25 percent. An alternative approach is to increase ventilation (either voluntarily, or by inhaling a CO_2 mixture), and note the resultant increase of oxygen consumption. The cost bears a nonlinear relation to ventilation, being 0.5–1.0 ml of O_2 per litre of ventilation during quiet breathing, but increasing to as much as 5 ml/litre at the respiratory minute volumes encountered in maximum exercise. This raises the question whether the oxygen consumed by the respiratory muscles ever reaches the point where a further increase of ventilation would diminish the amount of oxygen available to other body tissues. Stated in mathematical terms, does the cost of a further increase in ventilation $(\Delta \dot{V}_{O_2(R)}/\Delta \dot{V})$ ever exceed the resulting gain in oxygen consumption $(\Delta \dot{V}_{O_2}/\Delta \dot{V})$? In a healthy young person, such a situation is unlikely, $\Delta \dot{V}_{O_2(R)}/\Delta \dot{V}$ does not equal $\Delta \dot{V}_{O_2}/\Delta \dot{V}$ until the respiratory minute volume is 130–140 litre/min BTPS, whereas the maximum exercise ventilation is typically 90–120 litre/min BTPS. The problem at high ventilation rates seems not so much an increase of $\Delta \dot{V}_{O_2(R)}/\Delta V$ as a precipitous decrease of $\Delta \dot{V}_{O_2}/\Delta \dot{V}$; because of the shape of the oxygen dissociation curve, any additional ventilation is very ineffective from the viewpoint of oxygen transport (Fig. 34). Exercising athletes sometimes develop a respiratory minute volume as large as 140–160 litre/min BTPS, but because they have a larger maximum cardiac output, it is still unlikely that they have reached the critical point where $\Delta \dot{V}_{O_2}/\Delta \dot{V}$ falls precipitously. On the other hand, the effort tolerance of older

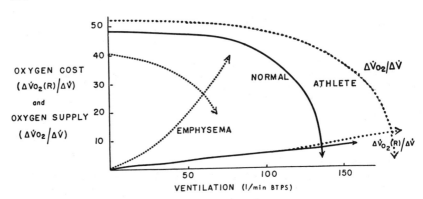

Figure 34. The concept of a critical cost of breathing, where the oxygen consumed by respiratory muscles $\Delta\dot{V}_{O_2}/\Delta\dot{V}$ exceeds the supply $\Delta\dot{V}_{O_2}/\Delta\dot{V}$.

subjects may well be limited by the work of breathing, particularly if they suffer from emphysema.

The optimum rate of breathing varies with the intensity of effort (Fig. 35). In a resting subject with a respiratory minute volume of 10 litre/min or less, the work of breathing is minimal at a frequency of fifteen to twenty breaths per min. At slower breathing rates, a substantial amount of work is performed against the elastic forces of the lungs and chest, and not all of this is recovered during expiration. At faster breathing rates, an excessive amount of work is performed against viscous forces. With physical activity, the respiratory minute volume increases, and the optimum frequency of breathing also rises; however, it is rarely more than forty breaths per minute, even in maximum exercise. It is remarkable that the breathing rate spontaneously selected corresponds closely with that required for minimum respiratory work over a wide range of respiratory minute volumes (Fig. 35).

The Respiratory Muscles

In normal, quiet breathing, the main responsibility for respiratory effort is borne by the diaphragm; however, the relative contribution of other muscles varies with posture. If inspiration is produced by descent of the diaphragm, it is necessary to displace the liver and other abdominal viscera in a

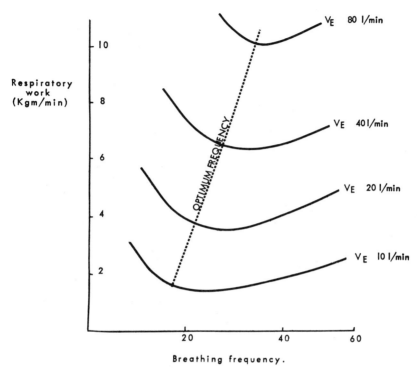

Figure 35. To illustrate the relationships between optimum frequency of breathing, respiratory minute volume, and work of breathing.

downward and forward direction, and this is most readily accomplished when a subject is sitting with his abdominal muscles relaxed, or is standing erect. Electromyograms commonly show activity of the external intercostal muscles during inspiration, and of the internal intercostals during expiration. However, it is uncertain how far this represents an active contribution to respiratory effort; it may merely indicate a passive adaptation to changing thoracic dimensions. As the respiratory minute volume is increased by exercise or voluntary hyperventilation, muscle groups are progressively recruited to the task of breathing. The abdominal muscles make an active contribution to expiration at respiratory minute volumes of 40 litre/min and above, and at this stage various "accessory" muscles such as the scalenes and the sternomastoids contribute to the inspiratory effort. The efficiency of the accessory muscles depends on the nature of the physical activity that is undertaken; for instance, they function more effectively if there is external fixation of the shoulder girdle (as when riding a bicycle). However, the maximum possible contribution from thoracic muscles is quite small, and if the thoracic cage is immobilized by a rigid binder, the maximum voluntary ventilation is reduced by no more than 20 percent to 30 percent.

Pulmonary Diffusion

Problems of Measurement

The pulmonary diffusing capacity, or transfer factor as it is sometimes called, expresses the number of ml of gas transported from the alveoli to pulmonary capillary blood per unit of pressure gradient (p. 107). Carbon monoxide is commonly used to measure diffusing capacity, since the mean pulmonary capillary pressure of oxygen $P_{\overline{pc},O_2}$) is technically difficult to determine. On account of differences in molecular size and water solubility, the oxygen diffusing capacity ($\dot{D}_{L,O_2}$) is 1.23 times as great as that of carbon monoxide ($\dot{D}_{L,CO}$).

It was originally hoped that because carbon monoxide had a very great affinity for haemoglobin, the "back-pressure" due to accumulation of this gas in the pulmonary capillary blood could be ignored when calculating diffusing capacity. Unfortunately, this is not the case. An ordinary city-dweller has about 1 percent carboxyhaemoglobin in his blood (the combined result of endogenous production and exposure to air pollutants—particularly car exhaust fumes). If the subject under investigation works as a traffic policeman or as an attendant in a parking tower, his blood may contain 2% or 3% carboxyhaemoglobin, and if he has the habit of introducing the exhaust pipe of a cigarette into his mouth, an average daytime value of 5% to 6% carboxyhaemoglobin may be anticipated. Unless account is taken of the initial pressure of carbon monoxide within the blood, the resting diffusing capacity of a smoker is underestimated by 20 percent to 30 percent.

There are two basic methods of measuring carbon monoxide diffusing capacity. In the single-breath method, a large volume of 0.1% carbon monoxide is inhaled, and the diffusing capacity is deduced from the change in alveolar carbon monoxide concentration over a ten second period of breath-holding. This form of test is used quite widely for clinical purposes, but the prolonged suspension of respiration is artificial even at rest, and is not practicable during vigorous activity. The alternative, steady-state procedure measures the uptake of carbon monoxide over a specified period of several minutes, and relates this to the pressure gradient between alveolar gas and pulmonary capillary blood. It is then necessary to determine an appropriate mean alveolar carbon monoxide pressure. Some authors have done this by measuring the CO content of expired gas, assuming a figure for dead space volume, and applying the Bohr equation (p. 120); in the resting state, the dead space can be predicted fairly accurately, but unfortunately it becomes more controversial during exercise (p. 122). Others have assumed that end-tidal gas samples are representative of alveolar carbon-monoxide concentration. This is not always the case; alveolar carbon monoxide levels vary widely over a breathing cycle, particularly if the respiratory rate is slow, and sometimes the average alveolar carbon monoxide pressure is closer to the midtidal than to the end-tidal reading. Reliance upon end-tidal sampling led to the erroneous conclusion that the slow, and deep pattern of breathing of the swimmer produced a large diffusing capacity. A third approach is to measure the CO_2 dead space by collecting arterial or "arterialized" capillary blood and to assume that the CO and CO_2 dead spaces are identical. This is acceptable for quiet breathing, but can lead to difficulties at the more rapid respiratory rates encountered in vigorous exercise. The perfect method of measuring diffusing capacity has yet to be devised, and careful account must be taken of possible artefacts in assessing information currently reported.

Response to Exercise

The resting CO diffusing capacity is about 25–30 ml/min/mmHg; this increases progressively with exercise, reaching a maximum of perhaps 60–70 ml/min/mmHg in a moderately athletic young man. Some authors have suggested that a "plateau" of diffusing capacity is reached before the maximum aerobic power is developed; others have been unable to confirm this, and some difficulty of technique seems responsible for such discordant views.

The diffusing capacity samples two functional components, one related to the characteristics of the alveolar membrane $(\dot{D}_M)$, and the other to the rate of reaction (θ) between carbon monoxide and haemoglobin within the capillary blood volume (V_c). The two components behave as series conductances:

$$\frac{1}{\dot{D}_L} = \frac{1}{\dot{D}_M} + \frac{1}{\theta V_c}$$

At rest, V_c lies in the range 50–100 ml, while the value of θ is about 0.6–0.7. Thus the terms $\dot{D}_M$ and θV_c have an almost equal influence on $\dot{D}_L$. Both terms increase with exercise, but because the measurements have a large experimental error, there is disagreement as to which term increases the more. At rest only about a fifth of the total alveolar surface of 70 m² is covered by patent capillaries. The increase of $\dot{D}_M$ reflects the expansion of existing capillaries to cover more of the available surface, and/or the opening up of new pulmonary capillaries. Both types of response also increase the value of V_c.

Practical Importance of Diffusing Capacity

Some authors have suggested that a large pulmonary diffusing capacity is an important asset to an athlete. This view probably arose in part from overestimation of $D_{L,CO}$ when measurements were made by the end tidal method (see above). Nevertheless, athletes have a slightly larger diffusing capacity than sedentary individuals and physical training leads to a small increase of diffusing capacity, roughly proportional to the gain of maximum oxygen intake.

The possible influence of diffusing capacity upon oxygen transport is indicated by the conductance equation (p. 105). The interaction between diffusing capacity and blood transport is given by the term $\left(\dfrac{B}{1-B}\right)\dfrac{1}{\lambda \dot{Q}}$, where $B = e^{-\dot{D}L/\lambda\dot{Q}}$. The corresponding pressure gradient ($P_{A,O_2} - P_{a,O_2}$) depends not only upon incomplete equilibration of alveolar gas and mixed venous blood, but also on inequalities of ventilation/perfusion ratio and frank venous-arterial shunts through channels such as the Thebesian vessels and the anterior cardiac veins. A total A-a gradient of some 10 mmHg is common at rest, but the major part of this is due to shunting; equilibration of blood within the lungs is virtually complete (see Fig. 23). In vigorous exercise, the A-a gradient increases to perhaps 20 mmHg; the arterial oxygen tension changes little, but there is a substantial increase of P_{A,O_2}. The percentage of shunted blood remains small (1%–2% of cardiac output), but because the oxygen content of venous blood is lower, a given shunt has a larger effect upon the A-a gradient. The transit time through an average pulmonary capillary decreases from 0.75 to 0.33 seconds. This is still adequate for fairly complete equilibration (Fig. 23), but in the shorter capillaries (where the transit time is less than average), there may be some residual gradient. Failure of equilibration is more extensive if vigorous exercise is performed at high altitude or underwater (where the total oxygen pressure is reduced by breath-holding); under these special circumstances, there may be a physiological advantage in having a large pulmonary diffusing capacity.

Blood Transport

Blood transport is essential for tissue respiration. If subjects have difficulty in developing a large cardiac output, whether as the result of congenital disease (for instance, pulmonary stenosis, a narrowing of the pulmonary valvular orifice) or secondary to rheumatic heart disease (for instance, stenosis of the mitral valve) a blueness of the extremities (cyanosis) and of the cheek (malar flush)* may be detected The determinants of maximum cardiac output are discussed in the previous chapter. Blood transport is limited equally by the maximum cardiac output and the oxygen carrying capacity of the blood (the solubility term λ). Adaptation to environmental problems such as high altitude and chronic carbon monoxide poisoning (the habitual smoker) are thus possible through an increase in the red cell count. Unfortunately, any increase in the number of red cells and thus the haematocrit carries the penalty of increasing blood viscosity and cardiac workload. The relationship between haematocrit and viscosity is nonlinear (Fig. 36), and through some mechanism yet to be elucidated, further production of red cells is restrained at the inflexion of the curve (haematocrit about 60%, red cell count 6.5×10^6 cells/mm^3).

The haemoglobin level of women (average 13.8 gm/100 ml) is 11 percent to 12 percent less than that of men (average 15.6 gm/100 ml), and this inevitably limits the maximum oxygen intake of the female by a corresponding amount. Clinical anae-

---

*The malar flush of the mitral stenotic reflects not only cyanosis but also a high venous pressure.

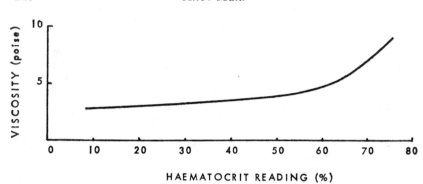

Figure 36. Relationship between viscosity of the blood and haematocrit reading.

mia is not usually diagnosed unless the haemoglobin level is below 12 gm/100 ml, but an athlete with a haemoglobin reading of 13 gm/100 ml will have a substantial handicap in terms of oxygen carriage. Athletic training normally increases the haemoglobin level; nevertheless, some athletes are anaemic, perhaps because of dietary fads, iron loss in the sweat, and an increased destruction of red cells in the circulation (p. 236).

Tissue Diffusion

There are no simple procedures for measuring the tissue diffusing capacity. However, the technique of Fig. 23 can be used to estimate the mean oxygen pressure within the capillaries of active muscle (P_{tc,o_2}, about 20–25 mmHg). The second value needed to calculate tissue diffusing capacity is the average pressure of oxygen within the active tissues. We are unable to do more than specify the range within which this pressure must fall. It is greater than the pressure at which metabolism falters in a tissue culture (1 mmHg), and less than the pressure in blood leaving the active muscles (6–10 mmHg); a reasonable estimate would be 5 mmHg, giving a gradient (P_{tc,o_2}–P_{t,o_2}) of 15–20 mmHg (see further page 108). In a sedentary young man with a maximum oxygen intake of 3 litre/min STPD, the corresponding diffusing capacity would be 150–200 ml/min/mmHg. This is three times the diffusing capacity of the lungs, and it is therefore most unlikely that tissue oxygen uptake is restricted by diffusion. In the conductance equation, the terminal pressure gradient is from venous blood to tissue oxygen tension; at most, this amounts to 1–12 mmHg, confirming that the interaction between tissue diffusion and blood transport does not limit oxygen intake significantly.

The maximum oxygen intake can be increased by involvement of a greater number of muscles in the test procedure. At a first glance, this seems at variance with our view that tissue diffusion is unimportant. The additional muscles are providing an increased capillary surface, and therefore a larger tissue diffusing capacity. However, closer examination of the problem suggests that the basis of the increased oxygen intake is an improvement of blood transport rather than tissue diffusion. If the proportion of active muscles is increased, then there are less regions where pooling of blood can occur. The central blood volume is better maintained, and a larger stroke volume can be developed. Further, the maximum oxygen intake can be reached without every fibre of the active muscles contracting continuously. There is thus opportunity for perfusion of fibres between contractions. The vascular basis of an apparent peripheral limitation of performance is particularly marked in patients with intermittent claudication. A very severe disabling pain is felt in the quadriceps muscle when walking. The immediate cause is a build-up of metabolites within the muscle, but the underlying pathology is an obliteration of the vascular supply to the limb (thromboarteritis obliterans). Often the blood flow to the limb is improved and the symptoms are relieved, at least temporarily, by cutting the sympathetic nerve supply.

The Transport of Carbon Dioxide and Acid/Base Regulation

If the conductance equation (p. 108) is applied to the transport of carbon dioxide, the two main terms are again alveolar ventilation and blood transport. The blood solubility factor λ is at least five times as great for carbon dioxide as for oxygen, and for this reason the overall conductance is also twice as great. Even in maximum exercise, the tissue CO_2 pressure does not exceed 70–80 mmHg, whereas the total gradient of oxygen pressure from the atmosphere to the working tissues is 150 mmHg. The elimination of carbon dioxide is more dependent on alveolar ventilation than on blood transport. Partly for this reason, and partly because the relationship between CO_2 pressure and content of the blood is relatively linear, overbreathing has more influence on CO_2 than on O_2 stores.

Because CO_2 is very soluble in water, it is often stated that no problem can arise in the diffusion of CO_2 across the alveolar membrane. There are several fallacies in this arguement, perhaps the most obvious being the composite nature of diffusing capacity; from page 138:

$$\frac{1}{\dot{D}_L} = \frac{1}{\dot{D}_M} + \frac{1}{\theta V_c}$$

The substantial water solubility of CO_2 ensures a large $\dot{D}_M$ reading, but it has no influence on θV_c; the latter is of the same order as for oxygen. $\dot{D}_L$ is thus only two to four times greater for CO_2 than for oxygen. Furthermore, the crucial factor in determining CO_2 exchange is not the magnitude of $\dot{D}_L$ but the ratio of $\dot{D}_L$ to $\lambda \dot{Q}$; since λ is five times as great for CO_2 as for oxygen, $\dot{D}_L$ must also be five times as great in order to permit comparable equilibration.

It is difficult to test A-a gradients because of respiratory fluctuations in alveolar gas composition. In vigorous exercise, the end-tidal samples often exceed arterial blood CO_2 tension by 2–5 mmHg, and a major part of this "negative" pressure gradient is undoubtedly due to an inappropriate choice of "alveolar" gas. However, there have been suggestions that part of the "negative" gradient is a real phenomenon, induced by a negative electrical charge on the walls of the pulmonary capillaries.

The substantial buffering capacity of the blood plays an important role in carbon dioxide transport; in the absence of buffer systems the metabolically produced CO_2 would cause a large shift in blood and tissue pH, with a disastrous effect on other chemical reactions. The main buffer systems are proteins (haemoglobin and plasma proteins), bicarbonate ions (HCO_3^-/H_2CO_3) and phosphate ions ($HPO_4^=/H_2PO_4^-$); of these, haemoglobin is the most important. Reduced haemoglobin is a weaker acid than oxyhaemoglobin, so that as oxyhaemoglobin is reduced within the active tissues, a substantial quantity of hydrogen ions can be accepted without a decrease in pH. In vigorous exercise, there is inevitably a greater reduction of oxyhaemoglobin, and this helps the transport of CO_2 and other acid metabolites away from the active tissues. Buffering may also be increased by the splitting of creatine phosphate to creatine and phosphate ions. If exercise is sufficiently vigorous for accumulation of lactic acid, then a "metabolic acidosis" develops. Initially, the blood pH falls somewhat ("uncompensated metabolic acidosis"), but as the change of pH is transmitted to the chemosensitive tissues of the fourth ventricle and the carotid bodies, there is a compensatory increase of ventilation. The blood pH is progressively restored to its normal value ("compensated metabolic acidosis") at the expense of a decrease in plasma bicarbonate concentration; the arterial CO_2 tension is also driven below the resting value while compensatory hyperventilation is occurring.

If a large dose of an "alkali" such as sodium bicarbonate is ingested, the converse situation ("metabolic alkalosis") develops. Initially, the pH of the blood rises ("uncompensated metabolic alkalosis"), and over the next fifteen to thirty minutes compensation occurs by a diminution of ventilation; a normal pH is restored with an increase of plasma bicarbonate level (Fig. 74). It has been suggested that human performance could be improved by the ingestion of sodium bicarbonate, both during the acute phase of increased pH, and also during the subsequent stage where blood buffering capacity is increased. This presupposes that the main factor limiting human performance is an accumulation of acid; while this may be the case in some forms of exercise, oxygen transport is normally the dominant factor. Unfortunately, by altering the body buffering systems we also alter the responsiveness of the ventilatory control mechanisms, and thus reduce oxygen transport. Partly for this reason, and partly because of the many body mechanisms that counteract alkalosis, it is difficult to demonstrate that performance is helped by bicarbonate. Other authors have proposed the use of organic buffers such as "THAM"; these are less readily eliminated from the body, but again the improvements in performance following treatment have been far from convincing.

Deliberate hyperventilation, whether in preparation for a contest or as a result of anxiety, leads to respiratory alkalosis, with diminution of plasma bicarbonate and an increase of blood pH. If the subject engages in vigorous physical activity, metabolic CO_2 production soon restores the situation to normal, but if this does not occur, compensation is achieved through a decreased excretion of hydrogen ions by the kidneys.

The Regulation of Ventilation

The Controlling System

The basic control unit is the respiratory centre of the medulla. This has an inherent rhythmicity even when isolated from the rest of the body. Normally, the basic pattern of rhythmic activity is modulated by a wide variety of afferent information, and appropriate efferent impulses are sent to the respiratory muscles (via the phrenic nerve, to the diaphragm, and the intercostal nerves, to the intercostal muscles).

The medulla is well supplied with blood vessels, and the respiratory centre is thus sensitive to changes in the general chemical environment of the body. Exposure to moderate concentrations of carbon dioxide (2% to 5% CO_2 in air) increases the activity of medullary centres, but they are depressed by high concentrations of CO_2 ($>10\%$). At one time, mixtures of CO_2 and oxygen were used for resuscitation, but it is now recognized that when an individual has stopped breathing, the concentrations of CO_2 within the brain are already reaching narcotic levels, and it is harmful to increase them further by adding CO_2 to the breathing mixture. In general, oxygen lack has a depressant effect on both respiratory and cardiovascular centres. However, if oxygen lack is severe, there is a rise of blood pressure, perhaps because the medullary centres are stimulated by increasing acidosis and release of catecholamines;

at this stage there may be some stimulation of respiration, with rapid shallow breathing.

Other regions of the brain modify the activity of the medullary centres. In man, the highest areas of the cortex maintain a considerable control over breathing. Overbreathing (hyperventilation) is seen in acute stress (such as an athlete prior to a contest or a fighter pilot engaged in a difficult aerobatic manoeuvre) and in chronic anxiety. Examples of the voluntary arrest of breathing are provided by the diver, the singer, and the soldier donning a "gas mask." Conditioned reflexes may give rise to an increase of breathing immediately before or coincident with the onset of vigorous physical activity. Irradiation of impulses from the motor cortex contributes to the increase of ventilation in the early stages of exercise. Impulses from the hypothalamus, relayed to the medulla via the pons, initiate an increase of ventilation with a rise of deep body temperature; in animals such as the dog, "thermal panting" is a particularly useful mechanism of body cooling following vigorous exercise. Finally, some irradiation of information may occur from the vasoregulatory centres, so that a sudden rise of blood pressure (injection or release of catecholamines, isometric effort may cause a momentary cessation of breathing; "adrenaline apnoea" is one well-known example of this phenomenon.

Specific areas of chemosensitive tissue are found in the lateral part of the fourth ventricle and in the carotid bodies. The main responsibility for correcting an increase of arterial CO_2 tension is borne by the ventricular receptors. However, their response time is relatively long, as CO_2 must diffuse from the blood stream into the cerebrospinal fluid and there induce a change of pH. The carotid bodies respond much more briskly to a change in either oxygen or carbon dioxide tension. If impulses are recorded from the branch of the glossopharyngeal nerve that innervates the carotid bodies, action potentials can be detected under normal resting conditions. These are abolished a few seconds following a single breath of pure oxygen, and there is an associated temporary reduction of tidal volume (Fig. 37). We may thus conclude that the normal arterial oxygen tension of 90–100 mmHg provides a small stimulus to the

Alive Man!

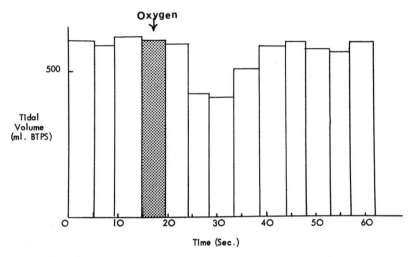

Figure 37. The reduction in tidal volume following inhalation of a single breath of pure oxygen. Each bar represents the volume of one breath. (Schematic, based on experiments by Dejours.)

receptors of the carotid body. However, the tension must be further reduced (to 60–70 mmHg) before there is a major increase of either impulse traffic in the glossopharyngeal nerve or ventilation (Fig. 38). Activity of the glossopharyngeal nerve is also increased by a sudden and substantial rise of arterial CO_2 tension (>10 mmHg), and there is an associated increase of ventilation. The carotid body may thus play some role in the immediate response to CO_2, but it has a much lower CO_2 sensitivity than the ventricular chemoreceptors, and is not normally concerned with long-term CO_2 homeostasis.

A wide range of peripheral receptors contribute afferent information to the respiratory centres in the medulla. Vagal fibres from the trachea and bronchial tree report the distension of the lungs, and exert an inhibiting influence on normal inspiration (the "Hering-Breur" reflex). They are stimulated to a greater extent by forced distension of the lungs (as may occur when the breathing pressure is increased without adequate counter-pressure), and are also activated by exposure to cold, dry air, irritant vapours and particles. Other fibres within the lung structure are stimulated by forced deflation, as may occur

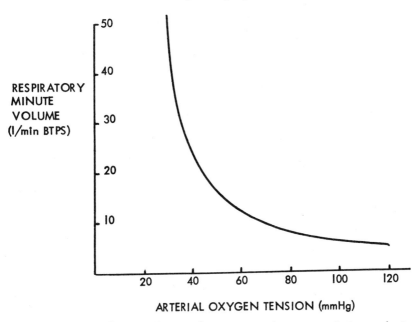

Figure 38. The influence of arterial oxygen tension on respiratory minute volume (other factors held constant).

during diving; these fibres enhance the activity of inspiratory neurones within the medullary centres. The muscles and joints both contain mechanoreceptors (p. 171). Those from the joints (and perhaps also those from the muscles) induce an increase of ventilation when they are stimulated by either voluntary or passive movement of the limbs. Examples of ventilatory drive from passive movement include a relaxed subject sitting on a bicycle ergometer driven by an electric motor, and a pilot subjected to intense vibration while flying a low-level military aircraft. Receptors in the skin induce a brisk hyperventilation in response to either cold (for instance, a 15° C shower) or painful stimuli.

Respiratory Control in Exercise

We have noted a close correspondence between ventilation and metabolic effort (p. 27), and it is thus tempting to explain the primary control of respiration during exercise in terms of changes in either oxygen or carbon dioxide tension. Large

changes of blood gas tensions are undoubtedly caused by vigorous exercise, but unfortunately, these occur on the venous
side of the circulation. Attempts to demonstrate chemosensitive
tissue either within the active muscles or in the great veins
have been uniformly unsuccessful. Early respiratory physiologists such as Haldane suggested that since there was only a
small increase of alveolar (and thus arterial) CO_2 tension during exercise, the receptors were extraordinarily sensitive to this
particular gas. Such an argument is perhaps tenable in moderate
exercise (where arterial CO_2 pressure increases from 40 to 41
or 42 mmHg) but it is difficult to reconcile with the situation
in very vigorous exercise (where CO_2 pressure drops substantially *below* the normal resting value). It is equally difficult to explain exercise ventilation on the basis of a decrease
in arterial oxygen tension; although the alveolar-arterial gradient is broadened by vigorous exercise (p. 138), the arterial
oxygen pressure changes very little, and certainly does not
fall to a level that would induce a brisk response from the
carotid chemoreceptors (Fig. 38). By analogy with other sense
organs, it is possible that the carotid body responds not to the
mean gas tension but to the rate of change of tension within the
blood stream. Exercise could conceivably increase oscillations
about the mean pressure, or alter the phase relationship between
inspiration and a change of tension within the receptor. Such
hypotheses have yet to be categorically disproved, but it seems
unlikely that substantial oscillations of gas pressure can be
transmitted from the lungs through the damping system offered
by the heart, the blood vessels and the chemosensitive tissues
themselves.

In very vigorous exercise, there is a substantial production
of lactic acid, and the increase of hydrogen ion concentration
then contributes to the ventilatory response. But in most circumstances, the dominant role is played by neural rather than
chemical stimuli. As with the cardiovascular system, the early
increase of ventilation is in part a conditioned reflex, and in
part a result of irradiation of impulses from the motor cortex.
As exercise continues, the respiratory drive is supplemented by
the stimulation of mechanoreceptors in the active parts, by

chemoreceptor stimulation (if lactate is produced), and ultimately by hypothalamic stimulation (if there is a rise of deep body temperature). If the systemic blood pressure is increased, there may also be some irradiation of inhibitory impulses from the vasomotor centres. Taken together, these several stimuli seem adequate to account for the magnitude of the ventilatory response to exercise. But the close matching of ventilation and metabolism remains a puzzle that challenges further research.

Breath-holding

The possible length of breath-holding varies markedly from one individual to another. At rest, the range is from thirty seconds to several minutes, and in maximum exercise five seconds is a common limit. The "breaking point" is reached when the sensations arising from an increasing CO_2 tension, a decreasing oxygen tension, and the absence of respiratory movements cannot be counteracted by voluntary inhibition of the respiratory centres. At one time, the duration of breath-holding and the somewhat related ability to hold a column of mercury at a pressure of 40 mm were used as tests of physical fitness, particularly for aircrew (p. 403). Unfortunately, tests of this type depend very much upon motivation. This is well-demonstrated if a subject is persuaded to watch a clock which is driven at an unnaturally slow speed; by this device, the breath-holding time can often be extended to twice the best previous effort. The duration of breath-holding is greater if the lungs are fairly fully inflated. This is partly because changes of arterial gas tension proceed more slowly, and partly because the medullary centres are inhibited via the Hering-Breur reflex. When the "breaking point" is reached, some relief can be obtained through the physical act of breathing, even if the gas mixture that is inhaled has no metabolic value (for instance, a nitrogen/carbon dioxide mixture). However, chemical stimuli play a significant role, and the possible length of breath-holding can be extended by preliminary inhalation of oxygen or hyperventilation. The latter is a common prelude to diving and can be dangerous. If a diver hyperventilates, he has removed the normal CO_2 stimulus to breathing, and is relying on oxygen lack to stimulate his carotid body and force him to surface. Unfortunately, the margin between a stimulant and a dangerous depression of O_2 tension is small. The oxygen pressure continues to fall as the diver is surfacing, and if the preceding exercise has been vigorous, consciousness may be lost before the surface is reached (p. 293).

Intermittent Breathing

Intermittent breathing is a distressing problem of respiratory regulation encountered in the early stages of acclimatization to high altitudes. The tidal volume waxes and wanes, and respiration may cease altogether for short periods. The basis of this phenomenon is an exaggeration of the normal "hunting" reaction that occurs in the respiratory centre, as in any other feedback regulating system. If the respiratory centres are presented with a sudden ("square wave") challenge such as the inhalation of a 5 percent mixture of carbon dioxide in air, the respiratory minute volume usually overshoots the equilibrium adjustment to this challenge, and shows some further minor oscillations before a new steady level of ventilation is reached. However, the fact that the main CO_2 receptor is located in the cerebrospinal fluid gives a measure of damping to the system, and oscillations are rarely excessive. On the other hand, if a subject engages in vigorous physical activity on first arriving at altitude, he may wash out so much carbon dioxide from the body that there is no longer an effective respiratory stimulus. Ventilation is now dependent on a hypoxic drive from the carotid bodies. These lie in much more intimate relationship with the bloodstream, and little damping of response is possible. When the oxygen tension falls in the receptors, vigorous breathing is induced, and this continues for several seconds until well-oxygenated blood from the lungs reaches the bifurcation of the carotid arteries. Ventilation is then suppressed for several seconds until the situation is reversed by arrival of a "slug" of poorly oxygenated blood. Intermittent breathing is particularly likely to develop if the individual has a prolonged circulation time from the lungs to the carotid bodies.

The Use of Oxygen

Oxygen Poisoning

It has been recognised for a long time that high pressures of oxygen are poisonous (p. 277). However, the same seems true of the prolonged use of 100% oxygen at normal ambient pressures. If small mammals are kept in oxygen for two or three days, the lungs show acute congestion, and a proportion of the animals die of bronchopneumonia. Military aviators have inhaled 100% oxygen for periods of six to twelve hours without dramatic effect; however, they also have had occasional complaints, including substernal soreness and collapse of the lungs, and twelve hours seems a desirable limit for the continuous administration of oxygen.

One important source of difficulty is a loss of the normal respiratory "strut" provided by nitrogen. If a small airway is occluded by mucus, the alveolar nitrogen pressure is so similar to that within the blood stream that absorption of the trapped gas proceeds very slowly. However, if the gas beyond the point of obstruction is pure oxygen, it is rapidly absorbed, thereby leading to a complete collapse of the affected lung unit. This tendency to collapse is enhanced by an inhibition of alveolar surfactant production, possibly a consequence of pulmonary vasoconstriction. High pressures of oxygen cause other more general problems. Sulph-hydryl enzymes (—SH groups) may be converted to their oxidized form, thereby preventing normal metabolic activity. The tissue oxygen requirements are met from gas dissolved in physical solution. Haemoglobin thus tends to remain in the oxy-form. This is a poor carrier of hydrogen ions, and CO_2 accumulates in the brain and other tissues. Cerebral accumulation of CO_2 is enhanced by a concomitant reduction of cerebral blood flow.

Oxygen and the Athlete

If an athlete is given oxygen to breathe during submaximal activity, the ventilation and pulse rate are each decreased by about 10 percent. The diminution of ventilation could reflect either a direct suppression of impulses from the carotid body, or (as some authors have found) a lesser production of lactate at a given work-load. In maximum exercise, where the oxygen cost of breathing makes a substantial charge upon the total oxygen intake, the use of increased oxygen concentrations leads to a small gain in performance (p. 133, 363). It is of course impractical for contests. Nevertheless, the development of lightweight portable oxygen equipment played a significant role in the white man's final conquest of Everest; it is interesting to note that the Sherpa, Tensing, had sufficient adaptation to high altitude that he found oxygen an unnecessary encumbrance.

Oxygen may be useful in recovery from athletic contests (p. 363). It leads to a slightly more rapid fall of pulse and ventilation rates, although apparently there is no alteration in the rate of repayment of any oxygen debt that has been incurred.

The inhalation of oxygen in preparation for a contest is more controversial. Many authors feel that oxygen is eliminated so rapidly from the body that no advantage could be gained. The main result of oxygen breathing is a 3.2 litre increase in the oxygen content of the lungs (Table II). However, other tissues

TABLE II

THE NORMAL OXYGEN STORES OF THE BODY, AND THEIR
MODIFICATION BY OXYGEN BREATHING

Site of Storage	Volume of Store (litre)	AIR BREATHING		OXYGEN BREATHING		Increase with Oxygen (ml)
		Unit Content (ml/litre)	Total Content (ml)	Unit Content (ml/litre)	Total Content (ml)	
Lungs	4	140	560	940	3760	3200
Blood—Arterial	1	195	195	215	215	20
—Venous	4	140	560	160	640	80
Myoglobin (Muscle)	24	10	240	11.5	276	36
Body Fluids (Physical Solution)	38	0.55	21	0.66	25	4

(blood, myoglobin, and the body fluids) also gain some 140 ml. of oxygen, and this advantage is not entirely dissipated until several minutes after oxygen breathing has ceased. The volume of oxygen involved is small relative to the oxygen debt (5 litres) and the aerobic power (3–6 litre/min); nevertheless, it could be a significant factor in a race won by a small fraction of a second.

Types of Equipment

Respiratory Equipment

Respiratory equipment may be worn by the diver to provide an underwater air-supply, by both the mountaineer and the aviator to provide oxygen at altitude, and by firefighters and others working in a toxic environment to provide a chemically safe breathing mixture of adequate oxygen content. Specific types of diving equipment are discussed on page 270. At altitude, devices range from a simple facemask to partial and full pressure suits that supply oxygen at supraatmospheric pressures. Firefighters commonly use a small self-contained rebreathing system with a built-in oxygen supply; other devices for contaminated environments include the war time "gasmasks" and ventilated hoods.

Respiratory Resistance

Resistance to breathing is the main obstacle when wearing most forms of respiratory equipment. If maximum effort is attempted, the limiting symptom is usually shortness of breath.

In some devices such as the "pendulum" type under-water breathing apparatus (p. 272), the resistance is similar during inspiration and expiration. However, if air is drawn through a filter or absorbent canister, the inspiratory resistance commonly exceeds expiratory resistance. We have noted the widely held view that an expiratory resistance is tolerated better than an inspiratory one (p. 129). Physiological "explanations" of this supposed phenomenon include the larger size of the expiratory portion of the pressure-volume diagram (Fig. 33), and possible collapse of the lungs and cardiac embarassment induced by what is in effect negative pressure breathing. However, if careful records of subjective preference are kept, an expiratory resistance is tolerated no more readily than an inspiratory resistance. Furthermore, the increase of intrathoracic pressure engendered by expiratory resistance causes a peripheral pooling of blood, and a restriction of cardiac output is at least as likely as when there is an increase of inspiratory resistance.

Standards of resistance vary with the type of equipment and the level of physical effort that is proposed. Military respirators ("gasmasks") are regarded as adequate if the inspiratory resistance does not exceed 10 cm H_2O at a steady airflow of 85 litre/min. The United Kingdom Ministry of Fuel and Power recommends a resistance of 2.5 cm H_2O at the same airflow; this is for a dust respirator to be used in light to moderate exercise. The most exacting standards are for resistances that are not noticeable subjectively (2 cm H_2O at 400 litre/min airflow) and produce no measurable decrease in maximum voluntary ventilation (0.7 cm H_2O at 85 litre/min). Some authors have argued these very exacting standards should be met by all breathing equipment used during maximum exercise. Unfortunately, it is difficult to design compact and effective filter/absorbent canisters that meet such specifications. The less perfect military standard is by no means pleasant to wear during all-out effort, but from the practical point of view it has a surprisingly small influence on the capability for brief periods of maximum work.

In the evaluation of diving equipment, account must be taken not only of bench tests* but also of the effects of increased ambient pressure upon the turbulent component of the total flow resistance. The pressure drop P under turbulent flow conditions is roughly proportional to gas density δ and a resistance that is well tolerated while breathing quietly at the surface may be quite intolerable when swimming at a depth of one hundred feet, where the gas density is increased fourfold.

The peak inspiratory flow is about 2½ times the average respiratory minute volume. Thus if the equipment is to be used at an exercise ventilation of 100 litre/min BTPS, it should be capable of meeting a peak demand of 250 litre/min BTPS. Peak requirements can be reduced if a capacity (a large hood or air-filled waistcoat) is incorporated into the system. The flow resistance is further minimised if air is fed to the mask or hood, using a line from a cylinder, or a small compressor is worn by the subject. It then becomes important to ensure that flow exceeds demand at all times, otherwise the subject breathes against the very large resistance of the pump or induces leakage at the margins of his facepiece.

Other Problems of Respiratory Equipment

Many other physiological problems arise when using respiratory equipment. Some types of apparatus, such as pendulum devices (p. 272) have a large dead space; the subject must then increase each breath by the volume of this added dead space in order to achieve his normal alveolar ventilation. In some situations, a considerable proportion of the total body heat is eliminated from the face; breathing equipment may thus impose a thermal stress. Communica-

---

* I refer here to engineering rather than exercise bench tests!

tion is also impaired by respiratory equipment; speech is difficult and distorted, the visual field may be restricted by goggles and canister, and the clarity of vision is impaired by fogging of the lenses. Fortunately, the last problem can be minimised by use of anti-dimming compounds and appropriate channelling of airstreams. If a facepiece is worn frequently, dermatitis may develop; rubber and its various additives must be carefully screened for their allergenic properties. Lastly, careful maintenance of the equipment is vital. The necessary standards of performance are exacting—leakage must be less than 1% in an oxygen mask, less than 0.01% in an anti-chemical respirator and less than 0.0001% in an antibacterial respirator; absorption of carbon dioxide must also be virtually complete in all closed-circuit equipment. This degree of efficiency can only be attained by frequent adjustment of harnesses, regular inspection of valves for deterioration of rubber and accumulation of dirt, and replacement of absorbent canisters at carefully calculated intervals.

Pressure Breathing

The breathing pressure may exceed atmospheric (positive pressure breathing) if a subject surfaces suddenly from a dive without exhaling; positive pressures are also used by the aviator at altitudes above forty thousand feet (p. 98) and intermittent positive pressure is applied when assisting ventilation (p. 98, 159).

The main hazard of sudden surfacing is lung rupture (p. 292) High altitude pressure breathing creates circulatory problems (p. 98); also, unless counterpressure is applied to the exterior of the chest, the thoracic cage expands to a volume determined by the applied pressure and the compliance of the system. Unless a full-pressure suit is worn, it is difficult to apply counterpressure to the neck, and a dramatic expansion of the airway may occur in this region. This leads to a forcible stimulation of stretch receptors, which may contribute in turn to the ultimate loss of consciousness. There is some evidence from industry (for example glassblowers) that frequent exposure to high pressures leads to a permanent stretching of the upper airway.

Artificial Respiration

General Principles

Artificial respiration may be needed in drowning (p. 295), following electric shock, and in other situations where natural respiration has ceased. Because of the limited viability of the brain (p. 50), it is essential that measures to restore ventilation (and if necessary, the activity of the heart) be undertaken as rapidly as possible.

The essence of artificial respiration is to carry out—manually or mechanically—pressure/volume work previously performed by the chest muscles. Often, the work of breathing is increased by the emergency; bronchospasm is initiated by inhalation of water and/or vomit, and the compliance of the lungs is reduced by vascular congestion and collapse of areas of lung. The optimum technique of artificial respiration is one that provides the necessary ventilation, without impeding the circulation of blood through the lungs.

All methods of resuscitation are dependent on patency of the airway. Time must thus be taken to clear the mouth of vomit and other possible obstructions. The head must then be positioned in such a manner that further vomit does not accumulate, and the tongue does not fall backwards to block the airway in the back of the throat; the usually recommended position is to tilt the head sideways and backwards, while at the same time pulling the angle of the jaw forwards.

Older Manual Methods

The chest volume is modified by pressure on the thorax, lifting the arms, or a combination of the two procedures. In the Silvester method, the victim lies supine, and the rescuer alternates rhythmically between thoracic pressure and elevation of the arms. The main disadvantage of this technique is that both hands of the rescuer are fully occupied, and it is impossible to prevent airway obstruction by traction on the angle of the jaw. In the Schafer method, the victim lies prone, and the rescuer compresses the rib-cage beyond the normal position of relaxation, allowing it to expand subsequently by elastic recoil. Respiration is thus confined to the unfavourable part of the pressure-volume curve (Fig. 29), and the rescuer must work exceedingly hard to achieve a respectable tidal volume. The normally small expiratory reserve volume is further compressed in the prone position, and there is the added disadvantage that the reduced lung volume enhances the tendency to collapse of the lungs. The Holger-Nielsen method combines certain features of the other two methods, being carried out in the prone position, and using both back-pressure and arm lifting to produce ventilation. Each method has enjoyed periods of popularity among life-saving societies; currently, it is appreciated that the prone position does not obviate airway obstruction, and the Silvester technique is now the preferred manual method.

All three procedures have been successful in resuscitating a substantial number of patients with respiratory arrest. Laboratory evaluation has been carried out on conscious subjects whose breathing has been arrested temporarily by hyperventilation. Under such circumstances, all three methods have yielded more than adequate tidal volumes (500–1000 ml). However, their adequacy is less certain when a general loss of muscular tone permits obstruction of the airway. If carried out too vigorously, they also carry a risk of rib fracture and damage to underlying viscera; rupture of the liver or spleen and the development of a pneumothorax are well recognized complications of overenthusiastic treatment.

Mouth-to-mouth Resuscitation

Mouth-to-mouth resuscitation has been practised intermittently since the time of the prophet Elisha. In 1958, it was recommended as the method of choice by the United States National Academy of Sciences. Their decision followed a comparison of mouth-to-mouth and manual methods on a panel of anaesthetized volunteers.

There seems little question that larger tidal volumes can be achieved by the mouth-to-mouth technique, particularly when the rescuer is ventilating an unconscious subject. With the manual methods, figures of 500–700 ml are attained, but with mouth-to-mouth ventilation volumes of 1000–1500 ml are readily achieved. This in itself would not provide grounds for abandoning the manual procedures A tidal volume of 500–700 ml, produced twelve times per minute, is equivalent to at least a normal respiratory minute volume (6.0–8.4 litre/min BTPS). The main advantages of the mouth-to-mouth method are (a) the hands are left free to overcome airway obstruction, and

(b) any increase in resistance to airflow is readily sensed both by the reduced outward movement of the victim's chest and also by the increased loading of proprioceptors in the rescuer's chest muscles. In the early stages of resuscitation, a large tidal volume may also help to reverse collapse and compensate for a poor matching of ventilation and perfusion.

The tidal volume must be increased if expired air is used in resuscitation. However, the added gas volume is less than might be supposed, since the first 150–200 ml of insufflated air comes from the rescuer's dead space (20.93% oxygen, 0.03% carbon dioxide), while the final 150–200 ml of gas with the lowest oxygen and highest carbon dioxide content remains in the victim's dead space. The recommended pattern of mouth-to-mouth resuscitation commences with four 1500 ml breaths and continues with 1000 ml breaths twelve times per minute.

Reference to the pressure-volume diagram (Fig. 33) shows that a strong and healthy young rescuer could exert a dangerous pressure on the lung structures of an unconscious victim. Normally, this pressure is dissipated as the lung expands. However, if inadequate time is allowed for the chest to empty between inflations, damage may occur. Because of this risk, some authors recommend mouth-to-nose resuscitation for very young patients; the nose provides an additional resistance, minimizing the possible pressures developed within the chest of the victim.

The main physiological objection to the mouth-to-mouth technique is that intermittent positive pressure has an adverse effect on the circulation. Mechanical respirators that do not include a "negative" pressure phase depress cardiac output, particularly if the heart is weakened by an initial period of oxygen lack, and this is equally a limitation of the mouth-to-mouth technique not adequately considered by its proponents. Frequent attempts at mouth-to-mouth resuscitation also expose the rescuer to a serious risk of cross-infection.

Other Simple Techniques

Eve introduced a "rocking" technique in 1932; the victim was strapped to a board, and rocked twelve to fifteen times per minute through an angle of 120–180°. Ventilation occurred because the weight of the abdominal viscera created a "negative" intrathoracic pressure in the foot-down position, and a positive pressure in the foot-up position. The method was at one time popular with the British navy. As with other manual procedures, an adequate tidal volume can be achieved if the airway resistance and compliance are normal, but it is difficult to maintain an unobstructed airway while rocking is being carried out.

A number of bellows resuscitators are commercially available. The majority of these suffer from the defect that one hand is needed to operate the bellows, and the second must seal the mask on the face, leaving no means of manipulating the jaw. The Porton resuscitator has a specially moulded facemask that enables the operator to pull the jaw forwards while holding the mask. Most bellows have a capacity of 1000–1500 ml, and they are fitted with a "blow-off" valve which prevents the operator from developing a pressure of more than 20–30 cm H_2O. An anaesthetist who is accustomed to holding a facemask can achieve a very good tidal volume with a bellows resuscitator, but ordinary mortals often produce indifferent results, mainly because air leaks between the mask and the face. If inflation is carried out rapidly, the combined elastic and nonelastic resistance of the victim may exceed the "blow-off" pressure, and gas is then lost through the relief valve.

Mechanical Devices

Any form of manual ventilation is very exhausting for the rescuer, and if adequate natural respiration does not recommence within a few minutes, a mechanical respirator should be sought. These are of two basic types—pressure and volume-cycled respectively.

In a pressure-cycled device, gas is supplied to the facemask until a predetermined pressure is reached. The gas flow is then interrupted until "zero" or a specific "negative" pressure is developed, when the cycle recommences. Venturi ducts mix preselected proportions of air and oxygen, and spring-loaded valves control the cycling procedure. The entire apparatus can be quite small, and it will operate at distances of up to one hundred feet from the oxygen supplying cylinder (for instance, when injury occurs in the hold of a ship). The incorporation of a negative-pressure phase is helpful as far as the circulation is concerned. The output of a heart weakened by oxygen lack is 40 percent to 50 percent greater with a mask that cycles between $+15$ mmHg and -10 mmHg than with a comparable device operating over the pressure range 0–25 mmHg. The main disadvantages of the pressure-limited device are (a) that if a poor seal is achieved at the facepiece, the cycling pressure ($+15$ mmHg) may never be developed, and (b) if the airway is obstructed, the cycling pressure is reached too soon, giving very rapid, shallow, and ineffective ventilation.

The volume-limited device is essentially a mechanized bellows resuscitator. It can be adjusted to deliver a tidal volume of 500–1500 ml fifteen or more times per minute. It is easier to operate than the pressure-limited machine, since it continues to cycle at the intended rate despite minor leakage at the facepiece and changes in airway resistance.

Devices for Teaching Artificial Resuscitation

Failures of artificial ventilation are usually due to obstruction of the airway in the neck, and (in the case of mouth-to-mouth resuscitation) a certain reluctance on the part of the rescuer to make the necessary oral contact with a cold, clammy, and possibly vomiting victim. To minimise the incidence of failures, a number of teaching devices are now available. These can be used to learn not only mouth-to-mouth, but also mouth-to-nose, bellows, and mechanical ventilation of the lungs. Some of the models have remarkable physical realism, but most are unrealistic in terms of physiological parameters such as resistance and compliance. Considerations in the choice of a teaching device include hygiene (ease of cleaning or replacing "skin" and "airway," routing of expired gas away from the rescuer), realism in the texture of the "mouth" and "nose," accuracy of the "head" and "neck" mechanisms, realism in the extent of chest movement, and accuracy of the airway resistance and compliance settings.

Some devices incorporate simple pressure cuffs, to permit training in techniques of cardiac massage.

References

Shephard, R.J.: The oxygen conductance equation. In *Frontiers of Fitness.* Springfield, Thomas, 1971.

Haldane, J.S., and Priestley, J.G.: *Respiration.* Oxford, Clarendon Press, 1935.

Comroe, J.H.: *Physiology of Respiration.* Chicago, Year Book Medical Publishers, 1965.

Hugh-Jones, P., and Campbell, E.J.M.: Respiratory physiology. *Brit Med Bull., 19:1–89,* 1963.

Caro, C.G.: *Advances in Respiratory Physiology.* London, Arnold, 1966.

Fenn, W.O., and Rahn, H.: *Handbook of Physiology.* Section 3: Respiration. Vol. 1–2, 1964.

Comroe, J.H., Forster, R.E., Dubois, A.B., Briscoe, W.A., and Carlsen, E.: *The Lung. Clinical Physiology and Pulmonary Function Tests.* Chicago, Year Book Publishers, 1955.

Cotes, J.E.: *Lung Function. Assessment and Application in Medicine.* Oxford, Blackwell, 1965.

Bates, D.V., and Christie, R.V.: *Respiratory Function in Disease.* Philadelphia, Saunders, 1964.

Bartels, H., Bücherl, E., Hertz, C.W., Rodewald, G., and Schwab, M.: *Methods in Pulmonary Physiology.* New York, Hafner, 1963.

Varhga, G., and Kovats, J.: *Pulmonary Function Tests and their Clinical Application.* Budapest, Akademiai Kiado, 1968.

Howell, J.B.L., and Campbell, E.J.M.: *Breathlessness.* Oxford, Blackwell, 1966.

Dickens, F., and Neil, E.: *Oxygen in the Animal Organism.* New York, MacMillan, 1964.

Cunningham, D.J.C., and Lloyd, B.B.: *The Regulation of Human Respiration.* Oxford, Blackwell, 1963.

Brooks, C. McC., Kao, F.F., and Lloyd, B.B.: *Cerebro-spinal Fluid and the Regulation of Ventilation.* Oxford, Blackwell, 1965.

Torrance, R.W.: *Arterial Chemoreceptors.* Oxford, Blackwell, 1968.

Davies, C.N.: *Design and Use of Respirators.* Oxford, Pergamon Press, 1962.

Gillies, J.A.: *A Textbook of Aviation Physiology.* Oxford, Pergamon Press, 1965.

Nunn, J.F.: *Applied Respiratory Physiology With Special Reference to Anaesthesia.* London, Butterworths, 1969.

Shephard, R.J.: Devices for the teaching of expired air resuscitation. *Med Services J, Canada, 22:273–284,* 1966.

6

THE NEUROMUSCULAR SYSTEM

The Structures Involved in Muscular Activity

Gross Structure and Function of Muscle

If the skeletal muscles are regarded as a single functional unit, then the resultant "organ" accounts for 40 percent of body weight (some 28 kg in a 70 kg man). At least 20 kg of the total muscle mass are active during exercise that develops an individual's maximum oxygen intake (for instance, treadmill running, stair climbing, bicycle riding or swimming); some muscles find employment in moving the limbs, while others maintain the stability of joints, balance the body, support its weight, and develop the necessary associated respiratory effort. In other less demanding and more localized activities, it is possible to identify a few muscles that are primarily responsible for a given movement (the *prime-movers*), others that assist in its performance (the *synergists*), and yet others that control or oppose the movement (the *antagonists*). A given division of functional responsibility is peculiar to movement in one particular direction; thus, if the activity changes (for example, from flexion to extension of the forearm), the role of individual muscles is largely reversed.

It it customary to distinguish "isometric" and "isotonic" contractions. These terms have rather different meanings for the physiologist and for the physical educator. The physiologist thinks in terms of the "pure" situation of an isolated frog gastrocnemius/sciatic nerve preparation. When such a preparation undergoes isometric contraction, shortening is prevented by a rigid lever. In an isotonic contraction, on the other hand, the load is supported by a stop until the muscle has developed sufficient tension to lift it. Thereafter, contraction is recorded by an ultra lightweight pen which permits the muscle to shorten without further increase of tension. The isometric activity of the physical educator involves simultaneous contraction of prime-movers and their antagonists, and thus coincides quite closely with a physiological isometric contraction. However, weight-lifting is often described as "isotonic" work, although it involves substantial static (postural) effort, and there are also large changes of tension in many of the limb and shoulder muscles as the activity proceeds. Human work is rarely isotonic; it may even be desirable to abandon the term, and merely distinguish dynamic and static contractions.

Let us now review the gross structure of a typical muscle. It is surrounded by a sheath of connective tissue, the perimysium. This connective tissue penetrates into the interior of the muscle, dividing it into a number of "fasciculi." As buyers of meat will appreciate, the number and thickness of the connective tissue "septae" vary from one individual to another, and there is some evidence that muscular training is associated with an increase of septal tissue. There is also a variable amount of fat within the muscle belly. Account must be taken of "dilution" by fat and connective tissue if the bulk of muscles is assessed by measurements of external circumference or by soft-tissue radiographs.

Each fasciculus consists of several hundred muscle fibres, from 1 to 40 mm in length, and from 10 to 100μ ($1\mu = 0.001$mm) in breadth. The diameter of the individual fibres increases somewhat with appropriate forms of muscular training; however, a limit is set to such development by the oxygen requirements at the centre of the fiber. Other factors being equal, the oxygen tension is inversely proportional to the square of the distance over which diffusion must occur; thus hypertrophy of a fibre reduces the oxygen tension at its centre, and a limit of growth is soon reached, beyond which metabolism cannot be sustained.

In some muscles, such as those of the hip and shoulder girdle, power is more important than speed or range of movement. Individual muscle fibres are then inserted angularly into the main tendon (the so-called *"pennate"* form of arrangement). In other muscles such as those producing arm movements, power requirements are subordinate to the demands of speed. The fibres are then arranged longitudinally (the so-called *"fusiform"* arrangement).

A further rather obvious difference between muscles is the relative pigmentation of their fibres. *"Red" muscles* are mainly concerned with maintenance of posture and they contain large quantities of myoglobin. *"White" muscles* are mainly concerned with rapid voluntary movements and they have a much lower myoglobin content. Myoglobin is an oxygen-binding pigment that is structurally similar to haemoglobin. However, it has very different oxygen binding properties. The haemoglobin curve is of a sigmoid shape, with half-saturation at an oxygen pressure of 24 mmHg, while the myoglobin curve is a hyperbola, with half-saturation at an oxygen pressure of 6 mmHg (Fig. 39). These differences of oxygen affinity are related to the fact that myoglobin contains only one atom of iron and one heme molecule, whereas haemoglobin contains four heme molecules. The characteristic absorption spectrum of myoglobin

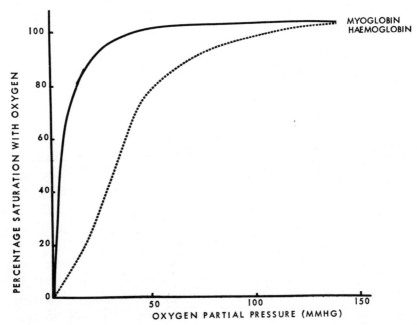

Figure 39 A comparison of the oxygen-binding properties of hemoglobin and myoglobin.

permits an assessment of oxygen pressure within the contracting muscles. Much of the pigment is in the reduced state, and the oxygen pressure thus cannot exceed 3–5 mmHg; this is within the range previously suggested (p. 63, 169) for tissue oxygen tension. The separation of haemoglobin and myoglobin dissociation curves is important in maintaining the flow of oxygen from the blood stream to the active tissues, particularly at the venous end of the capillaries.

There are other gross microscopic differences between red and white muscle (Table III). Normally, the physiological properties coincide with gross appearance, but there are a few muscles that have a rather pale colour, and yet show the slow contraction pattern of a "red" muscle; considerable research on such "intermediate" fibre types is currently in progress.

TABLE III
A COMPARISON OF "RED" AND "WHITE" MUSCLE

	Red	*White*
Myoglobin Content	High	Low
Glycogen Content	Low	High
Fat Content	High	Low
Mitochondrial Content	High	Low
Speed of Contraction	Slow	Fast
Duration of Twitch	100 msec	10 msec
Liability of Fatigue	Low	High
Usual Function	Postural Control	Rapid Movement

Microstructure of Muscle

The microstructure of muscle has been greatly clarified by electron microscope studies. Each muscle fibre is bounded by a membrane, the sarcolemma; this contains the sarcoplasm, a viscous fluid in which are found many nuclei and mitochondria, and about five hundred myofibrils. The outer layers of the sarcolemma are collagenous, and merge with the connective tissue of the septae and tendons. The inner part of the sarcolemma comprises a few molecular layers of lipid and protein; it is in fact a typical cell membrane.

The sarcoplasm contains the pigment myoglobin and various energy stores—ATP (adenosine triphosphate), creatine phosphate (CP), fat and glycogen. The immediate energy requirements of a muscular contraction are met by the splitting of high-energy phosphate bonds from ATP. (Fig. 40). Each gram-molecule of ATP yields 10–12 kcal of energy. Unfortunately the total ATP content of the sarcoplasm is small, about 5×10^{-6} gram molecules per gram. Since the usage of ATP can be as great as 10^{-3} Moles/gm/min, stores are exhausted in less than half a second. Creatine phosphate also contains a high energy phosphate bond, and this provides a basis for the resynthesis of ATP. Creatine phosphate stores again are very limited (about 15×10^{-6} gram molecules per gram of sarcoplasm), and the available CP is used in about two seconds of vigorous activity. Thereafter, energy must be derived from the breakdown of fat and/or carbohydrate. The metabolism of fat requires oxygen, but glucose and glycogen can be converted to lactic acid in the absence of oxygen; if oxygen later becomes available, part

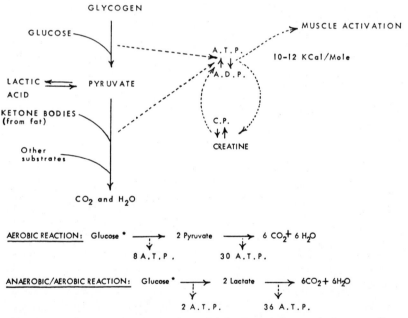

Figure 40. The chemical reactions involved in activation of a muscle.

* One molecule of ATP is used in the initial reaction of converting glucose to glucose-6-phosphate. The total yield from glucose (38 moles of ATP per mole) is thus less than the yield from the equivalent portion of the glycogen molecule (39 moles of ATP per mole).

of the lactate is oxidized to CO_2 and water, while the remainder is reconverted to glycogen in the liver. Anaerobic metabolism is much less efficient than aerobic; for each molecule of glucose that is broken down anaerobically, only two molecules of ATP are synthesized, whereas the complete oxidation of glucose to CO_2 and water yields thirty-eight molecules of ATP (Fig. 40). The chemical efficiency of aerobic metabolism is about 63 percent.

During vigorous activity, the fat and glycogen stores of the sarcoplasm are depleted, and the extent of such stores is one factor limiting sustained performance (see p. 37 and 195). The muscle fibres also draw upon glucose and free fatty acids supplied by the blood stream. During the recovery phase, circulating foodstuffs are used to replenish glycogen and fat stores, and if the blood sugar level is high or insulin is provided, the glycogen content of the sarcoplasm may rise above the preexercise level.

When viewed under a light microscope, the myofibrils seem to consist of alternate light and dark structures, named (after their optical properties) the I ("isotropic") and A ("anisotropic") bands. Electron microscopy shows that this appearance is produced by the interdigitation of long-chained protein filaments, predominantly actin and myosin (Fig. 41). When activated by ATP, the actin fibres slide over the myosin and

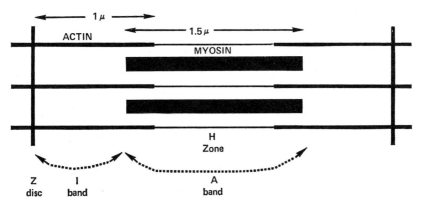

Figure 41. Diagrammatic representation of the electron microscopic appearance of skeletal muscle.

toward each other; there is also a structural bonding of the two types of filament (formation of "actomyosin"). During relaxation, these changes are reversed. Shortening or folding of the individual filaments does not occur, unless the muscle undergoes extreme shortening. However, a substantial viscous resistance is encountered as the filaments slide over one another, and for this reason work is performed within the muscle as it contracts; indeed, during isometric activity, this is the sole basis of energy expenditure.

Vascular Supply

Some aspects of the vascular supply to skeletal muscle have been discussed previously (p. 93). Blood flow is normally expressed per 100 ml of tissue volume. At rest, muscle has a fairly low flow (1–2 ml/min/100 ml). During rhythmic (isotonic") activity, flow increases to 20–30 ml/min/100 ml. However, this still may not be enough to meet metabolic demands, so that lactate accumulates. With moderate work, any inadequacy of blood flow occurs mainly in the first two or three minutes of exercise, being related to the slow "on-transient" of vascular adjustments. In consequence, the blood lactate rises initially, but returns towards the resting level of 5 to 10 mg/100 ml as exercise is continued (Fig. 42). On the other hand, with near maximal work lactate accumulation continues until the maximum tolerated level (100–150 mg/100 ml) is reached. It must thus be concluded that the blood flow remains inadequate in part or all of the contracting muscle throughout vigorous effort. This is borne out by detailed study of blood flow patterns (p. 95). If activity is rhythmic, more flow occurs between contractions than during contractions, and there remains a substantial blood flow debt that is repaid in the first few minutes following cessation of activity (Fig. 21). With isometric activity, there are no pauses when the blood flow debt can be repaid; the maximum duration of an isometric contraction is thus determined largely by the effects of the activity upon blood flow. If the force of contraction is less than 15 percent of maximum strength, there is no significant impairment of blood flow, and the contraction can be sustained

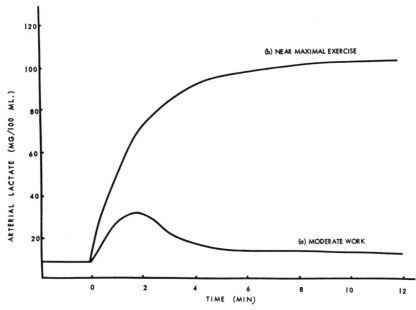

Figure 42. Course of blood lactate accumulation during (a) moderate and (b) near maximal rhythmic work.

almost indefinitely. However, if stronger contractions are induced, blood flow is progressively impaired (Fig. 43) and there is a corresponding decrease in the maximum time over which the effort can be sustained. If the force of contraction is more than 70 percent to 80 percent of maximum, blood flow is occluded completely; the maximum duration of contraction is then short, and is uninfluenced by deliberately occluding the limb circulation with a sphygmomanometer cuff.

The increased blood flow of rhythmic exercise is associated with a great increase in the number of patent capillaries within the muscle (see also p. 102). Since the gradient of oxygen pressure from the capillaries to the active tissues is inversely proportional to the square of the distance over which diffusion must occur, the extraction of oxygen from blood perfusing the muscles is much more complete in exercise than at rest. The oxygen tension of blood leaving the muscles may drop from a resting value of 40 mmHg to 5 mmHg or less; this implies that

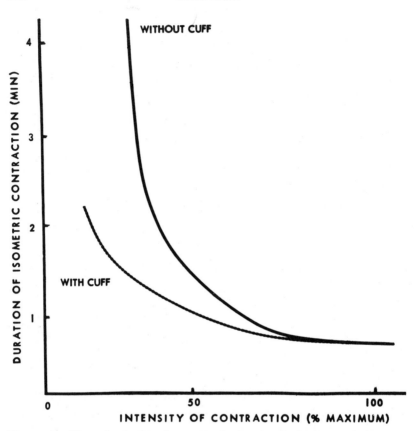

Figure 43. The relationship between intensity and duration of isometric contractions (handgrip). The prior interruption of the circulation by a cuff inflated above arterial pressure has little influence on the duration of contractions at more than 70% of maximum force.

the oxygen content has dropped from the usual venous value of about 14 ml/100 ml to around 1 ml/100 ml.

The exudation of fluid into the muscles (p. 102) is greatly increased during exercise, and a 20 percent gain of tissue weight is by no means uncommon during prolonged activity.

The Nerve Supply of Muscle

Sensory Nerves. The sensory nerve supply of skeletal muscle has many functions, but perhaps the most important is to detect changes of tension in the muscle and its associated tendinous

structures during contraction, relaxation and forcible stretching movements. The *"Golgi organs"* are simple sprays of fine
nerve terminals distributed throughout the connective tissue
of the tendons. They have a relatively high threshold, being
stimulated by a substantial increase of length such as accompanies a general rise of tension within the tendon. Through
their central connections in the grey matter of the spinal cord,
they initiate relaxation of the corresponding muscle (the
"antimyotatic" reflex). This reflex minimizes the risk of developing an excessive tension in the system. *"Muscle spindles"* are
cigar-shaped organs a few millimetres in length, embedded
between normal muscle fibres, and functioning in parallel with
them (Fig. 44). Each muscle contains many spindles. The
individual spindle has an outer connective tissue sheath enclosing two types of modified muscle fibre, a single "nuclear
bag" and four or five "nuclear chain" fibres. The *"nuclear bag"*
has striated polar regions and a central swelling containing
up to a dozen nuclei. Originally, it was held that myofibrils
were confined to the polar regions but most authorities now
believe that some fibrils traverse the central swelling. Sensory
nerve terminals are coiled around the central swelling, forming
an annulo-spiral ending. The polar regions are innervated by
fine (gamma) motor fibres that terminate in typical motor
end-plates. The *"nuclear chain"* fibres have nuclei distributed
along their length. The sensory receptors consist partly of
distinct annulo-spiral endings and partly of finer branches that
join the sensory nerve emerging from the nuclear bag fibre.
The motor supply to the "nuclear chain" again consists of fine
(gamma) efferents, but these terminate as diffusely branching
"trail" endings. The muscle spindles play a vital role in maintaining the normal resting tone of muscle; they also serve as
a sophisticated feedback mechanism that regulates the intensity
of any given muscular contraction. The spinal connections of
the spindle receptors are such that when stimulated—whether
by a passive stretch (knee jerk) or by activity of their own
γ motor fibres—the contraction of the corresponding muscle
is facilitated. During normal muscular activity, there is a parallel
discharge of impulses through the α fibres, to the muscle proper,

Alive Man!

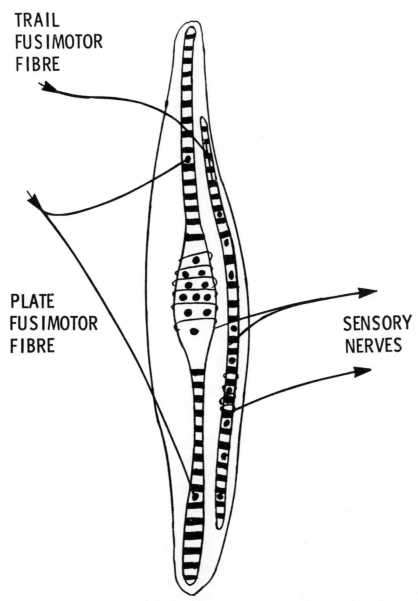

TRAIL
FUSIMOTOR
FIBRE

PLATE
FUSIMOTOR
FIBRE

SENSORY
NERVES

Figure 44. Nuclear chain and nuclear bag fibres within a muscle spindle. For clarity, one nuclear bag and one nuclear chain fibre are shown in this schematic drawing; however, mammalian spindle receptors usually contain four or five nuclear chain fibres.

and through the γ fibres to the spindles; the muscle as a whole shortens, and this rapidly relieves tension within the spindle. However, the feedback mechanism continues to facilitate activity of the α motor fibres if an unexpected external resistance limits shortening of the muscle. The system detects "length-tension inappropriateness." Feedback regulation of this type does not depend on conscious voluntary control. Nevertheless the spindle mechanism permits very sensitive conscious proprioception, and a subject can learn to report quite small differences of external resistance. Thus, in respiratory experiments, it is possible to detect an added elastic load equivalent to a water pressure of 10–15 mm (2.5 cmH$_2$O/litre), while the threshold for detection of viscous resistance is even smaller (0.6 cmH$_2$O/litre/sec, equivalent to a water pressure of about 3 mm).

> Engineers interested in servo-mechanisms have speculated on the advantage to the body of a dual system of receptors—the fixed response, high threshold Golgi organs, and the low threshold spindle receptors with adjustable sensitivity. One reasonable suggestion is that the former report static changes of tension, while the latter indicate the rate of change of tension. The design of the receptors is such that the relative proportions of "static" and "dynamic" information can be varied by activity of the γ efferent fibres. Engineers use a similar technique of "phase-advance" to minimise oscillations in a mechanical servo-system, and it is likely that the body uses this approach to counteract the instability introduced by long neural loops.

If spindle receptors do indeed detect the rate of change of tension, then they are particularly likely to be stimulated by bouncing and jerky movements. Such forms of activity should be avoided in "warming up" and in exercises designed to improve flexibility. Gains of flexibility are more likely to result from a sustained stretch of sufficient intensity to stimulate the Golgi receptors, thereby relaxing the corresponding muscle group.

Motor Nerves. The motor nerves contain many fibres, each of which arises from a single cell within the ventral horn of the spinal cord. The smallest functional unit comprises those muscle fibres innervated by a single ventral horn cell; it is known as a "motor unit" (Fig. 45). In some smaller muscles, such as the external muscles of the eye, the motor unit may activate no more than a single fibre, but in other areas such as the large muscles of the leg as many as 150 fibres may be activated by one ventral horn cell.

Motor units may be called into activity by impulses travelling through simple spinal reflex arcs (Fig. 45, receptors in the skin and muscle), or by volitional impulses travelling from the motor cortex of the brain, via pyramidal and extrapyramidal pathways. Granit distinguishes two types of motor unit, the

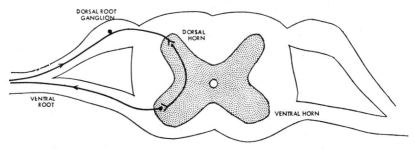

Figure 45. Typical segmental reflex arc in spinal cord. Sensory fibres enter via the dorsal root, and their cell bodies are located in the dorsal root ganglion. They terminate in the dorsal horn of grey matter, whence an internuncial neurone connects to the motor neurone in the ventral horn. The motor fibre leaves via the ventral root.

In the example illustrated, there are two synapses; this is typical of the flexion reflex that follows contact with a painful stimulus. The stretch reflex is monosynaptic, the internuncial neurone being omitted.

tonic and the phasic. The tonic is characterized by a low threshold, a slow rate of firing, and prolonged activity; the nerve fibres concerned have a relatively slow rate of conduction (50–80 m/sec), and they innervate slowly contracting "postural" muscles such as the soleus. The phasic motor unit has a higher threshold, a faster rate of discharge, and only transient activity; the nerve fibres concerned have a rapid rate of conduction (> 90 m/sec), and innervate rapidly contracting muscles such as the gastrocnemius.

The motor nerves terminate in a series of "end-plates," one per muscle fibre. These are situated in one or more troughs of the sarcolemma, about half-way along the length of the fibres. Signals are transmitted from the nerve to the muscle by the release of a neurotransmitter (acetylcholine) at the end-plate.

The Physiology of Muscular Contraction

Electrophysiology

Under resting conditions the interior of the muscle fibre has a negative potential of 50–100 millivolts with respect to the extracellular fluid. This difference of potential is attributable to metabolic activity at the cell membrane; a "sodium pump" actively extrudes sodium ions and maintains an excess of potassium ions within the cell.

When acetylcholine is released at the neuromuscular junction, the properties of the sarcolemma are altered locally. It becomes freely permeable to both sodium and potassium ions and the negative potential is progressively lost. The depolarization of the membrane ("end-plate potential") develops until a critical value is reached. The disturbance is then propagated over the entire length of the fibre as a muscle action potential. Some three or four milliseconds later, contraction occurs (Fig. 46). Recovery is associated with a destruction of acetylcholine by the enzyme cholinesterase, and a progressive repolarization of the membrane through the continuing activity of the "sodium pump." "Nerve-gas" and a number of organophosphorus insecticides inhibit the action of cholinesterase. This has adverse effects in many parts of the body. In the muscles, it leads first to fibrillary twitching, and subsequently to a sustained depolarization that effectively paralyses transmission at the neuromuscular junction. Other poisons such as tubocurarine "occupy" sites on the sarcolemma that are normally responsive to acetylcholine; again, neuromuscular transmission is blocked.

The basis for the coupling of electrical and chemical events within the muscle is currently being explored. It is thought that ionic currents first pass through a transverse tubular system in the region of the Z discs (Fig. 41). Calcium ions are thereby released into a second tubular system (the sarcoplasmic reticulum), that runs parallel with the myofibrils. The calcium ions in turn activate an

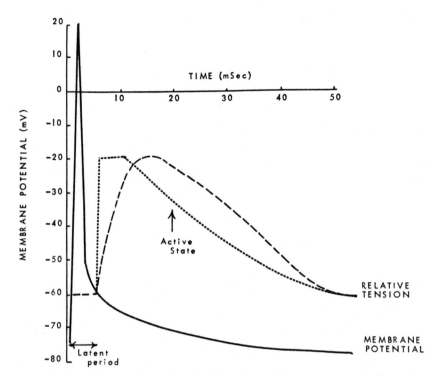

Figure 46. Illustration of (1) the latent period between a typical muscle action potential and the development of contractile tension, and (2) the discrepancy between the active state and the development of tension. The time course of the active state is indicated approximately by the *rate* of change of tension during contraction.

enzyme ATP^ase that is closely associated with the protein myosin. In the presence of magnesium ions, ATP^ase then catalyses the breakdown of ATP to ADP, orthophosphate and free energy that can be utilized in muscular contraction.

Muscle shortening involves a combination of actin and myosin, this reaction is reversible and can proceed outside the body. If ATP is added to a solution of actomyosin in 0.6 molar potassium chloride, the complex splits into its constituents, actin and myosin, with a decrease in viscosity of the solution. The myosin could in turn function as the enzyme ATP^ase, converting ATP to ADP, with the release of energy and reformation of actomyosin; however, the realization of this potential enzymic function is dependent upon appropriate ionic conditions. ATP thus performs two functions *in vivo*. At rest, it converts actomyosin to actin and myosin, keeping the muscle supple and extensible. After stimulation, on the other hand, it is broken down to ADP, with the liberation of energy that can be applied to muscular contraction.

Immediately following stimulation, the muscle may show a slight "latency relaxation." This is followed by a phase of increased rigidity, the "active state." Externally recordable tension is developed and lost more slowly, because various elastic elements are arranged in series with the muscle. A single twitch of a white muscle may persist for 7–10 milliseconds, while a twitch duration of 100 milliseconds is common in red muscle. In both types of fibre, the twitch duration is influenced markedly by the local temperature.

Muscle Heat Production

The time course of muscle heat production is technically difficult to study, since most methods of temperature recording have a rather slow response rate. Investigation has usually been based on isolated muscle preparations where contraction was slowed by cooling the muscle and exposing it to a hypertonic bathing fluid. Four phases of heat production are distinguished.

There is first the *activation heat*. This is associated with the breakdown of high energy phosphate compounds such as ATP, and the development of an active state within the muscle fibres. In an isometric contraction, virtually all of the initial heat production occurs in this phase. In an isotonic contraction, there is now a phase of *shortening heat*, dependent on the extent of shortening and the form of the force/velocity curve (Fig. 48). If the load lifted by the muscle is removed, there is no further initial heat production. However, if the load is lowered as the muscle relaxes, the potential energy stored in the load is liberated as heat within the muscle—the *relaxation heat*. Finally, there is a *delayed heat*, associated with the resynthesis of high energy phosphate bonds.

The overall efficiency of aerobic contraction (the ratio of work performed to energy consumed) is about 25 percent. We have already noted that the efficiency of ATP generation by the oxidative breakdown of glycogen is 63 percent. This implies that the forward reaction (coupling of the ATP energy to actin and myosin with the performance of external work) has an efficiency of $(25 \times 100/63)$, or about 40 percent. Direct measurements support this view. Under anaerobic conditions, the initial energy yield per mole of hexose is only $\frac{1}{19}$th of that for the aerobic reaction (Fig. 40). Some 90 percent of the lactate is later reconverted to glycogen, using energy derived from oxidation of the remaining 10 percent. Thus the overall efficiency of a muscular contraction that involves generation and repayment of an oxygen debt is $25\% \times \frac{1}{19} \times \frac{10}{1} = 13\%$; the efficiency of glycogen resynthesis is effectively $\frac{13}{25}$, or about 52 percent.

Tetanic Contraction

Let us suppose we have a frog nerve-muscle preparation, and that our stimulating coil is set to provide its maximum voltage. If a second maximum stimulus is applied to a motor unit within a few milliseconds of the first, there is no additional response—the muscle is said to be in a "refractory state." However, because of the phase difference between the active state and the tension within the muscle (Fig. 47), it is possible to select a longer stimulus interval such that the muscle will respond while the series elastic elements are still under tension from the initial contraction. Less of the energy of the second contraction is dissipated by the series elements, and the resultant tension is increased—*summation* is said to have occurred. If a series of maximal stimuli are applied, a tremulous contraction, or *subtetanus* is seen. If the stimulus interval is now shortened, fusion of the individual twitches becomes more complete, and at a frequency of about sixty stimuli per second, *tetanus* is fully developed. The force developed is now three or four times as great as during a single muscle twitch (Fig. 47).

Tetanic contractions are frequently used in performing normal physical activities. However, a tremulous movement is not seen because during voluntary effort motor units fire asynchronously, and individual tremors cancel one another out.

Length-tension Relationships

As with heart muscle (p. 54), the force developed during an isometric twitch depends upon the initial fibre length. A modest lengthening can increase force, but if the muscle is

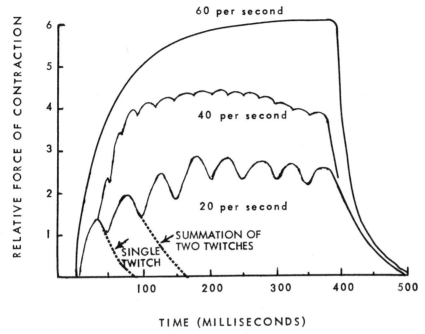

TIME (MILLISECONDS)

Figure 47. Illustration of summation and tetanus. The response to a second maximal stimulus is increased if it follows soon after the first. With repetitive stimuli, a partial tetanus is obtained at moderate stimulus frequencies (20–40 per second) and complete tetanus at frequencies of more than 60 per second.

stretched further, the resting tension increases without a parallel gain in the force that can be added by isometric activity (Fig. 48).

In most natural activities, a muscle shortens as it contracts. The contraction is then described as *"concentric."* However, there are situations where a muscle is lengthened during tetanic contraction; one good example of this is the use of the biceps muscle to control the rate of descent of the body following a "chin-up." The contraction is then described as *"eccentric."* The tension developed during an eccentric contraction can exceed the expected static reading (line c, Fig. 48). This is due in part to a change in the contractile properties of the stretched myofibrils, and in part to a reversible storage of energy in the series elastic elements.

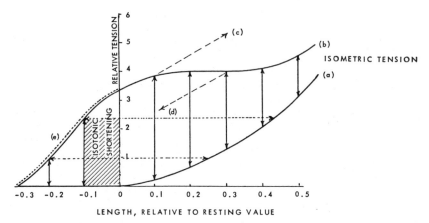

Figure 48. Length-tension relationships of muscle. (a) resting state; (b) maximum isometric contraction; (c) combination of forced lengthening and maximum isometric contraction; (d) combination of forced shortening and maximum isometric contraction; (e) isotonic contraction. The shaded area corresponds to the external work performed when the muscle develops a tension of 2.3 units, and then shortens from the resting length to −0.1. Solid vertical bars show potential isometric force at different initial muscle lengths. Interrupted horizontal bars show potential isotonic shortening at different initial tensions.

In the converse situation, a muscle may be forcibly shortened as it contacts. The tension that is developed is then considerably less than the expected static reading for an equivalent fibre length (line d Fig. 48).

During isotonic contraction, the length/tension relationship closely parallels the left-hand part of the isometric curve (Fig. 48). The abscissae indicate the shortening that occurs, and the corresponding ordinates the maximum load that can be sustained under these conditions. The external work performed is the product of shortening and load. The potential shortening is greatest at low tensions (25% or less of maximum), but the area of the tension/shortening diagram is greatest at about 60 percent of maximum tension. Unfortunately, one cannot use all of the area shown in Fig. 48 to perform external work. In order to achieve the full potential shortening, it would be necessary for the muscle to undergo an initial gross and passive elongation. When a man intends to lift a heavy weight, it is more usual for him to follow the pattern indicated by the shaded part of the diagram. Tension is developed isometrically until the torque (product of force and leverage) reaches the value required to support the weight. Subsequent shortening is outwardly isotonic, but if account is taken of the varying leverage presented to both the weight and the contracting muscles, it is obvious that further frequent changes of tension must be made throughout the period of activity.

The force of contraction is influenced by the speed of shortening (Fig. 49). At zero speed, we are in the condition of isometric contraction, and force is maximal. If there is no external load, we are in the situation of a "free" isotonic contraction; the speed is then maximal. The form of the relationship is a hyperbola, described by the equation

$$V = \frac{(Po - P)b}{(P + a)}$$

where V is the velocity of shortening, Po is the maximum isometric tension, P is the observed tension, a is a constant with the dimensions of force, and b is a constant with the dimensions of velocity.

> The rate of performance of external work is given by the product of P and V, while the rate of performance of internal work is given by the product of a and V. The English physiologist Hill showed experimentally that the sum of $(P + a)V$ decreased in proportion to the applied load $(Po - P)$; the constant b thus describes the relationship between work performed and external loading.
>
> Although the total rate of working decreases in proportion to loading, at light loads a high proportion of the work performed is attributable to internal work (aV); the maximum rate of external working is thus achieved at about 30 percent of maximum isometric tension. Well-designed machines operate at about this tension. Thus if the gearing is appropriately adjusted on a bicycle, the quadriceps muscle is functioning at some 30 percent of its maximum isometric force.

Some authors extend the graph to the left of the ordinate. This takes account of the situation where the muscle is forcibly lengthened as it is contracting. As in the static length/tension diagram (Fig. 48), the force to which the tendon is exposed is then substantially in excess of a normal isometric contraction.

This has some practical importance in that the elastic limit of the tendon may be exceeded before the Golgi receptors inhibit activity. Injury of the tendon or its attachment may then occur.

The rate of internal working (aV) is dependent on tissue viscosity, and thus on muscle temperature. The force/velocity curve is thus displaced to the right by a preliminary warm-up, this effect being most marked at the lighter loads.

Force Developed by Whole Muscles

Behaviour In-vivo. Individual motor units respond in an "all or none" manner; if the ventral horn cell receives a stimulus of sufficient intensity, a single twitch occurs in all the fibres

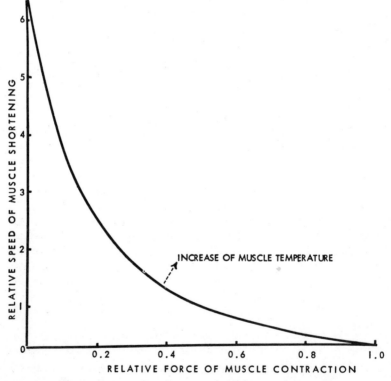

Figure 49. Relationship between speed and force of muscle contraction; the curve has the same general form for single fibre preparations and for contraction of the muscle as a whole.

of the associated motor unit. However, there is an infinite gradation of force during gross body movements. This is achieved in several ways: (a) the rate of discharge of individual motor units is varied up to and including the development of tetanus, (b) the number of active motor units is increased, (c) the speed of muscle shortening is varied (Fig. 49), and (d) the resistance offered by antagonistic muscles is reduced. Leverage has an important influence upon the externally measured force, and for many purposes it is convenient to think in terms of the torque rather than the force developed at a given joint (Fig. 50).

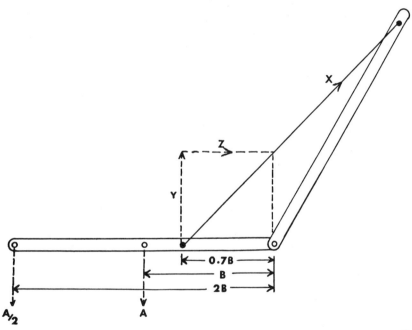

Figure 50. Illustration of the principle of leverage. A muscle exerts a pull of X kg in the direction indicated by the arrow. This can be resolved into two smaller components Y kg at right angles to the lower lever, and Z kg in parallel with the lower lever. The distance from the fulcrum of the lever to the lower insertion of the muscle is 0.7B cm. The torque developed is thus 0.7YB kg cm. The force is recorded by two harnesses at right angles to the lever, B, and 2B cm from the fulcrum; the torque at both sites is AB kg cm = 0.7YB kg cm, but the recorded forces are A and A/2 respectively.

In general, the lever systems of the human body are designed for rapid rather than for powerful movements. To achieve this objective, the distance between the fulcrum and the muscle insertion is kept short relative to the leverage exerted by the weight of the part and any external load. Thus the olecranon provides a very short lever for the triceps; the resultant throw is fast but lacking in power. By way of contrast, we may look at the ankle joint. Here, the calcaneum provides the gastrocnemius with a substantial lever, since this muscle is often required to lift the entire body weight.

We have noted that an individual muscle fibre develops its maximum tension when stretched a little beyond its resting length (Fig. 48). The same principle holds for an entire muscle, and if it is necessary to develop a large force in the course of an athletic event, it would seem reasonable to put the muscle under slight tension. However, this is not always advantageous. Sometimes the resultant posture results in unfavourable leverage. The best results are obtained through an intelligent combination of the length-tension relationship (Fig. 48) and the principles of leverage (Fig. 50). In many events, account must also be taken of the force/velocity relationship (Fig. 49). The optimum speed of muscle shortening depends on the relative requirements of power and speed of movement.

> The technique currently recommended for the lifting of heavy weights in industry has been criticised on the grounds of poor leverage. The worker is trained to maintain a rigid spine, and to lift by extension of the knees. However, if the load is lying on the floor or a low platform, the knees must initially be fully flexed. The extensor muscles then operate at a very poor mechanical advantage, and the average person is unable to develop sufficient force to lift legally permitted weights*—at least if he adheres to the recommended technique. One remedy is to raise the height of the loading platform, thereby improving leverage. Momentum may also be used to carry the load past positions where the spine is under heavy stress (the so-called "dynamic" technique of lifting). Inertial effects are minimized by relatively slow lifting. If the load gains an excess of kinetic energy, effort is expended both in producing this acceleration, and also in stopping motion when the final resting place is reached.

* The International Labour Office has recommended a limit of 40–50 kg for men, and 15–20 kg for women.

Minimization of inertial losses is important not only with external loads, but also with the movement of body parts; the avoidance of sudden accelerations and declerations is an important component of skill (p. 219).

Assessment of Muscle Development. The simplest method of assessing muscle development is to measure the circumference of the limbs, either at the broadest point of a muscle belly or at a level fixed in relation to a bony protuberance (for instance five inches above the condyles of the knee). The weakness of this approach is that a broad limb may reflect large muscles, large bones or an accumulation of fat. Accuracy can be improved if corrections are applied for the thickness of subcutaneous fat (as estimated by skinfold calipers, p. 433) and the breadth of the long bones (as assessed by intercondylar dimensions).

The same type of procedure can be carried out more accurately if soft-tissue radiographs are obtained in the anteroposterior and lateral planes. Precise positioning of the limb with respect to the X-Ray machine is important, and the apparent bulk of a muscle can be increased by oedema, intramuscular fat, changes of muscle tone, and other technical factors. Nevertheless, for any given muscle there is a rather consistent relationship between crosssection and strength; indeed, this holds over the entire period from early childhood to adult life.

A third general approach to the assessment of muscularity is to calculate the lean body mass (see p. 486). In the adult, an increase of lean body mass during training can reasonably be equated with an increase of muscle bulk.

The isometric strength of individual muscle groups is conveniently measured by a series of dynamometers and tensiometers. These may be either mechanical or electrical in type. The mechanical systems are simpler and more rugged, and the only real advantage gained from an electrical system such as a strain gauge is a continuous record of the tension developed. With the mechanical handgrip dynamometer, the subject exerts his maximum grip against a strong spring, and the force developed is recorded by movement of a unidirectional pointer over a suitable scale. It is important to adjust the size of grip to a convenient length for the palm of the subject, to choose the dominant hand, and to allow several preliminary practice attempts; if these precautions are observed, the test is relatively independent of technical factors. Cable tensiometers are used to measure the torque developed about other joints. These devices were originally intended to test the tension in cables bracing the wings of biplane aircraft. For the purposes of exercise physiology, a harness is fitted about a limb at a predetermined level, and a cable runs from this harness to a rigid external support. The tensiometer is applied to the cable indicating the tension developed during a maximum isometric effort. Unfortunately, the answer obtained from a tensiometer test is somewhat fallible. Unless very good techniques are used to immobilize the rest of the body, the subject may call upon various accessory muscles to increase the tension in the measuring cable. The precise result is also influenced by the positioning and angulation of the harness, and by the angulation of the joint (Figs. 50 and 51).

Because of the technical difficulties of tensiometry, it is interesting to examine how far the easier handgrip reading is representative of general body strength. Obviously, some occupations lead to a specific development of the wrist muscles;

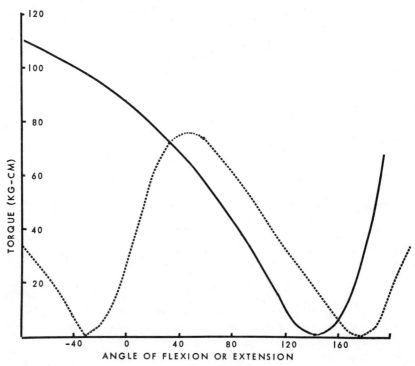

Figure 51. The influence of angle of flexion or extension on the torque developed by two parts of the deltoid muscle. Adapted from a study by Hvorslev, 1928.

this is particularly true of the anaesthetist and the professional tennis player. Some authors have found a rather poor correlation between grip and general strength, but Clarke, who has perhaps the greatest experience with the cable tensiometer sets the coefficient of correlation at 0.69; in other words, about half the variation in grip strength reflects general muscularity.

Isotonic strength has traditionally been measured using weights and pulleys. More elaborate torque generators are now available for this purpose. Some can be arranged to measure dynamic forces not only during shortening, but also when the muscles are extended beyond their resting length. However, the assessment of isotonic strength is still a technically difficult matter. The necessary loadings must be established by trial and error, leading to a variable amount of fatigue, while further complications are introduced by the influence of speed on the force of contraction (Fig. 49). Unfortunately, there seems little relationship between isotonic and isometric strength.

> Whether isometric or isotonic strength is to be determined, the use of maximum effort tests is not always desirable. In many instances, performance is limited by psychological rather than physiological factors; furthermore the rise of blood pressure that accompanies maximum effort (p. 88) could be dangerous, particularly for elderly patients and those recovering from myocardial infarction. There seems some possibility that *quantitative electromyography* may permit assessments during submaximum effort. The electromyograph is basically a record of electrical activity obtained over (plate electrodes) or within (needle electrodes) a given muscle belly. Needle electrodes are more specific to a given muscle and are thus invaluable to the kinesiologist. However, the plate electrodes give a better estimate of total activity about a given joint. The information collected consists of a series of "muscle spikes"; for the purpose of quantification, the number of spikes per second may be counted by a suitable scaling unit, or the root mean square of the signal voltage may be recorded. In any given muscle, there seems a close relationship between the tension developed and the intensity of electrical activity; further, if subjects of differing strength are compared, the electrical activity associated with a given external tension varies according to the strength of the subject (Fig. 52).

Variations in Gross Strength. Age and Sex. We have noted that the growth in strength from childhood to adult life is

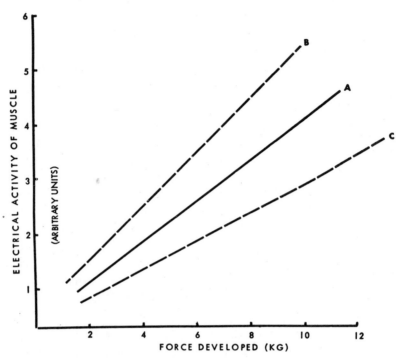

Figure 52. The relationship between electrical activity and muscle tension. Maximum isometric force 50 kg (subject A), 35 kg (subject B) and 65 kg (subject C).

closely related to the gain in cross-sectional area of a given muscle. There is little evidence that the quality of muscular tissue alters during the process of development. In the male, strength continues to increase throughout the adolescent period. The European men studied by Asmussen grew in strength until they reached the age of thirty, and there was a subsequent decline of no more than 15 percent to 20 percent to the age of sixty. In North America, the average man reaches a peak earlier (about 17 years), maintains a rather constant strength to forty-five years, and shows a decline of about 15 percent over the next twenty years (Fig. 53). Very young girls have a similar strength to that of boys; the rate of development is initially similar for the two sexes but with the onset of puberty, the girls show little further increase of strength. Adult women are only 55 percent to 65 percent as strong as men, and no

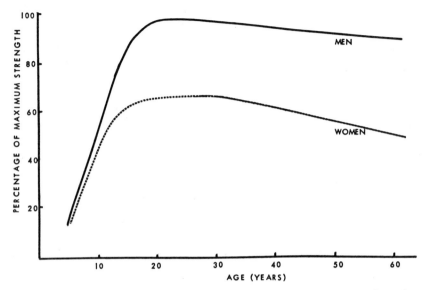

Figure 53. The relationship of grip strength to age. Based on data for Canadian men and women, obtained by Howell (Edmonton) and present author (Toronto).

more than a half of this relative weakness can be attributed to their shorter height.

Body Build. Because muscle strength is related to the square of a linear dimension (cross-sectional area), we might anticipate that tall people would be stronger than those who are short. In practice, this is not always the case, as tall people tend to be of the ectomorph type, with rather poor muscular development. Muscle strength is greatest in those with a mesomorphic body build (p. 485).

In assessing the practical significance of the strength recorded by the tensiometers, account must also be taken of (a) body weight (which influences the effort required for most tasks) and (b) differences of leverage afforded by long and short limbs.

Temporal Factors. Grip strength apparently shows a diurnal rhythm, being greatest during waking hours, and least in the small hours of the night. Body temperature shows a rather similar diurnal pattern, and it is tempting to ascribe the changes of measured strength to alterations of muscle viscosity that accompany "warm-up." Certainly, grip strength can be increased by immersion of the arm in hot water, and it is diminished by immersion in cold water. However, other factors such as differences of cortical arousal probably contribute to the diurnal changes of strength.

Psychological Factors. We have noted the problem that the observed isometric strength is limited more by psychological than by physiological factors. Psychological considerations also account for a large part in the difference of strength between the sexes. Steinhaus has shown that the recorded strength can be increased 5 percent to 10 percent by various forms of encouragement, and even larger gains (25%) can be achieved by hypnosis (p. 363). It is thought that positive suggestion helps remove cortical inhibition of effort. On the other hand, hypnotic suggestion of weakness can reduce the recorded force by up to 30 percent.

Warm-up and Warm-down

Physiological Effects of Warm-up. It is difficult to devise satisfactory experiments to test the practical effects of warm-up on athletic performance. Most athletes have rigid views on the appropriate routine that they should follow prior to a competition, and they are understandably reluctant to modify this regime in the interests of science. However, certain favourable changes of muscle physiology are produced by a warm-up period.

An increase of local muscle temperature reduces the viscosity of the system; the speed of a single twitch is thus increased, and a greater force can be developed at a given velocity. An appropriate warm-up regime should thus improve performance involving vigorous contractions. Other potential advantages of warm muscles include a greater relaxation of antagonists (thereby reducing the incidence of injuries), an increased rate of local metabolic reactions, an increased local blood flow, and a displacement of the haemoglobin dissociation curve leading to a greater (and more rapid) release of oxygen at a given pressure.

Techniques of Warm-up. Some of the differences in experimental results reflect not only the psychological impact of a familiar warm-up routine, but also differences in the techniques adopted to warm the body tissues.

If the warm-up involves a mild form of the intended exercise, then performance may be influenced by recent practice. If the warm-up is produced by external heating (hot baths or diathermy), then the metabolic consequences are less than if the heating is produced by local or general physical effort. A limited accumulation of metabolites within the muscle is probably helpful in speeding the circulatory "on-transient"; on the other hand, more prolonged or intense preliminary activity can lead to an excessive accumulation of metabolites and exhaustion of food reserves, thereby impairing the subsequent "definitive" performance. The optimum intensity and duration of warm-up varies from one individual to another. If a subject is athletic, he will find it profitable to warm-up for longer, and at a higher absolute intensity than if he is unfit. Because of the interaction of muscle strength and lactate accumulation at a given percentage of aerobic power (p. 87), the athlete may also find it an advantage to warm-up at a larger percentage of his aerobic power than a more sedentary person.

If local heating of the active part is carried out, then a large proportion of the blood flow may be diverted from the muscle to the skin. This can have an adverse effect on performance.

Objective evidence of the warm-up induced by various techniques can be obtained if intramuscular temperatures are recorded by needle thermocouples. The temperature within the active muscles rises by $2°–3°C$ in the first five to ten minutes of moderate activity, and thereafter remains relatively constant. The general body temperature, as measured by intraoesophageal or rectal thermocouples, rises more slowly over the first thirty minutes of activity. The extent of general body heating varies with environmental temperature and the state of training of the subject, but is usually not greater than $0.5–1.0°C$. Most authors consider warm-up as related more to muscle than to deep body temperature; five to ten minutes of moderate activity thus seems a suitable routine warm-up for the average person.

Muscle Tears and Injuries. One big advantage claimed by advocates of a preliminary warm-up period is a reduction in the incidence of subsequent muscle tears and injuries.

Vigorous rhythmic activities (sprinting, treadmill running, cycling, performance of a step test) may require leg movements to occur one hundred fifty to two hundred times per minute. The total duration of each contraction is then about 150 milliseconds. This still exceeds the duration of twitch for a white muscle by a factor of five to ten, but it is rather close to the twitch time for a red muscle. If injuries are to be avoided, it would seem important not only that the minimum twitch time is not exceeded but that there should be a rapid return to the relaxed state as soon as the antagonists commence to contract. Tears are normally attributed to contraction of the antagonists while the agonists are still under tension, and warm-up should reduce such dangers by speeding the relaxation process. However, there is little experimental evidence relating the incidence of injury to the presence or absence of warm-up.

Improvements of Performance. The measurement of maximum oxygen intake is usually preceded by a warm-up as a precaution against muscle and tendon injuries. Some comparisons have shown a slightly larger maximum oxygen intake under "warm" than under "cold" conditions; in such forms of maximal exercise as bicycle ergometry, where the main "limiting factor" is a local metabolic change within the active muscles (p. 413), the warm-up could conceivably improve performance by slowing the accumulation of anaerobic metabolites.

Performance times for speed events are materially improved by warm-up. Asmussen and his colleagues in Copenhagen found a close parallel between the rise of intramuscular temperature and the decrease in time required for a sprint. The maximum gain in performance was about 10 percent, most of the improvement occurring with the first ten minutes of warm-up. Activities requiring dynamic or explosive strength (such as throwing and vertical jumping) also benefit from a preliminary warm-up; however, the gains are generally less than 10 percent.

Perhaps because the temperature of most swimming baths is below the thermally neutral figure of 33–34°C, warm-up also offers a well-documented advantage of 1 percent to 2 percent in swimming contests of one to five minutes duration. In other forms of cardio-respiratory endurance activity, performance depends on the balance that is struck between the development of a faster circulatory "on-transient" and adverse effects of accumulating metabolites. Most authors find little change of endurance performance in response to a warm-up.

The cooling of the body following warm-up is a slow process, occupying an hour or more, and the beneficial effects on performance of the raised body temperature also seem to persist. If local facilities are restricted, there may thus be some advantage to athletes in warming-up away from the immediate vicinity of a contest.

Warm-down and Muscle Stiffness. Muscle stiffness or soreness is a common complaint for one to two days following unaccustomed exertion. Immediate stiffness is due to accumulation of fluid within the muscle (p. 102); this makes the fibres thicker, shorter and more resistant to stretch.

Soreness is due to stimulation of pain receptors. The immediate basis of pain may be a local accumulation of metabolites, but this cannot explain effects that persist for several days. The half time for the oxidation of lactate is ten to fifteen minutes, and most metabolic processes are restored to normal in three to four hours. Soreness which lasts for more than one day is generally thought to reflect minor injury, a rupture of some of the muscle or tendon fibres. Some workers have advanced an alternative hypothesis that immediate oxygen lack in the muscle brings about a painful spasm, which in turn perpetuates the oxygen lack. Experimental evidence adduced to support the spasm hypothesis has included a demonstration of increased electrical activity in a sore muscle, and reduction of this activity coupled with relief of soreness following passive stretching. However, the spasm could be a response to minor trauma, and the beneficial effects of passive stretching and light activity do not really resolve the question. On the other hand, there is little question that with gross injury, the spasm is worsened rather than improved by passive stretching.

Soreness and stiffness are important negative factors reducing interest in and enthusiasm for an exercise programme. It is thus vital that their incidence should be held to a minimum. The preventive value of warm-up has been noted. Warm-down is also important; gentle activity following a contest promotes circulation through the previously active tissues, assisting in the removal of metabolites, and helping return fluid to the central circulation. Sudden cessation of activity while standing may lead to circulatory collapse (p. 97).

The delayed relaxation of fatigued muscle fibres (vide infra) increases the likelihood of injury. It is thus important to plan a suitable rate of progression in any training programme. In the early stages, excessive stretching of the calf muscles may arise from the use of running shoes with a flatter heel than that normally worn; the absence of accustomed ankle support may also increase the stress on the tendo achilles, as may running or exercising on an unyielding concrete surface (the sidewalk or the basement floor). The recent introduction of vinyl-padded running tracks may minimise such injuries. Particular care is necessary when the pattern of exercise is changed (for instance, replacement of outdoor jogging by indoor running on the spot at the beginning of wintry weather). In such circumstances, it is advisable to lower the intensity of training for a few days, until the newly active muscle groups have developed a measure of conditioning.

Some types of exercise seem particularly prone to induce soreness; these include vigorous contraction of an already shortened muscle, sudden jerky movements performed by an inadequate number of motor units, prolonged repetition of a specific movement, and contraction of a forcibly elongated muscle (as in stopping a ballistic movement).

As with other medical problems mentioned in this text, if in doubt a physical educator or trainer should refer a man to his physician. This is particularly true if muscle pain is severe, if it is accompanied by deformity, swelling, or inflammation and if it fails to resolve in a few days.

Fatigue

Fatigue of Isolated Muscle. If an isolated nerve-muscle preparation is stimulated repeatedly, the maximum shortening diminishes. This is largely due to an incomplete relaxation between contractions—a state of "contracture" is said to develop. The electrical potentials in the nerve and muscle fibres remain normal, and it is presumed that a combination of oxygen lack, accumulation of metabolites, and lack of ATP lead to a loss of fibre elasticity.

Human Fatigue. When a man is making maximum "isotonic" contractions on a weight-lifting machine, a superficially similar phenomenon can be seen. The magnitude of the contractions diminishes progressively as fatigue occurs. However, the basis of the diminished shortening seems psychological rather than physiological since the full initial contraction can be restored by suitable incentives such as cheering or a sudden emergency. It is possible that under such circumstances, performance is restored by the recruitment of motor units not initially involved. However, there is also evidence that some of the fatigue is occurring in the brain rather than in the local reflex arc. In submaximum effort, an alteration of activity between adjacent motor units considerably extends the time to fatigue. However, the fact that individual muscle fibres are developing progressively less tension is suggested by the increased total electrical activity of the muscle.

Exhaustion of Glycogen Stores. A further factor in fatigue is the exhaustion of glycogen stores. The total glycogen content of muscle is about 400 gm, or 1.4 gm per 100 gm of tissue. When a man performs maximum aerobic work, he is drawing upon some 20 kg of muscle, or 280 gm of glycogen. This is equivalent to an energy expenditure of 1120 kcal, enough to sustain an expenditure of 20 kcal/min for almost one hour. Recent biopsy studies by Hultman and his associates show that the glycogen stores of the quadriceps muscle are exhausted by sixty to ninety minutes of vigorous effort.

We have seen (p. 181) that in maximum aerobic exercise, the tension developed by the most active muscles is about 30 percent of their maximum isometric force; however, it is also probable that the muscle fibres concerned are acting at close to their maximum power (Fig. 48). During a sustained isometric contraction, the glycogen is metabolised anaerobically, and the energy yield (Fig. 40) is about 33 kcal per mole of hexose (3 ATP molecules) as compared with the aerobic figure of 429 kcal per mole (39 ATP molecules). Other factors being equal, one would thus expect glycogen stores to suffice for four to five minutes of anaerobic work. In fact, the total time for which a maximum isometric contraction can be held is about one order shorter (0.5 minutes). Part of the discrepancy in tolerance of aerobic and anaerobic work can be explained by the fact that in the usual maximum oxygen intake test not all muscles are operating at maximal power (30% of maximum isometric contraction). Alternative substrates (fatty acids, fat, and blood glucose) are also available during aerobic activity. However, the discrepancy between the observed and the expected time to anaerobic fatigue is large, and it may well be that exhaustion of glycogen stores makes no significant contribution to isometric fatigue.

Applications in Industry and in Athletics. Rest pauses are an important means of counteracting physical fatigue. In the rare forms of industrial activity that still demand heavy physical effort, a formal allowance of perhaps ten minutes rest each hour is invaluable in minimizing both the accumulation of lactate within the body, and the accompanying toll of a steadily rising ventilation and pulse rate, with consequent exhaustion and a reduction in the quantity or quality of output. An even more effective approach is to redesign the task, so that the rest pause is added to each individual operation; for instance, a worker may lift a heavy box, and then recover while addressing the shipping label.

Interval work is commonly adopted as a technique of physical training (p. 449). The phase of vigorous activity may vary from fifteen to sixty seconds, depending on the type of event for which an athlete is training. With very brief bursts of activity (10–15 seconds), the immediate metabolic demands are met from stored ATP, creatine phosphate, and oxygen; if the recovery intervals are of sufficient length, no lactate accumulates. With sixty second bursts of activity, there is a progressive accumulation of lactate even if recovery intervals as long as four minutes are allowed. The general philosophy of interval training is to accustom the body to accumulation of lactate, both subjectively (by habituation to discomfort), and physiologically (by an increase of buffering capacity). Thus, the recovery period must be brief if the intended build-up of lactate is to be achieved.

Posture and Movement

General Comments

Although there is some allocation of function between red (postural) and white (voluntary) muscles, all movements are superimposed on a background of postural tone, and most movements involve a disturbance of normal equilibria with an increase of postural work. The extent of postural work depends upon body weight, the position of the centre of gravity* within the body, and the clumsiness of the individual. Inter-individual variations in postural work lead to substantial differences of mechanical efficiency from one person to another. Partly for this reason, predictions of oxygen consumption based on mea-

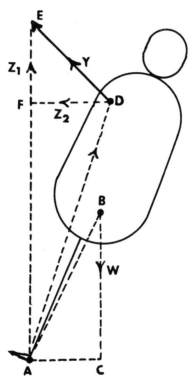

Figure 54. To illustrate the principle of the centre of gravity. A subject leans backwards, holding his legs as a rigid pillar, and pivoting about his heels (A). The body mass W behaves as if concentrated at point B, and exerts a torque W(AC) tending to cause the body to fall. In this example, falling is resisted by the arms, exerting a counterforce Y in the direction DE; this may be resolved into components Z_1 and Z_2 acting respectively in the axes EF and DF. For equilibrium, Z_1 (DF) must equal W (AC), and Z_2 must be opposed by an appropriate friction between the heels and the ground.

* The point within the body at which the total mass may be thought as acting without altering the responses to gravitational acceleration (see Fig. 54).

surements of the work performed are subject to an error of 5 percent to 10 percent (p. 209).

The extent of postural activity is reduced by learning, with a corresponding reduction in the oxygen cost of a given activity; one of the tasks of both the physical educator and the ergonomist is to teach patterns of movement that minimise postural work.

Physiological Basis of Muscle Tone and Posture

The Stretch Reflex. The fundamental basis of both muscle tone and posture is a simple reflex arc (p. 174 and Fig. 45). Stimulation of the muscle spindle receptors immediately initiates an increased activity of the corresponding motor units through this mechanism ("stretch reflex"). In postural control, a frank stretching may occur. At many of the body joints, there is a slight oscillation about the equilibrium position. As equilibrium becomes unstable, the muscles on the opposite side of the joint ("antigravity" muscles) are stretched, and a compensatory contraction is initiated. If compensation is excessive, overshoot again occurs and the oscillation is maintained; however, damping is possible through phase advance (p. 173). As with any compound pendulum, the frequency of oscillation is determined by the length of the moving parts, being as low as two to three cycles per second for the arms and legs, and as high as eight to ten cycles per second for the fingers (p. 218).

Muscular tone can be maintained independently of external stretching of the muscles. It then reflects the inherent elasticity of the muscle, and can exist in the absence of demonstrable electrical activity. Some authors maintain that in a well-relaxed subject, normal muscles show quite long phases of electrical silence (2 minutes or more). However, in most situations, the resting tone depends upon a "rotation of duty" among the many motor units that make up an anatomical muscle. The intensity of such activity seems dependent on phasic variations in the sensitivity of individual spindle receptors, controlled through the "gamma loop" mechanism (p. 173). The γ motor fibres are activated by centres in the reticular formation of the brain (Fig. 55). The activity of the reticular cells in turn reflects an individual's wakefulness or "arousal." Hence, both muscle tone and the sensitivity of stretch ("myotatic") reflexes are increased when a person is aroused (for instance, an athlete prior

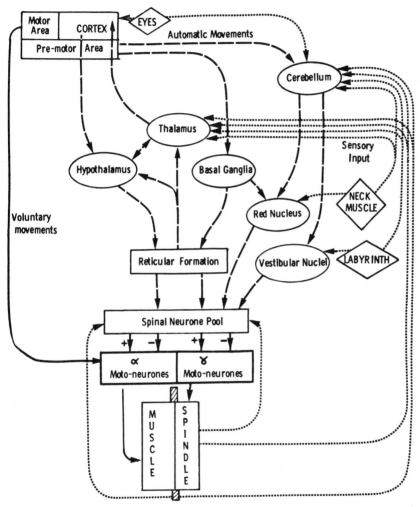

Figure 55. Simplified schematic of factors controlling the activity of α and γ motoneurones.

to a contest or an examination candidate who is "scared stiff"). As we have seen from the length-tension diagram (Fig. 48), there is an optimum resting tone. This is usually achieved by a happy and alert individual. Fear gives an excess of tension, while sadness and depression lead to a loss of tone, with a slouching gait and "half-hearted" physical effort.

The "facilitatory" effect of increased reticular activity is normally counteracted by inhibitory impulses from the basal ganglia of the brain. However, degeneration of the basal ganglia sometimes occurs in middle-age, and gross rigidity then develops (Parkinson's disease).

Other parts of the reticular formation also have an inhibitory influence on the γ loop. The input to these areas is derived from the cerebral cortex and the cerebellum, and the output plays an important role in ensuring an appropriate relaxation of antagonistic muscles during the performance of complex movements. It has recently been suggested that movements such as walking and running, which have become "automatic" are brought about largely through facilitation and inhibition of appropriate γ loops.

The Assessment of Muscle Tone. The assessment of muscle tone is a common clinical procedure. The subject is asked to relax, and the observer then senses the firmness of the muscle to palpation, the resistance to movement about a given joint, and the "briskness" of stretch reflexes such as the response to a tap on the patellar tendon.

De Vries has devised an apparatus for quantitative palpation of a muscle. It resembles the tonometer used by ophthalmologists. The main difficulty in its use is that the force recorded depends as much on the thickness of the subcutaneous fat as on any inherent "passive" turgor or elasticity of the muscle belly.

Electromyography permits a quantitative assessment of electrical activity. However, there are considerable technical problems when recording resting behaviour. Surface electrodes are used, since it is necessary to know the overall state of the muscle. The voltage recorded is then severely attenuated by overlying tissues (fascia, fat, and skin), and instead of a single well-defined action current the signal consists of a series of highly irregular and summated potential changes. During deliberate contraction of a muscle, there is substantial electrical activity and the magnitude of the signal can be closely correlated with the tension developed (Fig. 52). However, in the resting state, the voltage is small, and the true signal is difficult to distinguish from various forms of "noise."

Other dynamic approaches to the assessment of muscle tone include the recording of grip pressure from an idle hand, the recording of the pressure on a writing stylus, and measurements of blood lactate level.

The Art of Relaxation. Since resting muscle tone is influenced by anxiety, the tension measured by the integrated emg diminishes as the subject becomes familiar with the laboratory and the equipment used (habituation p. 444). The recording of resting muscle tone is sometimes useful in teaching a patient techniques of relaxation. One approach suggested by Jacobson is to train the individual to recognise progressively decreasing levels of voluntarily-induced tension. When his perceptive powers have been improved in this way, he becomes able to recognise and relieve involuntary tension.

The practice of yoga is a second method of reducing involuntary tension. The expert practitioner is said to be able to reduce the resting oxygen consumption by as much as 50 percent through Shavasana, the yogic technique of relaxation.

Athletes are able to reduce the integrated resting emg more readily than sedentary subjects. This is partly a question of practice, since sedentary people trained in the art of relaxation can often accomplish a greater reduction of muscle tension than athletes. However, there is some evidence that vigorous exercise can reduce muscle tension, particularly in those individuals where muscle tone is initially high.

Concepts of Posture. Posture is defined by the Oxford English Dictionary as carriage, or an attitude of the body or mind. From the physiological point of view, posture involves three elements:

1. *The static body position,* requiring a varying amount of muscular exertion and circulatory support, depending on whether the individual is standing erect or is lying in a recumbent posture.

2. *A dynamic pattern of neuromuscular coordination,* which serves to maintain the existing posture against gravity and other external forces, permits the accomplishment of current voluntary activities, and adjusts the body position in anticipation of future activities.

3. *A personal attribute* expressing the general character of the individual, his attitude to a given task and to life in general.

Man is one of the few animals that is not a quadruped. The assumption of the erect position is an important evolutionary advance, since it frees the arms and hands for manipulative tasks, and this in turn permits the reshaping of the mouth in a manner that allows the use of complex speech. However, the standing position has a number of disadvantages in terms of equilibrium, circulation and respiration.

Maintenance of Equilibrium. A body remains in a state of

stable equilibrium as long as the centre of gravity (Fig. 54) remains within the vertical projection of the area bounded by its supports. This condition is likely to be observed if the area of support is large, and if the centre of gravity is low. Unfortunately in man, the area bounded by the feet is small, and the centre of gravity is high. Thus even a minor displacement of the trunk moves the centre of gravity outside the area of support, creating an unstable equilibrium. Tall individuals with an unusually high centre of gravity are at a particular disadvantage in this respect.

The tendency to fall is resisted by a number of skeletomuscular mechanisms. Where possible, the joints are positioned to form rigid supports. Thus when standing, the knee joint is "locked" by an outward rotatory movement. If mechanical locking is not possible, the joint must be braced by continuous muscular activity—either unilateral contraction against the gravitational field, or a simultaneous contraction of agonists and antagonists. In the latter case, there is commonly a slight oscillation about the position of equilibrium (p. 197).

A given static posture may be maintained for long periods, and the muscle responsible must thus be resistant to fatigue. The high myoglobin content, long contraction period, and other peculiarities of the red muscle (Table III) are important in this regard. Fatigue reflects largely an impairment of blood flow, and may be anticipated when contractions are sustained at more than 15 percent of maximum voluntary force (p. 87). Postural requirements normally do not reach this level. However, they can do so if (a) an "awkward" posture is maintained, with bad alignment of the centre of gravity of the various body parts, (b) if the supporting muscles are weakened through disease or lack of physical training, and (c) if the subject is supporting a heavy load or is himself obese.

The primary control of static posture is at the level of the *spinal cord* through the stretch and other segmental reflexes (p. 174). This can be demonstrated in a cat whose spinal cord has been deliberately severed in the lower lumbar region. Such an animal is capable of supporting the weight of its hind quarters for several minutes. However, if stance is to be maintained for a longer period, more coordination is necessary than can be achieved at a segmental level.

Coordinating centres are located in a part of the midbrain known as the cerebellum. This receives impulses from the eyes, the inner ear, the neck, and the soles of the feet; such information is weighed against the state of activity in the segmental stretch reflexes, and the segmental response is suitably modified by facilitatory or inhibitory impulses from the reticular system. The importance of the cerebellum in modulating spinal reflexes is shown by the effects of disease and injury. An individual with cerebellar injury shows *ataxia* (clumsy, slow, and incomplete movements), *asthenia* (weakness) and *atonia* (loss of muscle tone). The muscles also fail to act in a coordinated manner (*asynergia*), and there is a coarse tremor because the mechanism for damping body oscillations (p. 173) has been lost. There is some evidence that the role of the cerebellum extends beyond simple coordination of postural information, and that it can also learn and "store" movement patterns that are particularly effective in restoring the balance after equilibrium has been disturbed. A footballer who slips on a muddy field, or a boxer who receives a staggering blow both recover more quickly than would an untrained person. Information is probably stored in the form of appropriate γ loop settings that can be recalled to initiate automatic movements (see further, p. 214).

A healthy individual has a fair impression of his body position even if the eyes are closed. However, *visual sensations* are much more important to the maintenance of posture if other receptors are no longer functional. The eyes play a particularly vital role in rapid movements; visual stimuli from the retina are supplemented by information from the stretch receptors in the ocular muscles and the attachments of the lens, as convergence and accommodation occur. Paralysis of accommodation leads to a surprising loss of postural control; one common example of this is the incoordination of the ophthalmic patient treated with an atropine mydriatic prior to examination of the eyes.

The *labyrinth* of the inner ear contains organs that sense both dynamic changes of posture (the semicircular canals), and also the static orientation of the head (the otolith organs, saccule and utricle). The discharge from the receptors of the semicircular canals is proportional to the acceleration of the head, and if a steady rotation is maintained the neural activity ceases within about thirty seconds. The otolith organs are stimulated by tilting the head through 2.5° or more; the saccule detects a lateral tilt and the utricle a fore and aft tilt. The intensity of discharge is proportional to the angle of tilt, and the receptors show little "adaptation," continuing their discharge for as long as the head remains tilted. Individuals with a good sense of balance are thought to have a greater sensitivity of their labyrinthine receptors. There is some evidence that sensitivity is also increased by frequent stimulation, and that it is reduced or lost in the absence of normal gravitational acceleration (as in space voyages). Overstimulation of the receptors (by whirling or tumbling movement, and by various forms of travel) leads to dizziness, nausea, and impairment of balance—the familiar picture of "motion sickness." The problem is essentially related to head rather than body movement, and if the head can be kept still, sickness does not develop. In travel, a firm shoulder harness is helpful, while in dancing and in figure skating the experienced athlete learns to watch a distant point until the neck can no longer be turned comfortably, finally moving the head quickly to "fix" the eyes on a second distant point. Training greatly reduces the liability to dizziness, and a champion figure skater often performs manoeuvres that would cause an incapacitating labyrinthine reaction in a novice.

Stimuli received by the eyes and the labyrinth normally tend to maintain an appropriate orientation of the head during tumbling or falling. This increases the tension in the neck muscles, and the attitude of the rest of the body is then adjusted by the *neck reflex*. In springboard diving and gymnastic tumbling, a slight error in the positioning of the head greatly reduces the precision of body movement.

Finally, much information on body posture is derived from the deep pressure endings in the soles of the feet. The cerebellum compares the intensity of discharge from different parts of the feet, sensing a loss of balance from the increased discharge on the side towards which tilting has occurred. The relevant sensory impulses travel up the spinal cord in the dorsal columns of "white matter." Degeneration of these columns may occur in the late stages of syphilis (the clinical condition of "tabes dorsalis"). Affected patients are able to maintain their balance while the eyes are kept open, but once the eyes are closed compensation is no longer possible, and they soon fall over. A common complaint is of tumbling into the basin when washing.

Cardiovascular Problems. Substantial cardiovascular adjustments are necessary on moving from the recumbent to the upright posture, and vice-versa. When standing, the pressure in the leg veins is 80 to 90 mmHg. In consequence, their vascular capacity (Fig. 17) is realised, and substantial pooling of blood occurs, with a corresponding reduction of central blood volume. This leads in turn to a fall of diastolic filling pressure, stroke output (Starling's law, p. 55), and systemic blood pressure. The decrease in impulse traffic from the aortic and carotid sinus pressure receptors then initiates several compensatory mechanisms, including tachycardia, peripheral vasoconstriction, and constriction of the leg veins. However, in some situations these adjustments are inadequate, and fainting can occur, particularly

1. after exercise, when the body is hot, and the muscle vasculature is widely dilated.
2. in a hot environment, where the capacity vessels are further relaxed, and blood volume is depleted by sweating.
3. in poorly trained subjects with a low blood volume, and/or diminished reflex adjustments to gravitational stress ("vasoregulatory asthenia").
4. in men exposed to weightlessness for long periods, so that the normal reflex adjustments to gravity have been "forgotten."

A number of the older circulatory tests of fitness such as the Crampton Index and the Schneider test are based on the briskness of the reflex response on moving from the supine to the vertical position (p. 402).

The upright position increases the capillary pressure in the dependent parts, thus favouring effusion of fluid. Prolonged standing leads to a tiring swelling of the limbs, especially on a hot day (when capillary permeability is increased). The peripheral pooling and diminution of central blood volume can compromise renal flow. This is reflected in a loss of protein in the urine (the so-called "orthostatic proteinuria," generally regarded as a normal phenomenon).

The body normally finds little problem in adapting to the increased central blood volume on lying down. However, if the output of the left side of the heart is impaired, as in such pathological conditions as stenosis of the mitral valve, acute breathlessness may develop.

Respiratory Problems. The importance of posture to ventilation has sometimes been overemphasized. The upright position (standing, and especially sitting with a relaxed abdominal wall) is associated with a higher proportion of diaphragmatic breathing. At one time, this was thought to improve ventilation of the lower part of the lungs. However, this is unlikely, as changes of pressure are distributed rapidly throughout the pleural cavity. The compliance of the lungs is increased by the reduction of central blood volume; in consequence, the various static lung volumes are increased by up to 500 ml. Greater expansion minimizes the tendency to collapse of dependent lung regions, but this benefit is largely offset by an increased gradient of pressure in the pleural fluid. Perfusion of the upper parts of the lung is also more difficult when standing; pulmonary arterial pressures (25/10 mm Hg) are small relative to the height of the average thorax.

Assessment of Posture. It is difficult to provide a general description of good or bad posture, because the optimal standing position varies according to body type (ectomorph, mesomorph, or endomorph, see p. 485). There are also marked individual differences in the structure of the vertebral column and in the centre of gravity of different body segments. The ideal posture minimises static work. A caricature of "bad" posture is shown in Fig. 56. The initial fault is thought to be a hyperextension of the knee-joints, possibly due to overflexible joints or lack of tone in the hamstring muscles. This defect is compensated by a hollow back, an increase of the pelvic angle, and a protruding abdomen. These changes lead in turn to a rounding of the shoulders and a thrusting forward of the head (poke-chin).

Many defects of static posture such as those illustrated, can be detected by *simple observation.* In the anteroposterior view, account should be taken of tilting of the head, differences of shoulder height, differences in prominence of the hip bones and of the two halves of the rib cage, alignment of the legs (knock-knees, bow legs, inward rotation of the thighs) and deformities of the feet (pronation/supination, hallux valgus, and hammer toes). A *plumb-line* is also helpful in making a simple overall assessment of posture. If the stance is good, the lobe of the ear should be in line with the middle of the shoulder tip, the middle of the great trochanter of the femur, the back of the patella, and the front of the fibular malleolus.

More detailed study of the spine and other bony structures should include radiographic examination. A number of mechanical devices for the study of spinal curvature have enjoyed some popularity among those who do not have access to X-Ray equipment. In general, they do not add greatly to subjective rating. The "*conformateur*" consists of a stand carrying a series of horizontal probes that are advanced until they make contact with the spine. The "*spinograph*" has a rigid probe that follows the spine, and is linked

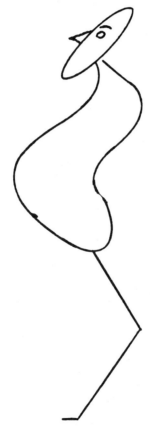

Figure 56. A caricature of bad posture. Note the forward thrusting ("poke") chin, rounded shoulders, hollow back, increase of pelvic angle, protruding abdomen, and hyperextension of the knee joint.

to a pen writing on a chart or blackboard. *Silhouette photographs* have also been used to rate posture; the silhouette is sometimes partially illuminated to show bony protruberances and the state of development of the body muscles.

Some faults of dynamic posture can be detected by observation. More detailed information can be obtained from a frame by frame analysis of cinematograph film. The dynamic efficiency can be assessed in physiological terms, such as the oxygen cost of a given activity, and the corresponding load imposed on the heart (pulse-rate curves), the ventilatory system, and the postural muscles (electromyography). The cumulative effects of poor posture can be investigated in terms of blood lactate levels, oxygen debt, and the delayed recovery of pulse rate and ventilation following effort.

Harmful Effects of Bad Posture. At one time, various abdominal complaints were attributed to bad posture (for example, "dropped kidney" and "visceroptosis"). It is now recognized that surprisingly large displacements of the abdominal organs can occur without harmful effects, and such terms as visceroptosis have been discarded by the medical profession.

The main justification for an improvement of static posture is undoubtedly cosmetic. A better appearance can in turn have beneficial effects on personality and the attitude to minor aches and pains. As long ago as 1743, Audry called sitting upright a "good posture," and sitting in full flexion a "bad posture." In the latter position, the back was "crooked and round," and the body form was "ungraceful."

Improved posture reduces static work. There is thus less tendency to accumulation of lactate, and if a given body position must be maintained for a long period there is less likelihood of fatigue. Bad dynamic posture is also aesthetically displeasing. An awkward performance leads to an excessive expenditure of energy, and loss of accuracy. It may also contribute to organic injuries such as prolapse of an intervertebral disc.

Both static and dynamic posture are largely a matter of habit. The reflexes involved are acquired at an early age, and good posture should thus be taught from early childhood. Bad habits are not only hard to eliminate, but may also lead to organic changes in muscle, cartilage and bone. Ultimately, less energy may be required to sustain a "bad" than a "good" posture.

Some Practical Applications

Efficiency of Effort. The mechanical efficiency of effort E is normally reported as a net figure:

$$E = \frac{\text{Work Performed}}{\text{Total Energy Expenditure—Resting Energy Expenditure}}$$

The resting value may be measured directly, or alternatively the "basal" energy expenditure (p. 9) may be subtracted. This amounts to some 0.67 kcal/m² body surface area in a young man. If the subject is truly basal, the energy expenditure is perhaps 1.0–1.1 kcal/min. When lying in a resting but not basal condition, it is 1.2 kcal/min, and on standing it rises further to 1.6–2.0 kcal/min. The additional 0.4–0.8 kcal/min represents the cost of maintaining the upright position, and if ignored, it can lead to a substantial error in the calculation of mechanical efficiency. Most forms of laboratory exercise such as the step test and bicycle ergometry include an element of postural work that varies with body weight.

Optimum Working Height. The energy cost of industrial and domestic tasks varies with the level of the working surface. The optimal height varies with body build and the nature of the task to be performed, but is commonly about thirty-six inches. If the bench height is increased, the body weight can no longer be used to assist in performing the task. On the other hand, if the bench is too low, the worker must stoop continually, and a substantial postural effort is required. In one specific example studied by J.R. Brown, energy expenditures were as follows:

Height of Work Surface	Energy Cost
(cm)	(kcal/min)
69	4.1
93	2.8
162	3.1

In many commercial tasks, reaching and bending are involved, and then work is performed in lifting and lowering the centre of gravity of the body. This is well illustrated by Brown's data for housewives:

Sitting (e.g. sewing, cooking)   1.6 kcal/min
Standing (e.g. dishwashing, ironing)   2.3 kcal/min
Reaching up (e.g. dusting, polishing, 4.1 kcal/min
        window cleaning)
Bending down (e.g. bed making)   5.6 kcal/min

Walking with a stoop may increase energy expenditure by as much as 30 to 50 percent; the effects of awkward posture are seen particularly when men must work in cramped quarters (for instance, miners cutting a very shallow seam of coal).

Specific Problems of Lifting. Back injuries are a tremendous and apparently an increasing hazard of modern employment. In the Province of Ontario (population some 7 million), the total loss to the economy from back injuries has been set at about $15 million dollars per year. A proportion of the injuries are due to external trauma or psychoneurosis, but the most common cause is an internal trauma, arising from faulty techniques of lifting and carrying heavy weights. Often there are contributory factors— an uneven or slippery floor surface, a twisting motion while lifting, general fatigue, and organic abnormalities of the spine. But on many occasions a painful back injury causing prolonged disability may have no other outward cause than the lifting of an excessive weight. The commonest anatomical form of injury is a "slipped disc," a forward herniation of the central spongy portion of the intervertebral cartilage. This presses upon the spinal cord, causing acute pain and/or paralysis.

Injuries are perhaps most common in industries where lifting is not a regular occurrence. Presumably, in these circumstances the back muscles are less well-developed and the task is less formalized; the worker concerned is unlikely to have learnt "tricks" for minimising the stress imposed on the vertebral column, and will have received no formal instruction in lifting techniques.

Jones has recently summarized some principles of safe lifting. He notes that the spine has a greater resistance to compression than to tension, shear or torsion. Curvature of the column creates a bending moment, and thus lowers the resistance to compression. The back is more stable when locked in a given position than when in process of changing its curvature. In considering the mass to be lifted, account must be taken not only of the external load, but also of body weight and momentum. The momentum of the load and/or the body can be used to move the system through positions where the muscles are acting at a poor mechanical advantage and/or the curvature of the spine is changing.

The classical technique of lifting involves extension of the flexed knees while the back is rigidly locked in a straight position. Because of unfavourable leverage, this method is impracticable if a heavy load has to be lifted from the floor. Jones is currently suggesting use of a "dynamic" lifting technique. The momentum of the body and load assists in the lifting process, and the back is positioned to provide the required support and thrust at different stages of the operation. The spine is not necessarily straight, but the curvature is altered only when the applied load will safely permit this. The practical benefit from the new approach has yet to be seen, but at least it conforms more closely to the intuitive pattern of lifting adopted by those who have had many years of experience with heavy loads.

Moderate loads can be lifted slowly and deliberately, but the very large loads manipulated by professional weight-lifters require the simultaneous contraction of all motor units in the active muscles. Such intense activity can only be sustained for very short periods—hence the usual lifting technique of a "clean and jerk."

Postural work is minimised if the load is held close to the body. For this reason, it is much more exhausting to carry a bulky package than a compact box of equal mass.

The lifting process is usually accompanied by a dramatic rise of systemic blood pressure. This is in part a reaction to a Valsalva manoeuvre (expiration against a closed glottis, raising the intrathoracic and intraabdominal pressures). The Valsalva manoeuvre presumably provides countersupport for the spine and fixation points for the active muscles of the limbs and shoulder girdle. A second factor leading to hypertension is the accumulation of anaerobic metabolites in the active muscles. The work of the heart is greatly increased by the rise in blood pressure (p. 66).

The mechanical efficiency in performing an average lifting task (such as loading 50 pound boxes onto a truck) is quite low (2% to 4%); this is because a large proportion of the total work is performed against the body mass rather than the external load. Efficiency is greatest over the range twenty to forty inches above the ground, and falls markedly if stooping or reaching is required. When reaching, the effort is sustained by a relatively small muscle mass, and the pulse rate for a given oxygen consumption is much higher (see Fig. 2). The poorest efficiency figures are yielded by obese subjects.

Body Movement

Reflex and Voluntary Movement. A *reflex* movement is an involuntary reaction to an immediate external stimulus. A good example is provided by the "knee jerk," a response to a tap on the patellar tendon. The nature of the resultant movement is dependent upon the site and—with some reflexes—the intensity of the stimulus. A gentle stimulation of the sole of the foot gives an extensor thrust, part of the normal reflex of walking. More painful stimulation of the same area leads to an involuntary withdrawal of the limb.

Reflexes such as the knee jerk, extensor thrust and flexor withdrawal are coordinated at the spinal level. However, some reflexes involve the higher centres of the brain; an example of a centrally coordinated reflex would be the turning of the head towards a sudden loud noise. The reflex is then "conditioned" by the cumulative experience of the individual. If the noise is the slam of a door, and it is invariably followed by the appearance of a pretty girl in a mini-skirt, the reflex may well persist. However, if the noise is the slam of a door closing, and there are no interesting sequelae, the reflex may be progressively extinguished; deconditioning or habituation has occurred.

"*Voluntary*" movement is also in a sense reflex, since there is invariably some identifiable external stimulus. However, the pattern of response depends not only on the nature and intensity of the immediate stimulus, but also on information stored in the cortex as a result of a lifetime of favourable and unfavourable experiences. Unfamiliar voluntary movements require considerable concentration and thought. A person who is not accustomed to typing or to playing a piano must watch carefully where each finger is placed. But with repetition of the task, the appropriate settings of the various γ loops are "learnt" and stored; the movement becomes automatic, or what some authors call rather confusingly a *"reflex act."*

Many classical neurophysiologists such as Hughlings Jackson held the view that the motor cortex of the brain (Fig. 57) had represented within it neural connections corresponding to com-

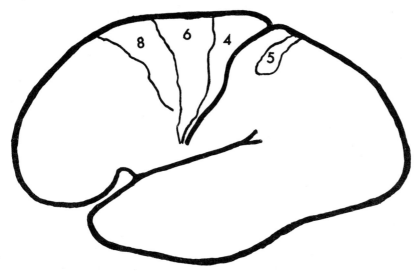

Figure 57. Illustration of areas of the brain concerned in motor activity. Zones 4, 5, 6, and 8 correspond with the system of numbering proposed by Brodman.

plex movement patterns. Impulses arising from an appropriate group of "upper motor neurones" ("area 4" in Brodmann's nomenclature) travelled via the pyramidal nerve fibres to a corresponding group of "lower motor neurones" in the ventral horn of the spinal cord, and thus initiated a well-defined movement.

More precise techniques of electrical stimulation have now contradicted this view. The upper motor neurones each control a relatively small and highly specific group of muscle fibres, usually on the opposite (heterolateral) side of the body. The gross muscles are represented in inverse order, those of the foot being controlled from the uppermost part of the motor cortex (area 4). The number of fibres controlled by a single upper motor neurone is least in the case of those muscles concerned with fine movements. In consequence, a relatively large part of area 4 is concerned with the muscles of the mouth and the fingers and much smaller areas are allocated to the control of the leg and trunk muscles.

As a task is learnt, and becomes automatic, control is passed from the motor cortex to the premotor cortex (area 6, and to a lesser extent areas 5 and 8). Efferent fibres now pass via the extrapyramidal pathway, and instead of travelling direct to the ventral horn cells, they are relayed to the reticular formation of the brain stem, and thence modify the settings of the γ loop (Fig. 55). The cerebellum now plays a most important role. While the movement is programmed and initiated by the premotor cortex, the strength, duration and range of the resultant movement is modulated by impulses from the cerebellum. This receives a continuous input of information from the eyes, the labyrinth, and the proprioceptors, compares this information with previously stored settings, and adjusts the discharge to the γ motor fibres accordingly.

The process of learning is accompanied by an increase of mechanical efficiency. With repetition, the oxygen cost of such simple tasks as treadmill running, stepping, and riding a bicycle ergometer may decrease by 5% to 10%. This facility is lost as a subject fatigues. The function of the premotor/cerebellar control system deteriorates, perhaps because of exhaustion of the sensory receptors, and movement patterns become clumsy and inefficient.

Description of Movement. The movement patterns needed to perform a given activity have many characteristics that are common from one individual to another. However, they also embody features peculiar to the individual and his specific situation at the time of observation. We are looking at the γ loop settings stored over the individual's lifetime, and the manner in which these are modified by the immediate environment. Careful observation and description of movement patterns is important to those engaged in the teaching of motor skills, and a number of systems of "shorthand" such as those of Hunt and of Jokl are available to assist in recording the characteristics of activity.

Aspects to be considered include:

Breadth of movement vocabulary—training may broaden the possible range of movement patterns, while injury induces a temporary restriction of vocabulary.

Quality of movement—in some situations, a movement may be tense or inhibited, reflecting an increase of resting tone; at other times, movement may be exuberant, with exertion that is excessive relative to the task that must be performed, or forceful, with a large proportion of the available motor units called into play to meet an external resistance.

Skill of movement—skill can improve markedly with training, and equally can deteriorate with fatigue; this is shown by the general form of movement (clumsy or neat), by the overall mechanical efficiency (large tasks) and by specific measures of accuracy (fine tasks). See further page 221.

Dimensions of movement—a correct *tempo* is very important to athletic success. The optimum tempo varies with external factors such as temperature, altitude, and fatigue. If an athlete competing in Mexico City adopts the same rate of breathing and the same pace of swimming as used in Toronto, he will undoubtedly accumulate an exhausting oxygen debt before the end of an endurance event.

Posture has an important bearing on both the cost of activity (p. 209) and also the effectiveness of "righting reflexes" (p. 204). Description should also be given of the *size* of a movement, its *direction, speed* and *force*, the type of *rhythm* (even, or irregular), the *body parts* that are active and the *consistency* of activity.

Movement and Personality. Movement patterns reflect the personality of an individual. This is perhaps most obvious with regard to the small muscles that control the appearance of the face. It does not take great powers of observation to pick out a cheerful or an anxious person from the habitual movements of his facial muscles. Posture is also influenced by an individual's feelings regarding his personal appearance, his success in a particular situation, and his apparent role in society; the pompous stride of the professional diplomat, the stiff bearing of the military man, and the slouch of the high-school drop-out all reflect the body image of the individual concerned. The same can be said of many of the sexual differences in activity that develop in the preadolescent period. There are few physiological differences at this stage, but the growing girl is taught to feel "unladylike" if she runs to school; her role in the community is to walk with a languid droop.

Movement patterns are profoundly modified by the temperament and culture of the community as a whole. The Latin temperament finds it necessary to reinforce conversation with numerous gestures, and the manner of talking of a Southern European is in marked contrast to the quiet restraint of a typical Anglo-Saxon.

There may also be a more immediate interaction of personalities. A nervous apprentice may suffer a temporary loss of all his acquired skills when closely watched by his supervisor; on the other hand, many athletes are unable to develop their best efforts in the absence of a cheering crowd.

Learning of Movements. While analysis of movement patterns may be helpful in correcting specific faults of performance, the body tends to think of a movement as a whole, rather than as a series of isolated muscle contractions. As a task is learnt, and becomes "automatic," the main site of control is shifted from the cortex (where individual muscles are represented) to the cerebellum (where information on the sensory consequences of movement is stored); the sole role of the cortex is now to call the movement into play in response to an appropriate external stimulus (Fig. 55). A shift of attention from the elements of a task to the initiating signal is the essence of motor learning. At one time, it was common to train athletes awaiting the starter's gun to think of the initial movements (the technique of "motor set"). However, Henry has shown that most individuals respond more quickly if they direct attention to the initiating signal. He interprets the faster response to a "sensory set" in terms of reliance upon existing programming of movement. Attempts to reprogramme arise with a motor-set, and the response is thereby slowed.

Most movement patterns are established by the age of three years, and it is relatively difficult to learn new skills in middle-life. Thus if the reflexes concerned with maintaining body balance are poorly established as a child, it will take much perseverance to become even a moderate skater at the age of thirty-five or forty years.

If a task is learnt by the dominant limb, there is a considerable "cross-education" of the opposite limb; this is shown by an increase not only in skill, but also in strength and endurance. However, training of the nondominant limb has relatively little effect on the dominant limb. The physiological basis of cross-education has yet to be fully explained. Training must involve the "overload" condition, and in these circumstances there may well be some involuntary tensing of muscles on the opposite side of the body; one possible anatomical factor is that 15 percent to 30 percent of the fibres from the motor cortex travel to the same rather than the opposite side of the body. The augmentation of force in a weak or tired muscle by contraction of the homologous muscle in the opposite limb ("cocontraction") has also been explained on this anatomical basis.

> If the muscles normally responsible for a specific movement are weakened or paralysed by a disease such as anterior poliomyelitis, the body learns by a process of trial and error techniques for the use of alternate muscles. Thus if the leg muscles are affected, walking is achieved by the trick of swinging the hip bones, using the quadratus lumborum. Once these abnormal patterns of activity are established and the corresponding γ loop settings are stored in the cerebellum, they in turn become "automatic," and are difficult to eradicate if there is later a recovery of normal muscle function. It is necessary to reeducate the patient, restoring normal movement patterns as soon as possible. If this is not done, further wasting of the unused muscles may occur, possibly associated with shortening of tendons and the development of permanent deformities.

Types of Movement. The limbs are lightly pivoted, underdamped, and relatively long levers. They must have many of the features of a compound pendulum, including a natural frequency of oscillation that is proportional to the square root of the distance separating the centre of gravity from the pivot; the extended lower limb vibrates at 2–3c/sec, while the fingers vibrate at 8–10c/sec. The extent of tremor is increased by an increase of muscle tone; examples are provided by the excessively aroused person who is "shaking with fright" and cases of Parkinson's disease (where normal inhibition of the γ loop via the basal ganglia is weakened).

For practical purposes, the limiting frequency of movement

is set by the natural frequency of a body part, although a very fatiguing *forced* vibration can be initiated at somewhat above the resonant frequency. Rapid movements such as shaking or tapping are initiated by a sudden rise of tension in the concentric muscles; this reveals the natural frequency of the part.

A ballistic stroke can be viewed as a single oscillation of the relatively slowly moving pendulum formed by the arm or forearm. Movement is initiated by a sudden contraction of the concentric muscles. Thus, if the elbow is flexed, the biceps shows a very vigorous and sustained burst of activity until acceleration of the forearm has been completed. The arm then travels under its own momentum; at this stage, both the biceps and the triceps are quiescent. Finally, there is a burst of activity from the triceps to decelerate the forearm, preventing overshoot. One advantage of a ballistic movement is that little muscle shortening occurs during the active phase; for this reason, the muscle is able to develop almost its full isometric tension. The main disadvantage of a ballistic movement is that once initiated it cannot be modified.

A reciprocating movement (such as running) is essentially a series of ballistic strokes. The decelerating contraction of the antagonistic muscles continues for sufficient time to reverse the movement and initiate a ballistic stroke in the opposite direction. If the natural frequency of the limbs is exceeded, the movement becomes much less efficient. Resonance thus limits the rate of running. Once the maximum frequency is attained, greater speed can usefully be developed only by lengthening the stride.

A controlled movement such as the careful manipulation of a lever involves damping of the limb by the contraction of antagonistic muscles. Let us suppose the movement involves wrist extension; the extensor muscles contract continuously, but excessive acceleration of the wrist is prevented by bursts of activity in the flexor muscles. These fire out of phase with natural oscillations, at a frequency of 8–10c/sec.

The electromyograph is most useful in delineating different types of movement. It also exposes the wasteful use of muscles when performing a particular movement. Excessive electrical activity is a striking feature of the electromyogram in a man who has been performing heavy manual work for some hours and is suffering from physical fatigue.

Skill and Agility

Development of Skill

The development of skill is particularly important in activities requiring brief bursts of maximal effort. The achievements of a given individual can be greatly enhanced by learning appropriate techniques of movement. In submaximal work, lack of skill leads to awkward and apparently exhausting effort, with consequent early fatigue; thus at a given water-speed, an unskilled swimmer may expend four or five times as much energy as a well-trained individual. The secrets of the reduced energy expenditure of a skillful performer include:

1. development of balance and coordination, thereby minimizing postural work.
2. elimination of unnecessary and exuberant movements.
3. modification of necessary movements to ensure that these occur in the right direction, with a uniform speed that minimizes loss of kinetic energy.
4. more effective use of muscles, including choice of the most efficient prime-movers and a better coordination of agonists, antagonists and synergists; a minimum of energy is spent in initiating the movement, while antagonists present a minimum opposing resistance and exert the minimum necessary force to terminate the movement.
5. the replacement of controlled movements by ballistic strokes (p. 218).

In the specific example of swimming, a novice allows the speed of arm movement to vary widely, but the arms of an expert move forward in a smooth and graceful curve at an almost constant velocity. In running, a well-trained performer brings his thighs forward at close to the maximum speed permitted by resonance,*

* The maximum speed of leg alternation in the sprinter is 3–5 c/sec. Higher frequencies are possible in cycling (5–7 c/sec) because the length of the "compound pendulum" has effectively been shortened by increasing movement at the knee joint.

and he takes a stride that may be eight inches longer than that of a novice. The increased speed requires a more intense contraction of the agonists, the longer stride a greater relaxation of the antagonists. Dynamic posture is also better in the trained runner; in particular, he permits less lateral oscillation of his hips and trunk.

Acquired skills are in general highly specific. Thus a season of badminton, far from improving performance at tennis, may actully lead to a deterioration of skill for the second sport.

The novice attempts to compensate for lack of skill by using greater strength. However, this is an exhausting and largely ineffective substitute. Although the successful performer achieves far more than the novice, he may use *less* forceful muscular contractions in carrying out the specific activity.

Measurement of Skill and Agility

A variety of psychomotor tests are available to measure skill, agility, and dexterity. Some assess the *overall performance* of a physical task. A subject may be required to thread as many bolts as possible in a metal plate over a one minute period; this measures the dexterity of his fingers, and the test response is adversely affected by exposure to cold. A subject may be required to transfer ball-bearings from a tray to a series of depressions in an inclined and rotating turntable, using a pair of forceps; this test again depends on manual dexterity, and is adversely affected when there is lack of hand steadiness. A third formal task requires a subject to match the movement of one pointer or dial with a second pointer or dial, using a control knob or lever. This is known as a "tracking" or "pursuit" task. The movement of the target pointer may be continuous or discontinuous. Performance can be represented as the discrepancy between the two pointer readings (Fig. 58). With a discontinuous task, there is an initial "response time" before the subject notices the target reading has changed, a period of "travel," when the control level is being moved rapidly and a final phase of "manipulation" as the subject attempts to match the target position. Finally, a certain level of accuracy is accepted. Slight depression of the central nervous system (mild oxygen lack, a small dose of alcohol) decreases cortical control of the movement (Fig. 55). The initial response time is shorter, and travel is more rapid but the matching of the two pointers is less accurate. Greater depression of the brain leads to slowing of all phases of the reaction. Usually, the tracking task is controlled by manipulation of a knob or a light lever, but in one form developed by the applied psychology unit at Cambridge University, the control level is heavily weighted.

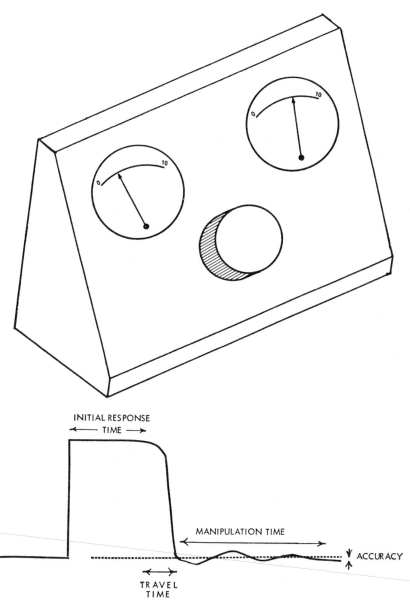

Figure 58. A discontinuous tracking task. (*Top*) The apparatus. A series of readings is presented on one voltmeter, and the subject must manipulate a control knob to produce a corresponding set of readings on a second voltmeter. (*Bottom*) The output of the machine, showing initial response time, travel time, manipulation time, and final accuracy of matching of the two dials.

Other forms of psychomotor test sample a specific attribute of performance. The *reaction time* may be measured if an electrical timer accurate to 1/100th sec is started coincident with a cue (such as a noise or a light) and if the timer is stopped as soon as the subject responds by touching a suitable key; a good example of this test is the brake reaction time device available at many driving schools. More complex reaction tasks may be devised, where the subject is presented with one of several possible cues, and must make a choice before initiating his response. *Travel or movement time* can be gauged by the interruption of a series of light beams; the task may be "terminated" if it ends in striking an object, but usually the final timing mechanism is also operated by a light beam, so that "nonterminated" tasks with a "follow-through" can be studied. *Hand steadiness* can be tested by passing a brass probe through a small hole in a brass plate. Every time that the subject hits the edge of the hole, an electrical contact is made, and this detracts from his ultimate score. *Balance* can be assessed by a stabilometer; with this device, the subject stands astride a board, pivoted at its centre, and endeavours to prevent it rotating. The total angular rotation in a thirty second period is scored against him. *Kinesthetic* sensitivity can be assessed by measuring the minimum displacement of limbs and joints that can be detected under different conditions.

Limitations of Skill

Body Build. Specific limits of skill are set by the general characteristics of the human body and by the genetic endowments of the individual.

A *tall* person has a high centre of gravity, and for this reason has difficulty in maintaining his balance (Fig. 54). Height is an important handicap in many sports. However, there are a few activities where a tall person has the advantage. In running, stride length is roughly proportional to leg length L, whereas the natural frequency of oscillation varies as $\sqrt{\frac{1}{L}}$; a tall runner can thus take longer if slightly slower strides. In basketball, also, the tall player may use his long reach to guide the ball through a substantial part of its total trajectory.

A *heavy* person is usually less skillful than one who is lighter. Subcutaneous fat may physically impede movement; further, the moment tending to cause loss of balance is directly proportional to body mass.

Kinesthetic Sensitivity. The sense of *balance* depends in part on the inherent sensitivity of the receptors in the inner ear; however, the performance of any given individual is probably improved by training. The γ loop settings needed for the rapid restoration of equilibrium are presumably learnt and stored within the cerebellum. Balance deteriorates with acute over-stimulation of the labyrinth (motion sickness) or chronic under-stimulation (weightlessness).

The cerebellum contributes to skill through the storage of *kinesthetic* information (the interpretation of muscle tension in terms of body position). When first playing tennis, a novice keeps his eyes on the position of his arms and racquet, making it difficult to watch either the target or its destination. With practice, the joint sensations corresponding to a given racquet position are learnt and stored in the cerebellum, and the eyes can then concentrate on following the ball. However, individuals vary in both their eye-muscle coordination (the ability to align the body in response to a visual signal provided by a moving target), and in their kinesthetic sensitivity. A defect of kinesthesis may occur at either the cerebellar (subconscious) or cortical (conscious) level. In the latter case, there is an impaired functioning of the association areas of the sensory cortex; the individual receives a normal range of sensory signals, but has difficulty in interpreting them. He may not recognise clearly which parts of the body are touched or moved, and he will have difficulty in predicting the weight, shape, size and texture of an external object that he cannot see.

The execution of all rapid movements depends greatly on *timing,* the ability to contract and relax individual muscles in a closely planned sequence; again, people apparently vary in ability to store such movement sequences within the brain.

Speed and Precision. The speed of performance in an athletic event depends on the rate of response to the starter's signal (a form of reaction time) and on the ability to accelerate the body mass and sustain its motion against (a) external resistance (particularly wind or water drag) and (b) continuing internal energy demands (gravitational work, acceleration and deceleration of the limbs and postural work).

The *reaction time* differs substantially from one individual to another, but like several of the factors already discussed, it is not clear how far this variation is an inherited feature, and how far it is a reflection of practice. Certainly, the reaction time can be shortened by training.* It reaches a minimum between the ages of twenty and thirty, and is shorter in men than in women. Athletes have a faster reaction time than nonathletes, and this difference is especially marked for contestants in "sprint" events. Reaction time also seems specific to a given body part; thus an individual may react quickly with his arms, and slowly with his legs. There seems little correlation between reaction time and the speed of subsequent movement, particularly if allowance is made for the common effects of age and sex upon the two variables.

Although we often think of an athlete as a "natural sprinter" or a "born distance man," *speed* is highly specific. One man may be good at accelerating, while another may have the ability to maintain speed. Acceleration is probably limited by the shape of the individual's force/velocity curve (Fig. 49), and thus muscle temperature, while maintenance of speed depends more upon the efficiency of neuromuscular coordination. Speed also shows intraindividual specificity. A subject may be capable of very rapid arm movements, but performance with his legs is relatively slow. He may also make a rapid forward swing of his arm, but show a rather slow backward movement.

One might anticipate that if a person performed a task inefficiently, speed could be maintained by use of greater strength. In practice, there is little correlation between speed and static strength unless the task involves the movement of heavy weights; however, there is a good correlation between speed and dynamic strength (the force exerted by a muscle group in accelerating an external load). Both isometric and "isotonic" training improve the speed of an individual's performance.

One might also anticipate that an improvement in flexibility would improve speed by reducing the internal resistance to

---

* The simplest forms of reaction time depend solely upon the length of the reflex arc and the number of intervening synapses; however, the reaction times of athletic interest are more complex and are thus susceptible to improvement by training.

movement. However, such experiments as have been conducted to date do not confirm this hypothesis.

Women perform most movements more slowly than men; this reflects partly their lesser relative muscular strength, partly the shorter lever length in their limbs, and partly differences of motivation between the two sexes.

> The *speed* and the *precision* of movement in any given individual depend on the direction of movement. Because of inertial effects, speed is greater for smooth, curved trajectories than for sharp, jerky movements. Again because of inertial effects, speed is reduced by any increase in the weight of the moving parts. Thus a heavy limb or an excessively weighted bat or racquet impairs this component of skilled performance. In general, a horizontal movement is performed more rapidly than a vertical one. Urging increases speed, but decreases accuracy; the mechanism seems an increase of arousal, and thus of tension in the active part (Fig. 55). There is an optimum tension for most activities, and excessive tension due to anxiety or other causes lead to awkward, stiff and jerky performance. The precision of movement is greater if the hand moves away rather than towards the body. It is also improved by the use of both hands rather than one, and by the increase of external loading (thereby increasing the stimulation of proprioceptive nerve endings). Both hands operate more precisely when moving towards the supine position; a right-handed movement is thus made best in a counterclockwise direction, while the reverse is true of a left-handed movement. Cricket provides a good example of this; the right-handed batsman finds it much easier to place the ball precisely on the left than on the right-hand side of the pitch.

Visual Factors. The acuity of the eyes is important in some sports. Assuming that there is no error of refraction at the lens, skilled performance is limited by the angle that the target subtends at the nodal point of the eye (where light is brought to a focus). The average individual can distinguish two objects that are separated by an angle of one minute (this is equivalent to a separation of 4.5μ on the retina). The more distant an object, the smaller the angle it subtends; hence, performance is enhanced if a nearby reference point is used (for example, the spot system in bowling). Many sports do not fully exploit visual acuity; for instance, a cricket stump subtends an angle of about fifteen minutes at a distance of forty yards. The batsman uses the kinesthetic sensitivity of his ocular muscles to assess the speed of the on-coming ball. As it approaches him, the eyes converge, stimulating the proprioceptors; information derived in this way is pooled with other sensory impressions such as increasing size and clarity, and the association areas of the sensory cortex then makes a judgment as to speed.

Flexibility

Static Flexibility. The static flexibility is simply the range of possible movement at any given joint. At some joints, movement is limited by opposition of soft tissues (for example, elbow flexion) or bony structures (elbow extension). However, at other joints movement is limited by the elastic resistance of the muscle sheath, tendon, joint capsule or supporting ligaments, together with the overlying skin.

Flexibility is generally greater in girls than in boys, and deteriorates with age. It is improved by warmth and habitual exercise. The conventional calisthenics used for the development of flexibility involve a wide variety of bouncing and jerking movements; typically, a body part is set in motion by one group of muscles, and is arrested at the end of the possible range of movement by a forcible stretching of the antagonists.

We have noted previously that a slow, "static" stress is more effective in inducing relaxation than a bouncy jerking movement. However, both techniques seem equally effective in improving flexibility. The main disadvantage of the jerky movement is the liability of producing an injury, either locally in the stressed tendon, or elsewhere in the body (for instance, a prolapsed intervertebral disc).

It is debatable how important flexibility is to the average citizen. However, a wide potential range of joint movement is essential to many types of athletic performance.

Dynamic Flexibility. The dynamic flexibility refers to the resistance encountered in moving a joint through its normal operating range. It has been studied much less fully than static flexibility, but obviously has greater potential influence on the speed and efficiency of movement.

Most of the dynamic resistance of the joint tissues is related to their elasticity and resistance to plastic deformation. Inertia, viscosity, and friction make a negligible contribution.

It is likely that dynamic flexibility deteriorates with age, and is increased by habitual physical activity.

Measurement of Flexibility. Static flexibility is commonly assessed by a *goniometer*. This is basically a large protractor with long measuring arms. The main difficulty when using the apparatus is to determine the axis of rotation for the joint, and to ensure the alignment of the goniometer in this axis. An alternative device is Leighton's *flexometer;* this is strapped to the moving limb like a watch; the pointer is kept vertical by a heavy weight, while the scale of the instrument rotates with the limb.

Some authors assess flexibility by means of performance tests such as "trunk flexion" or "sit and reach." Many of the failures on the Kraus-Weber test (p. 404) are attributable to limited flexibility, particularly difficulty in touching the floor without bending the knees. One would suspect that the ectomorphic type of individual, with long legs and a short trunk would have a substantial disadvantage in this type of test.

Dynamic flexibility is studied by attaching a recording goniometer to the joint, for instance, a slider moving over an arc of resistance wire. With this type of apparatus, changes in joint position are indicated by a change in electrical resistance, and if the signal is differentiated, the rate of angular motion may be deduced and related to the torque applied to the moving limb.

Other Features of Joints. The articular surfaces of joints are covered by a layer of *hyaline cartilage.* This plays an important role in ensuring smooth and relatively friction-free movement about the axis of rotation. The thickness of the cartilage layer is increased by habitual activity, and the entire layer may be lost as a result of injury; in the latter case, an abnormal proliferation of the exposed bone occurs (osteoarthritis), leading to stiff and painful joints.

White *fibrocartilage* is found in the attachment of ligaments and tendons to bone, in the intervertebral discs, and in the "cartilage" of the knee. It consists of a mixture of fibrous tissue and cartilage. In the articular cartilages, the fibres are arranged at right angles to the imposed stress; because of this histological arrangement, the tension resistance is about 0.2 kg/mm^2, while the resistance to compression is almost ten times as great. The articular cartilages are repeatedly deformed during activity, and regain their shape with rest. If the other supporting mechanisms of the joint fail due to fatigue, previous injury, poor coordination, an excessive external stress, or a combination of such factors, the deformation of the cartilage can exceed the elastic limit of the tissue so that tearing occurs.

The synovial fluid is normally a very thin viscous film that acts as a lubricant and shock-absorber. If the joint is injured or inflamed, it may accumulate in excessive amounts.

References

Ernst, E., and Straub, F.B.: *Symposium on Muscle*. Budapest, Akad. Kiadó 1968.

Ernst, E.: *Biophysics of the Striated Muscle*. Budapest, Akad. Kiadó, 1963.

Banister, E.W.: Energetics of muscular contraction. In Shephard, R.J. (Ed.): *Frontiers of Fitness*, Springfield, Thomas, 1971.

Hultman, E.: Muscle glycogen stores and prolonged exercise. In Shephard, R.J. (Ed.): *Frontiers of Fitness*. Springfield, Thomas, 1971.

Rohmert, W., and Jenik, P.: Isometric muscular strength in women. In Shephard, R.J.: *Frontiers of Fitness*. Springfield, Thomas, 1971.

Mottram, R.F.: Metabolism of exercising muscle. In Shephard, R.J.: *Frontiers of Fitness*. Springfield, Thomas, 1971.

Di Prampero, P.E.: Anaerobic capacity and power. In Shephard, R.J.: *Frontiers of Fitness*. Springfield, Thomas, 1971.

Lind, A.R., and McNicol, G.W.: Muscular factors which determine the cardiovascular responses to sustained and rhythmic exercise. *Canad Med Ass J, 96:* 706–713, 1967.

Rohmert, W.: *Muskelarbeit und Muskeltraining*. Gentner Verlag, Stuttgart, 1968.

Hettinger, T.: *Physiology of Strength*. Springfield, Thomas, 1961.

Clarke, H.H.: Muscular strength and endurance in man. Englewood Cliffs, N.J., Prentice-Hall, 1966.

Asmussen, E., Heeboll-Nielsen, K., and Molbech, S.: Muscle strength in children. In Jokl, E., and Simon, E. (Eds.): *International Research in Sport and Physical Education*. Springfield, Thomas, 1964.

Mathews, D.K.: *Measurement in Physical Education*. Philadelphia, Saunders, 1965.

Basmajïan, J.V.: *Muscles Alive. Baltimore*, Williams & Wilkins, 1967.

Broer, M.R., and Houtz, S.J.: *Patterns of Muscular Activity in Selected Sport Skills. An electromyographic study*. Springfield, Thomas, 1967.

Turner, M.: *Faulty Posture and its Treatment*. London, Whitefriars Press, 1965.

Grandjean, E.: *Sitting Posture*. London, Taylor & Francis, 1969.

Howell, M.L., Loiselle, D.S., and Lucas, W.G.: Strength of Edmonton schoolchildren. Unpublished report, Fitness Unit, University of Alberta, Edmonton, Alberta.

7

OTHER BODY SYSTEMS

This book makes no pretence to cover the physiology of all body systems; inevitably, in discussing the response to exercise, emphasis falls upon the heart, lungs, and neuromuscular systems. However, this chapter will consider briefly the exercise responses of other body regions, including the gastrointestinal tract, the liver and kidneys, the blood and body fluids, and certain of the endocrine glands.

Gastrointestinal Tract

The Stomach

In general, physical activity depresses the rate of emptying of the stomach; however, light activity may have a beneficial effect, and the response of the individual to a given absolute intensity of work thus depends on his physical fitness.

Animal experiments suggest that whether the stomach is in a fasting state or is stimulated by food or histamine, the rate of gastric secretion is reduced by exercise. The acidity of the secreted fluid is also lowered, but the enzyme secretion is apparently unchanged, and the incidence of histamine-induced gastric ulcers may actually be increased if animals are exercised immediately following the administration of histamine. Physical training also alters the resting response to a test dose of histamine. The enzyme secretion remains unchanged, but less acid is secreted, and the gastric juice contains more mucin.

The physiological basis of these various responses is uncertain. The marked influence of such emotions as fear and anger upon the character of the gastric secretions is known from observations made on the famous technician "Tom," whose gastric lining was visible through an old stomach wound. Other possible ways in which exercise could affect the stomach include an alteration in the balance of sympathetic and parasympathetic activity, a restriction of gastric blood flow, and the liberation of some circulating hormone. Support for this last concept has been obtained in some cross-circulation experiments.

The Intestines

Exercise apparently has no acute effect on the movements of the small intestine, although there is a very obvious blanching of the vasculature. There is some evidence from animal experiments that the chronic response to physical conditioning is an increase of motility, but it is less clear how far this is due to an alteration of eating habits, and how far it reflects changes in the balance of sympathetic and parasympathetic nervous activity.

In animals, at least, movements of the large intestine are stimulated during activity, and there is a phase of subnormal movement following exercise.

The effects of exertion upon the digestion and absorption of food from the intestines are unknown; in view of the reduction of splanchnic blood flow during activity, the acute response is probably a depression of absorption. Under resting conditions, the splanchnic region is substantially overperfused (p. 50), receiving as much as a quarter of the total cardiac output. If maximum exercise is performed in a hot environment, regional flow can be reduced by as much as 80 percent, thereby contributing 1.0–1.5 litre/min towards perfusion of the active tissues.

Timing of Meals

The timing and composition of meals prior to an athletic contest is discussed on page 481. Some authors have given athletes a light meal only half an hour before running and swimming events, apparently without adverse effects upon performance. However, a full stomach is uncomfortable during vigorous effort, and it also presents an obvious danger of vomiting to swimmers and those participating in contact sports.

Liver and Kidneys

Liver

The liver participates in the general reduction of splanchnic blood flow that accompanies physical activity. Depression of liver function is shown by a decreased elimination of substances such as bromsulphthalein blue. In some circumstances, tissue oxygen lack may reach the point where intracellular hepatic enzymes are liberated into the blood stream. The extent of oxygen lack and reversible cellular damage at any given intensity of effort is reduced by physical training. However, if the test exercise is held at a fixed percentage of aerobic power, it is less certain whether the extent of tissue injury is reduced by training; certainly, interindividual differences are much reduced if data on either blood flow reduction or functional impairment is compared at the same relative work load.

The reduction of hepatic blood flow persists and may even develop over an hour or more of sustained exercise. Nevertheless, there is little evidence of permanent harm to a healthy individual. During exercise, the oxygen consumption of the liver is increased by at least the amount that would be predicted from the general rise of body temperature (the "Law" of Arrhenius, p. 49), and transient nausea and gastrointestinal disturbances offer the only suggestion that an adverse effect may be carried over into the postexercise period. The safety of intense exercise is less certain in patients with a pathological restriction of cardiac output; repeated hepatic oxygen lack may contribute to the development of centri-lobular necrosis of the liver in such individuals.

As exhaustion is approached, there is a rapid breakdown of liver glycogen stores. The rate of glycogenolysis is such that there is a glucose output of 1–2 gm/min, from seven to fourteen times the resting value. Although often associated with hepatic oxygen lack, the "purpose" of the increased glycogenolysis may be to maintain the glucose supply to the brain.

Kidneys

The kidneys play a vital role in homeostasis, maintaining the blood composition within closely defined limits, and thereby permitting an even more precise regulation of the immediate milieu of the tissues.

Urinary Volume. Posture, central blood volume and exercise all modify the volume of urinary secretion against a background of diurnal phasic change. Urine secretion is less during sleep than when awake, and during the period of wakefulness the output of urine is increased either by assumption of a horizontal body position or by an increase of blood volume (such as may follow ingestion of fluids). Vigorous exercise brings about a dramatic decrease of urine secretion, and since this response is independent of the nerve supply to the kidneys, it probably reflects an increased secretion of antidiuretic hormone (ADH); this compound modifies the "water-proofing" of the distal convoluted tubules of the kidney, enhancing the reabsorption of fluid. ADH is secreted by the posterior lobe of the pituitary gland, and the trigger for its release may well be not exercise itself, but associated emotional stimuli. Release of ADH is certainly reinforced by excitement and such drugs as nicotine (which acts upon the pituitary gland); on the other hand, secretion of ADH is depressed by negative conditioning, and the output should thus fall as a subject becomes habituated (p. 444) to exercise.

Renal Blood Flow. The diminution of renal *blood flow* during intense exercise is well-documented. Perhaps because such circulatory adjustments are helping to meet the ever-increasing needs of heat dissipation, renal flow may continue to drop over at least an hour of sustained exercise, and the return to a normal rate of perfusion may be equally slow after effort has ceased. It is unlikely that the circulatory changes contribute to the reduced formation of urine. Glomerular filtration is reduced by renal ischaemia, but urine formation is virtually independent of blood flow. Renal function deteriorates in proportion to the intensity of the combined exercise/environmental stress and the duration of exposure. Urea clearance, one rough measure of renal function, may drop to 50 percent of normal when a man exercises in the heat; this reflects reduced glomerular filtration, and possibly an increased reabsorption of urea in the distal tubules.

Proteinuria. Exercise is associated with the appearance of protein, casts, and even red cells in the urine. This phenomenon is sometimes dignified by the name of "athletic pseudonephritis," and in the past was attributed to renal trauma.

However, it can be demonstrated following nontraumatic sports, and is more likely to reflect the combined effects of tissue oxygen lack and a rising blood acidity upon either the permeability of the glomerular intercellular "cement" or subsequent tubular reabsorption of protein.

Normally, the urine is free of protein. There is disagreement as to whether this indicates a complete lack of glomerular filtration of large molecules, or a moderate filtration with subsequent very efficient tubular resorption. Some authors describe a steady filtration and resorption of up to 360 gm of protein per day.

Exercise leads to a predominant loss of albumin, presumably because this has a smaller molecular weight than globulin. The urinary excretion of protein depends upon the intensity of effort relative to the aerobic power of the individual. Training decreases the proteinuria at a fixed work load, but has little influence upon the loss at a given percentage of maximum oxygen intake. Exercise proteinuria is a transient phenomenon and unless the activity is repeated, the urine is protein-free on the following day. It is thus unlikely that exercise is causing permanent damage to the renal system. Often, protein cannot be detected in the urine until exercise ceases, thus suggesting the possibility that flow to anoxic glomeruli is interrupted during vigorous activity.

> Is there additional renal trauma in contact sports? The question is not completely resolved. Most comparisons have shown rather similar urinary findings among participants in traumatic and nontraumatic activities. However, there are still occasional reports of substantial haematuria in boxers and in football players, and Kleiman has claimed a high incidence of hydronephrotic swelling of the collecting tubules amongst boxers.

Ionic Composition. Other changes of urinary composition include an increased excretion of ammonium and phosphate ions, and a decreased excretion of chlorides for some thirty minutes following a burst of vigorous activity. These alterations of ionic balance help to restore the normal acidity of the blood. The tubular cells accept carbon dioxide from the blood stream, and in the presence of the enzyme carbonic anhydrase, they convert this to carbonic acid (H_2CO_3). Ionization to H^+ and HCO_3^- then occurs. The hydrogen ions are subsequently neutralized in two ways. Some diffuse into the tubular fluid, where they combine with ammonia; the latter is produced from glutamic acid amide, by the action of an enzyme glutaminase, present in the tubular cells. The tubular epithelium is permeable to ammonia, but not to ammonium ions, and in consequence the ammonium ions are excreted from the body. The second mechanism of dealing with hydrogen ions involves buffering by disodium phosphate, already present in the tubules:

$$Na_2 HPO_4 + H^+ \rightarrow NaH_2 PO_4 + Na^+$$

Hydrogen ions leaving the tubular cells are replaced by sodium ions and since chloride resorption passively follows the movement of sodium ions, the chloride content of the urine inevitably falls.

Haemoglobinuria. Haemoglobin is sometimes excreted following prolonged marching. Haemoglobin, like albumin, is a protein of relatively low molecular weight (68,000), and it can pass into the urine if the kidney is suffering from oxygen lack. Normally, the small quantities of haemoglobin liberated into the blood stream combine with haptoglobins to form complexes of high molecular weight, and a substantial breakdown of red cells must occur before haemoglobin circulates as such. Loss of haptoglobins and frank haemoglobinuria have been associated with repeated minor trauma to the blood vessels of the feet—a heavy stride or marching upon hard surfaces; it may be that under such circumstances the red cells encounter sufficient pressure for a proportion to disintegrate. Urinary haemoglobin is seen in the first few hours after exercise, and must be distinguished carefully from urinary myoglobin; the latter is sometimes excreted one to two days following muscular trauma.

Blood and Body Fluids

Blood

Erythrocytes. The acute effect of vigorous exercise is commonly an increase in both the haemoglobin level and the red cell count. It is thus important that routine samples of blood are taken *before* any associated exercise tests. In some animals such as the dog, large changes of red cell count are induced by contraction of the splenic capsule. In man, the capsule contains little in the way of muscle, but red cells trapped in the splenic sinusoids may be released into the general circulation during physical activity. If protracted exercise is performed, haemoconcentration may also result from the fluid lost in sweat (up to 30 ml/min, in a hot climate), expired air (up to 4 ml/min) in a dry environment, and exudation into the tissues. Exercise increases the fluid content of the muscles by as much as 20 percent (p. 102), and if 20 kg of muscular tissue are active, exudation could theoretically reach the improbable total of five litres—certainly, the rate of exudation seems likely to match or exceed fluid lost by sweating.

The chronic effect of habitual exercise is to increase haemoglobin level and red cell count (p. 442). Similar changes are induced by chronic exposure to carbon monoxide or to high altitudes. The increased red cell count produces some increase of blood viscosity (Fig. 36), but over the normal range of change induced by exercise (an increase of haematocrit from 45 percent to 55 percent), the effect upon cardiac work load is not disastrous; indeed, exposure of the body to cold can have a much larger effect upon blood viscosity. In the large vessels, there is some tendency for plasma "skimming" and thus a lowering of effective viscosity. This is independent of blood flow rates. In the smaller arterioles and capillaries it is even more difficult to quote an appropriate figure for blood viscosity; the plasma moves relatively independently of the red cells, and during vigorous effort the effective resistance to blood flow is much lower than would be predicted from resting measurements.

As noted above, some forms of activity subject the red cells to mechanical trauma. The resulting breakdown of erythrocytes may be sufficient to outweigh the direct stimulating effect of exercise upon red cell production, and it offers a possible clue to the mild anaemia seen in some athletes.

Leucocytes. Exercise generally produces a substantial increase in the overall white cell count of the blood. This cannot be explained simply in terms of haemoconcentration. If the activity causes significant "stress," the eosinophil count shows an early increase, and a subsequent decrease associated with a rapid outpouring of hormones from the adrenal cortex. In the event that the adrenal gland becomes exhausted, there is a final increase of eosinophil count. However, it is rare for exercise to be pushed to this point except in an excessively hot climate.

Platelets. Light to moderate work is associated with an appreciable increase in the number of circulating platelets; their "stickiness" is also increased. In consequence, the acute effect of exercise is to increase the clotting tendency of the blood; with mild effort, the change is transient, but with heavier work it is more persistent, reaching a maximum in about thirty minutes.

The sympathetic nervous system may be involved in the release of platelets into the general circulation. Certainly, the effects of exercise can be mimicked by the administration of adrenaline, and they can be inhibited by agents such as ergotamine that block adrenergic receptor sites. The increase in "stickiness" of the platelets is thought due to an increase of Factor VIII; this plasma component accelerates the breakdown of platelets that have been in contact with damaged tissues, thereby forming more thromboplastin (Fig. 59).

Although clotting is accelerated, the bleeding time may be increased in exercise. When measuring the bleeding time, a small stab-wound is wiped clear of blood at fifteen second intervals. Under such circumstances, the duration of bleeding is

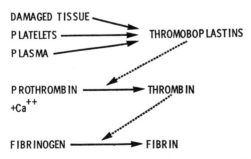

Figure 59. Simplified schema of blood-clotting mechanisms.

independent of clot formation, and reflects simply the tendency of damaged capillary vessels to retract. During exercise, there is an increase of capillary perfusion pressure. This probably holds the vessels open, thereby lengthening the bleeding time.

If these were the only effects of exercise, activity might seem a disadvantage to the coronary-prone individual. Certainly, he has no wish to increase the stickiness of his platelets. However, there is also an enhancement of fibrinolysis immediately following exercise; this seems due to release of an activator that converts plasminogen to the active, clot-destroying enzyme fibrinolysin. If the individual bout of exercise is unduly prolonged, there may be a secondary decrease of fibrinolysis as stores of the plasminogen activator are exhausted. Obviously, the "dose" of exercise needed by the coronary patient is rather critical.

Habitual activity also lengthens clotting times; this phenomenon has been demonstrated by comparing exercised with caged cockerels, and booking clerks with physically active railway "switchmen."

Body Fluids

Blood Volume. Information on changes in the body fluids during exercise has been presented at several points in this book; however, a brief coordinating review may be helpful. The blood volume is normally measured by a dilution technique (p. 424).

Brief exercise has little effect on the circulating volume, but because fluid is lost in sweat, muscle exudate and expired gas, sustained exercise causes a substantial decrease of blood volume. This has little effect on the maximum oxygen intake as measured over a period of a few minutes, but does influence the subsequent tolerance for extended periods of work. Exercise also alters the distribution of the available blood volume; leg work tends to increase the central blood volume, while arm work diminishes it (p. 26).

The chronic effect of exercise is to increase the circulating blood volume. One probable mechanism for this change is an alteration in the discharge of atrial stretch receptors. The resorption of fluid in the renal tubules is regulated by the antidiuretic hormone. Normally, secretion of antidiuretic hormone is inhibited by a stretching of the right atrium. The reflex is seen, for instance, following the infusion of a large volume of isotonic saline. With repeated exercise, one may presume that an adaptation of the receptors occurs in association with an increase of venous return, a displacement of the Starling Curve to the left (Fig. 9), and more complete diastolic emptying (p. 67).

Extracellular Fluid. The extracellular fluid accounts for 15 percent to 21 percent of body weight. It includes the plasma, cerebrospinal fluid, gastrointestinal juice, and interstitial fluid. The volume of extracellular fluid is estimated from the dilution of an injected marker substance. The answer obtained depends upon the completeness with which the extracellular fluid is penetrated and the extent to which marker substance enters the cells. The highest results are obtained with small molecules (radioactive sulphate ions, thiosulphate, and mannitol), and lesser volumes are estimated if sucrose, raffinose or inulin is used.

The chemical composition of the interstitial fluid is not known precisely, because the film of fluid lining the cells is normally too thin to collect. Analyses can be made of oedema fluid, but it is dangerous to assume that this is synonymous with interstitial fluid.

Factors that increase capillary permeability and thus the formation of interstitial fluid include tissue oxygen lack, a rise of body temperature, and an increase of capillary pressure. All of these factors are operative in exercise, together with a local accumulation of metabolites that increases the osmotic pressure of the extracellular fluid. We have noted elsewhere (p. 102) that a substantial swelling of the muscles accompanies physical activity. At the same time, the muscular contractions serve as a pumping mechanism to increase the return of fluid to the circulation via the lymphatic channels.

Intracellular Fluid. The volume of intracellular fluid cannot be measured directly; the standard approach is to measure the total body water, and to subtract from this figure the volume of extracellular fluid, determined by the methods described above. The total body water is determined by dilution of a marker substance such as urea, antipyrine, deuterium oxide (D_2O), or tritium oxide (^3H_2O). The last two compounds are perhaps the most reliable sources of information. The total body water ranges from 45 to 70 percent of body weight, averaging 62 percent in the male and 51 percent in the female. Since most tissues contain 75 to 80 percent water, it is possible to proceed from this information to the estimation of lean body mass, and thus percentage body fat (p. 486).

The increase of metabolism during exercise increases the osmotic pressure of the cellular contents, and other factors being equal, there is then an increase of intracellular fluid in an attempt to restore normal osmotic relationships.

Water Balance. The daily water requirement varies widely from 1.5 to 7 litres. Water is derived from ingestion of food (about 1000 ml), oxidation of food products (about 300 ml), and the deliberate drinking of fluids. Drinking habits are very variable, depending on both the intensity of effort and the thermal comfort of the environment; the intake ranges from perhaps a litre of fluid in a sedentary individual to five or more litres in a man performing hard exercise in a hot and humid environment (p. 231) or a cold and dry environment.

The daily water loss normally matches the intake fairly closely. A minimum "obligatory" urine secretion of 150 ml per day is set by the need to excrete waste products through renal tubules that have a finite concentrating power (p. 241). The urinary output is readily boosted to a litre per hour by the enthusiastic and bibulous celebration of success in a football match. Loss through the skin includes "insensible" perspiration and sweating. Insensible losses are relatively constant at 700 ml/day. Sweating is slight or nonexistent when a subject is seated in a thermally comfortable environment, but rises to 2 litres/hour if exercise is carried out under unfavourable climatic conditions. Losses of water vapour in expired air depend upon the absolute water content of the atmosphere and the respiratory minute volume. In the summer, the inspired gas may be almost fully saturated with water vapour at 30°C, giving it a water content of 30 mg/litre. Expired gas is fully saturated at 32°C, giving it a water content of some 33 mg/litre. Under such conditions, a man with a respiratory minute vol-

ume of 8 litre/min has a respiratory water loss of less than
1.5 ml/hour. In winter, there is a marked contrast. The inspired air is now perhaps 50% saturated at 0°C (water content 2 mg/litre), while the water content of expired gas is
almost unchanged at 33 mg/litre. The respiratory loss at a
ventilation of 8 litre/min is now increased to 15 ml/hour. During vigorous exercise, ventilation may amount to 80 litre/min,
and the loss rises proportionately to 150 ml/hour; it is easy to
appreciate from these figures how a combination of dry mountain air, vigorous exercise and oxygen hunger can lead to progressive dehydration. Faecal water loss is normally no more
than 100 ml/day. However, it can become quite large if there
is diarrhoea. Fluid losses secondary to a gastrointestinal dis-
tubance have sometimes led to poor performance when athletes have competed in unfamiliar parts of the world. The problem arises not from any well-recognized bacterial pathogen
such as the typhoid or paratyphoid bacillus, but from a host
of unfamiliar bacteria that have little effect upon the normal
resident of the country in question.

Water Deprivation. Problems of water deprivation in the marathon
runner and in the wrestler endeavouring to achieve a specific weight
category are discussed in later sections of this book (p. 316 and 490
respectively). In this chapter, we shall focus on the specific problems
of a wanderer lost in the desert or adrift in a small boat.

In this type of situation, neither drinking water nor water-contain-
ing foods are available, but a certain minimum loss of water from the
body is unavoidable. Urine production drops to the "volume obliga-
toire"; the required volume depends on the availability of foodstuffs.
Whereas 850 ml of urine must be excreted with a normal mixed
diet, 550 ml per day suffice for a fasting man, and if caloric requirements are met from sugar, as little as 150 ml of urine can be passed
per day. As dehydration develops, water is drawn from the extracellular fluid, and the osmotic pressure rises in this body compartment; this in turn tends to draw water from the intracellular
compartment. The renal excretion of electrolytes is increased, in an
attempt to restore the normal ionic composition of extracellular
fluid, and the mineral elements lost in this way must be restored
during subsequent treatment. The blood volume may change relatively little in the early stages of water deprivation; the decrease of
capillary and venous pressures and the increase of plasma osmotic
pressure both tend to draw water into the blood stream at the

expense of the extracellular space, and if reliance is placed upon estimations of haemoglobin level or plasma volume, there is a danger that the severity of a patient's condition may be underestimated.

If no water is available, the body initially loses about 1 kg of weight per day. The affected person is conscious of thirst and weakness, the skin becomes dry and the eyes are sunken. When some 4 kg of weight has been lost, both the kidneys and the circulation show signs of failure. Death usually occurs if the water loss exceeds 15 kg.

Can survival of a water-deprived mariner be extended by drinking sea-water? Much depends on the salt content of the ocean in question. Typically, sea water contains about three times as much salt as the plasma, and it is difficult for the ailing kidney to excrete the excess sodium ions. Thus, the drinking of sea water leads to a further increase in the osmotic pressure of both plasma and extracellular fluid; this in turn increases intracellular dehydration, and the survival time is shortened rather than lengthened.

Endocrine System

Sex Hormones

The administration of testosterone to experimental animals produces effects somewhat akin to repetitive muscular work. Changes include an increase of muscle mass, the growth of individual muscle fibres, and a decrease of body fat content. It thus seems possible that testosterone may play a role in both the normal development of muscular tissue and the enhanced growth that follows physical training. Certainly, adolescent boys show a sudden spurt of muscular strength coincident with puberty. Again, in middle-aged and older men the administration of testosterone enhances the response of the muscles to training, particularly following injury or immobilization of a body part. On the other hand, the response of a young man to a physical training regime is uninfluenced by testosterone— at least if this is administered as a "double-blind" experiment. Presumably, the circulating androgens of a young man are already at an optimum level for muscular development, and there seems little basis for the dangerous and unethical practice of administering such compounds to athletes.

Growth Hormone

Sustained and vigorous activity leads to an increased secretion of anterior pituitary growth hormone. The output of the gland reaches a peak with about one hour of continued effort. The release of the hormone is apparently related to a need for mobilization of depot fat as muscle glycogen is depleted and blood sugar levels fall. The anterior pituitary hormone not only serves as a linear amplifier of growth processes (p. 377), but also has an important sustaining role in metabolism. It inhibits the phosphorylation of glucose by hexokinase and increases the mobilization of fatty acids, conserving the remaining blood glucose for the needs of the brain. In proof of this hypothesis, the exercise-induced secretion of growth hormone is inhibited if an athlete is fed large doses of glucose or sucrose while he is active.

Posterior Pituitary Secretions

Vigorous exercise inhibits urine formation (p. 233). This probably reflects an enhanced secretion of antidiuretic hormone from the posterior pituitary gland, in response to either exercise itself, or associated emotional stimuli. Following exhaustive exercise, there is no change in the hormonal content of the primary secretory sites (the supraoptic and paraventricular nuclei of the hypothalamus), but stores of hormone in the posterior pituitary gland are depleted.

Adrenal Cortex

As with the posterior pituitary secretion, it is difficult to determine how far a change in the output of adrenal cortical hormones is due to exercise *per se*, and how far it is attributable to associated emotional factors. One crude index of adrenal cortical function is the eosinophil count; exhausting exercise induces a triphasic change in the number of circulating eosinophils (p. 237). A second crude index of adrenal activity is the urinary excretion of metabolic end-products such as the 17-ketosteroids. An increased output of such compounds shows that the adrenal glands are stimulated at some point during exhaustive exercise. Lastly, in animals at least, regular training increases the weight of the adrenal glands, while single bouts of exhaustive exercise depress plasma corticosteroid levels.

Surgical removal of the adrenals leads to weakness, and the work capacity can be improved in these circumstances by the administration of adrenal cortical hormones. However, it is difficult to dissociate such changes from related disturbances of electrolyte balance and carbohydrate metabolism (Fig. 60).

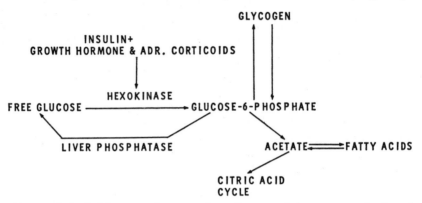

Figure 60. Probable sites of action of insulin, growth hormone, and adrenal corticoids.

Adrenal Medulla

The secretions of adrenaline and noradrenaline are not affected by moderate exercise. Exhaustive work leads to a two- to three-fold increase in plasma levels of noradrenaline, and a substantial decrease in plasma adrenaline. The source of the noradrenaline is still debated, but it may be released from the sympathetic nerve terminals rather than the adrenal glands; if so, the drop in adrenaline secretion suggests that the adrenal medulla is ultimately exhausted by vigorous effort.

Insulin Secretion

A programme of increased physical activity reduces the needs of a diabetic for insulin. Several mechanisms are involved, including the direct burning of sugar following a carbohydrate meal, an increased avidity of the muscles for glucose, and a sparing of functionally weak pancreatic islet cells following the ingestion of sugar (p. 495).

Menstrual Cycle

There have been numerous attempts to document changes of performance with the female menstrual cycle. The effects cited have been quite limited, and it has been difficult to dissociate a direct hormonal response from associated problems of personal hygiene. In general, skilled performance has deteriorated during the phase of premenstrual tension, and some items have been performed slightly better than normal during the phase of menstrual flow. Further research may clarify these changes. But in any event, a deterioration of function with menstruation is now rather an academic question, since the timing of the menstrual cycle can readily be adjusted by use of hormone preparations.

References

Rowell, L.B.: Visceral blood flow and metabolism during exercise. In Shephard, R.J. (Ed.): *Frontiers of Fitness.* Springfield, Thomas, 1971.

Stickeny, J.C. and Van Liere, E.J.: The effects of exercise upon the gastro-intestinal tract. In Johnson, W.R. (Ed.): *Science and Medicine in Sports.* New York, Harper, 1960.

Moore, R., and Buskirk, E.R.: Exercise and body fluids. In Johnson, W.R. (Ed.): *Science and Medicine in Sports.* New York, Harper, 1960.

Ulrich, C.: Women and sport. In Johnson, W.R. (Ed.): *Science and Medicine in Sports.* New York, Harper, 1960.

Rasch, P.T., and Wilson, I.D.: Other body systems and exercise. In Falls, H. (Ed.): Exercise Physiology. New York, Academic Press, 1968.

Keeney, C.E.: The effect of exercise in blood coagulation and fibrinolysis. In *Health and Fitness in the Modern World.* Athletic Institute, 1961.

Poortmans, J.R.: *Biochemistry of Exercise.* Basel, Karger, 1969.

PART TWO

MODIFICATIONS OF HUMAN PERFORMANCE

8

HIGH ALTITUDES

The peculiar problems of physical activity at high altitudes have fascinated man for many generations. In South America, the ancient Inca civilization enacted laws to prevent slaves from the coastal regions being worked to their death in the mountains. It was recognized that the difficulty arose from a decrease of ambient pressure. As early as 1608, Joseph de Acosta wrote "the harm comes from the quality of the air one breathes in and out, since it is so extremely thin and delicate," and in 1878 Paul Bert laid responsibility clearly upon the diminished partial pressure of oxygen.

Until recently, the physiologist has studied mainly the extreme altitudes encountered by the balloonist, the Himalayan explorer, and the aviator with limited oxygen equipment. However, the decision to hold the 1968 Olympic Games in Mexico City spurred investigation of the effects of more moderate altitudes; the Olympic stadium was some 7350 feet above sea level, with an average barometric pressure of 580 mmHg.

Physics of the Atmosphere

The percentage composition of the atmosphere remains essentially unchanged over the range of altitudes of interest to the physiologist, comprising 20.93% oxygen, 0.03% carbon dioxide, and a residue of inert gas (nitrogen, together with small quantities of argon, krypton, xenon and other "rare" gases).

There is a logarithmic decrement in the total ambient pressure with altitude, so that at eighteen thousand feet, the pressure is approximately halved (380 mmHg), and at 33,000 feet, it is only a little more than a quarter of the sea level reading (197 mmHg). The decline in total pressure inevitably reduces

249

the partial pressure of oxygen in inspired gas. Within the alveoli, both water vapour and carbon dioxide remain at relatively fixed partial pressures (47 and 35–40 mmHg respectively), and in consequence the partial pressure of oxygen is reduced even more markedly.

The *troposphere* extends from sea level to about 35,000 feet, reaching a greater height at the equator than at the poles. This zone is influenced by conduction, convection and radiation of the earth's heat, giving rise to variations in the temperature, moisture content and movement of the air.

The *stratosphere* extends beyond the troposphere to a total height of some twenty miles. It is characterized by a constant temperature (−55°C), and the absence of both moisture and air turbulence; there is also an appreciable formation of ozone by solar radiation.*
Most modern subsonic aircraft operate in the stratosphere in order to minimize fuel consumption and provide the comfort of turbulence-free travel. The cabin altitude of standard commercial aircraft is held to a maximum of eight thousand feet, but light feeder and charter planes may provide little or no cabin pressurization. Military aircraft are commonly pressurized to a cabin altitude of no more than 25,000 ft, a compromise between the problems of explosive decompression (should the fuselage rupture) and decompression sickness (which is rare at altitudes of less than 25,000 feet).

Beyond the stratosphere lie the cold *mesosphere* (−80°C), a region of warming (the *thermosphere*) and finally the *exosphere*, where temperatures may be as high as 2000°C. These zones are becoming increasingly known and understood as man explores space.

The atmospheric temperature normally decreases by 2°C per one thousand feet throughout the troposphere; hence the cold, dry air of most mountains. Occasionally, the temperature gradient is reversed for several hundred feet above the earth's surface. A temperature *inversion* is then said to have occurred. The hot air from factory chimneys fails to raise, and air pollution accumulates. If the inversion occurs in a geographical pocket such as a deep mountain valley, a dangerous concentration of atmospheric contaminants may develop. One example of this was seen in Donora, Pennsylvania—a small United States mining town set in a narrow ravine; eighteen people died in October, 1948, following a well-remembered thermal inversion.

---

* Concentrations of ozone in the cabins of commercial transatlantic aircraft may rise as high as 1 part per million. This is not dangerous to the occasional traveller, but may have an adverse effect on the pilots and stewardesses who are more regularly exposed.

The Acute Effects of Oxygen Lack

Fulminating Anoxia

The term fulminating anoxia is derived from the Latin fulmen = lightning. It is seen if there is a sudden disruption of an aircraft cabin during stratospheric flight, and also occurs experimentally on inhaling pure nitrogen. The partial pressure of oxygen in alveolar gas abruptly falls to near zero, and a reversal of the normal diffusion process robs blood of oxygen as it passes through the lungs; consciousness is thus limited to the time required to eliminate tissue oxygen stores. At thirty thousand feet, the average person remains reasonably coherent for forty seconds, and suffers a complete loss of consciousness in 2½ minutes. At forty thousand feet the total period of consciousness is no more than thirty seconds, and useful consciousness may be as little as ten seconds. It is thus very important that regulations requiring an aircraft pilot to wear an oxygen mask be carefully observed, and that passengers be given due instruction in the use of emergency equipment at the time of take-off.

In an emergency involving a commercial aeroplane, complete disruption of the cabin is unlikely; further, emergency blowers slow the rate of pressure loss, and the pilot dives to a lower altitude as rapidly as the condition of the aircraft will permit. Thus on most occasions, useful consciousness is longer than would be expected from chamber exposures to altitudes of thirty thousand to forty thousand feet.

The immediate response to oxygen lack is a rise of systemic blood pressure, induced by a massive release of catecholamines; subsequently, there is a fall of pressure and a decrease of peripheral resistance as the circulation fails. Muscular movements become incoordinated, with coarse tremors, jactitation (convulsive movements of the entire body), and loss of consciousness. The likelihood of death depends on the resistance of the circulation to oxygen lack. During World War II, the United States Air Force had at least thirty-six fatalities from acute oxygen lack; some occurred as low as 18,000 to 20,000 feet, but death was more common at 24,000 to 28,000 feet. The majority of aircrew who experienced oxygen lack recovered completely, even if consciousness was lost; however, in a few cases there was delayed or incomplete recovery of full cerebration.

Acute Anoxia

Acute anoxia was seen first by balloonists, as they allowed their vehicles to drift to progressively higher altitudes. More recently, the acute effects of oxygen lack have been studied by deliberate chamber exposures of air force personnel to low oxygen pressures, and by field observations on athletes who have been flown from sea level to high altitudes.

Effects on the Central Nervous System. The main effect of acute anoxia on the central nervous system is a loss of judgment. A lack of inhibition is coupled with an exaggeration of normal personality; often there is also a cheerful euphoria, so that the person involved does not realise his disability. In the early balloon voyage of Tissandier, Sivel and Croce-Spinelli (1875), Tissandier certainly realised that his arms were paralyzed and that he was unable to breathe from the primitive oxygen supply; nevertheless, he felt happy that the party had reached 25,000 feet and that the balloon was still rising. He then lost consciousness. He recovered as the balloon drifted down to about twenty thousand feet, and noted that his companions remained unconscious. Despite this unpromising circumstance, he let go more ballast and ascended for a further trip. Unfortunately, his two companions died. Physiology has many parallel tales of disturbed judgment, such as the great Haldane owlishly observing the colour of his face while looking into the wooden back of a hand mirror.

The time required for a deterioration in psychomotor performance (p. 220) depends upon the altitude, the health of the individual, and the sensitivity of the test that is used. Below ten thousand feet, it is difficult to demonstrate any change in a resting man. Until recently, the only known disturbance was a reduction in the acuity of the retinal rod cells. Apparently, the resynthesis of the rod pigment (visual purple) is markedly dependent upon the availability of oxygen. For this reason, military pilots are advised to breathe oxygen from ground level when flying at night. In the last few years, there have been occasional reports that quite modest degrees of tissue oxygen lack induced by the formation of carboxyhaemoglobin can impair other discriminant processes such as the ability to distinguish long and short auditory tones. If these observations are confirmed, then the chronic smoker should suffer a much greater decrement of performance than the nonsmoker at moderate altitudes. Typical psychological and psychomotor tests (flicker-fusion frequency, self-ratings of mood and liveliness, code-translation, tapping, hand-steadiness, reaction testers and pursuit meters) all show a decrement of performance with a few minutes of rest or light activity at eighteen to twenty thousand feet. Under these conditions the arterial oxygen saturation is 65% to 70%. Loss of consciousness is imminent when the saturation is less than 60 percent.

> All psychomotor changes are temporarily worsened when oxygen is restored (the *"oxygen paradox"*). Several factors contribute to this phenomenon. There is a general fall of systemic blood pressure secondary to dilatation of the pulmonary vessels, a vasoconstriction of the cerebral vessels, and a temporary inhibition of respiration secondary to removal of the hypoxic stimulus to the carotid body chemoreceptors. In consequence, the oxygen supply to the brain worsens in the first few seconds following administration of oxygen to an anoxic patient.

Disturbances of the central nervous system can be induced at much lower altitudes if the individual engages in vigorous physical activity. An unacclimatized person may develop permanent cerebral damage and even die if he undertakes strenous exertion at more than 15,000 feet. Partially acclimatized mountaineers have reported disturbances of vision, partial paralysis and other evidence of central nervous failure at altitudes of fifteen to twenty thousand feet and at the 1968 Olympic Games there were athletes who developed transient blindness of part of the visual field (scotoma) and temporary confusion during or immediately following their event.

Effects on Oxygen Transport. The carotid body chemoreceptors show a small discharge at normal sea-level pressures of oxygen. This increases somewhat as the altitude is increased, but first becomes marked when the arterial oxygen pressure has dropped to about 60 mmHg (Fig. 38). The medullary centres controlling respiration and circulation are depressed by oxygen lack, but nevertheless the immediate overall response is an increase of pulse rate both at rest and during submaximum work, with an increase in the rate (and to a lesser extent the depth) of breathing. The respiratory minute volume is increased not only in BTPS but also in STPD terms, and in consequence there is an excessive elimination of carbon dioxide from the body. This depresses both the chemoreceptors and the respiratory centres, diminishing the steady ventilatory response to a given reduction of arterial oxygen tension. It may also lead to intermittent breathing (p. 150), on account of the phase lag between stimulation of respiration (oxygen lack in the tissues of the carotid bodies) and depression of respiration (carbon dioxide lack in the tissues of the medulla). Intermittent breathing is most noticeable at night, when CO_2 production is low and the reticular activating system is depressed. It is a disturbing sensation, and can rob the newcomer to altitude of much sleep. The reduced CO_2 tension of arterial blood reduces cerebral blood flow, and for this reason an excessive hyperventilation may worsen psychomotor performance; there is an optimum respiratory minute volume for each combination of activity and altitude, but in general there is little advantage in reducing the alveolar CO_2 tension below 25–30 mmHg. The decrease of atmospheric density raises the critical velocity for a transition from laminar to turbulent airflow (p. 61); it also diminishes the resistance to turbulent air movement. The oxygen cost of a given BTPS ventilation is thus less than at sea-level, and the required STPD ventilation can be sustained at an approximately normal total cost. Unfortunately, oxygen lack commonly induces STPD hyperventilation; thus, there is a tendency for an increased consumption of oxygen by the respiratory muscles while at altitude.

The increase of heart rate tends to increase the cardiac output for a given level of submaximal work. Stroke volume may remain unchanged, but it often diminishes in the first few days at altitude. Hyperventilation in the cold, dry mountain air can lead to a substantial water loss, and exudation of fluid into the tissues is also increased. The haemoglobin content of unit volume of blood thus rises, at the expense of some increase in blood viscosity. Because of the shape of the haemoglobin dissociation curve (Fig. 39), a substantial reduction of alveolar oxygen pressure can occur with little change in the arterial oxygen saturation. At the altitude of Mexico City, for instance, the oxygen content of arterial blood falls by no more than 7% to 8%. In submaximum effort, this deficit can be made good by either a small increase in the cardiac output, or by a greater extraction of oxygen from the blood as it passes through the tissue capillaries.

While the diffusing capacity of the lungs presents little barrier to gas exchange at sea level (Fig. 23), it becomes more significant at altitude. The impedance term describing the interaction between diffusion and blood transport in the lungs (p. 108) includes the exponent $e^{-\frac{\dot{D}_L}{\lambda \dot{Q}}}$ The cardiac output $\dot{Q}$ is changed relatively little at altitude, but the solubility factor λ is increased, since the subject is now operating over the steep part of his oxygen dissociation curve (where a small increase in pressure gives a large increase in oxygen content). Further, if the diffusing capacity $\dot{D}_L$ is expressed in units of gas conductance (ml STPD/min per ml/litre concentration gradient) rather than the usual clinical units (ml/min per mmHg pressure gradient), then $\dot{D}_L$ decreases in proportion to the drop in ambient pressure. Equilibration of gas and blood is still fairly complete in the average alveolus, but in parts of the lung where the $\dot{D}_L/\dot{Q}$ ratio is low or the transit time through the pulmonary capillaries is shorter than average, saturation of pulmonary venous blood may be incomplete. The diffusion component of the A-a oxygen tension gradient is thus widened at altitude, particularly if the subject is exercising hard, and in this particular situation the individual with a large maximum diffusing capacity may have some advantage. At an altitude of 19,000 feet, West found that maximum exercise reduced the arterial oxygen saturation from 67% to 56%, and during short periods of "supramaximal" work, even lower oxygen saturations were recorded.

Two other components of the A-a gradient well recognised at sea level (inequalities of ventilation/perfusion ratio and "shunting" of venous blood past the lungs) become less important at altitude. Increased ventilation leads to a more uniform distribution of inspired gas, increased pulmonary arterial pressures lead to more uniform perfusion of the lungs, and the lower pulmonary venous oxygen tension reduces the effect of a given venous-arterial shunt on the oxygen pressure in mixed arterial blood.

It is difficult to estimate the change in aerobic power attributable to a given increase of altitude, because athletes and others visiting mountainous regions are immediately aware that their environment has changed, and many features of the new environment such as an altered climate, loss of sleep, and gastrointestinal infections contribute to the alterations of maximum oxygen intake that are observed. Most authors agree that aerobic power changes little at altitudes of six thousand feet or less; at greater heights, there is a progressive reduction, amounting to 7% to 8% in Mexico City, and increasing steadily to around 40% at eighteen thousand feet.

Below six thousand feet, it is relatively easy for the body to increase chest movements to the point where the STPD respiratory minute volume is restored. Some impedance to oxygen conductance develops at the lung membrane due to the increase of λ and the fall of $\dot{D}_L$; however, this is counterbalanced by an increase in blood oxygen transport ($\lambda\dot{Q}$) per unit of concentration gradient. At higher altitudes, these methods of compensation are no longer fully effective. Chest movements continue to increase until a large part of the maximum oxygen intake is being diverted to the muscles of respiration; however, it is no longer possible to maintain the sea level STPD ventilation. The effect of the diminishing $\dot{D}_L$ becomes more serious, and because the subject is already operating on the steepest part of his oxygen dissociation curve, there is no mechanism for a further increase of λ. Lastly, the maximum cardiac output falls; the reduction of stroke volume becomes more obvious, and there is also a decrease of maximum heart rate. Typical pulse readings of a young man drop from $\sim$195/min at sea level to $\sim$140/min at 24,000 ft.[*] This

---

[*] Somervell is an interesting exception to this. He reported a personal pulse rate of 160–180/min while climbing at an altitude of 27–28,000 feet.

decline in pulse rate may be an effect of oxygen lack on the myocardium, since in some subjects it is reversed by the administration of oxygen.

Chronic Oxygen Lack

Mountain Sickness. The clinical syndrome of mountain sickness first develops at an altitude of eleven thousand feet, and is well marked at seventeen to eighteen thousand feet. The symptoms include nausea, vomiting, muscular weakness and incoordination, fatigue, headache and irritability. Ventilation is increased, and arterial oxygen and CO_2 tensions are often low. The condition develops after the subject has remained a few hours at altitude. It reaches a peak at forty-eight hours, and regresses as the individual becomes acclimatized. It is not related directly to arterial oxygen lack, since symptoms are often worst when the arterial oxygen tension is recovering. It may be an expression of the combined effects of low intravascular oxygen and CO_2 pressures upon the tissue oxygen supply. Symptoms are reduced by prophylactic administration of acetazolamide, a carbonic anhydrase inhibitor, but this form of treatment does not improve the associated poor psychomotor performance.

Exceptional individuals, such as the Sherpa Tensing have conquered Mount Everest without oxygen, but eighteen thousand feet seems the limit of permanent adaptation for the average person. There are sulphur mines as high as nineteen thousand feet in Chile, but the workers prefer to live at 17,500 feet, complaining of loss of sleep, appetite and enjoyment of food when quartered nearer to the mines.

High Altitude Deterioration. Mountain sickness becomes progressively less apparent if the affected individual remains at an altitude of eleven to eighteen thousand feet. However, improvement of condition is not seen with sustained residence at a still higher altitude—indeed, the clinical status gradually worsens—"high altitude deterioration" is said to have occurred. The working capacity gradually declines, the appetite becomes poor, weight and sleep are lost, and the affected individual becomes increasingly lethargic.

Many factors undoubtedly contribute to the deterioration of physical condition. A large volume of water is lost from the body, due to vigorous ventilation in the dry mountain air, and sweating induced by the solar radiation* reflected from snow-covered glaciers. A daily intake of five to seven pints of fluid may be needed in order to avoid dehydration. It is surprisingly difficult to achieve this when snow must be melted over a primitive stove that is liable to set a climber's tent on fire, and the boiling point of the water is too low to make acceptable tea. The diet is commonly poor and unpalatable, and an energy expenditure of 4–5000 kcal per day may be matched by a food intake of no more than 1500 kcal. To these problems are added illness, intense mental and physical stress, biting cold, and lack of sleep. Hyperventilation may be so intense that a large part of the oxygen intake is diverted to the respiratory muscles, and the heat loss involved in saturation of the expired gas with water vapour may exceed the potential metabolic heat production.

Under such circumstances, deterioration of condition is hardly surprising. Preventive measures include provision of a high calorie diet and insistence on adequate replacement of fluids. Once the syndrome is established, the only practical remedy seems evacuation from the mountainous region.

High Altitude Oedema. An intense pulmonary oedema may develop from nine to thirty-six hours after reaching high altitude. This presents clinically as an acute shortness of breath (dyspnoea) with a blood-stained and watery phlegm (haemoptysis), chest discomfort and cough, nausea and vomiting. Confirmatory evidence includes the usual clinical signs of alveolar exudate, electrocardiographic signs of right heart strain (prominent R waves in leads V1 and V2, often with other abnormal features of these leads, including right bundle-branch block, depression of the ST segment and T wave inversion), and intense pulmonary vascular congestion on a chest radiograph.

Attacks are most common in those returning to vigorous activity following a period of relative leisure nearer to sea-level. Teenagers are frequently affected. However, a combination of youth and a last-minute return to work are common phenomena in the mining communities of the Andes. There is often a history of recent respiratory infection.

Fears were expressed that the very intense efforts of the Mexico Olympic Games might induce pulmonary oedema in some of the contestants. Fortunately, these anxieties proved groundless.

---

* Solar radiation may also cause problems of sunburn and snow-blindness.

In normal industrial and military activity, attacks do not occur below ten thousand feet, and are rare below twelve thousand feet.

> The causative factors remain uncertain. Various mechanisms predispose to pulmonary congestion at altitude, including peripheral vasoconstriction (secondary to carbon dioxide wash-out), pulmonary venous constriction (secondary to the reduction of alveolar oxygen tension), an increase in total blood volume (from previous acclimatization to high altitude), an increase in cardiac output (induced by a combination of effort and oxygen lack), and an increase of left ventricular diastolic pressure (secondary to myocardial oxygen lack). Pulmonary congestion in turn inevitably increases the transudation of fluid from the pulmonary circulation. The permeability of the pulmonary vessels may also be increased (due to infection or oxygen lack). The net result is a rapid and potentially fatal flooding of the lungs with oedema fluid.

Attacks are generally avoided if effort is preceded by appropriate preliminary acclimatization. Established cases should be treated by bed rest, oxygen, and antibiotics to avoid secondary infection.

Acclimatization to High Altitudes

If a person remains at altitude, a gradual process of acclimatization occurs. This has much in common with the processes of adaptation to effort, heat, and other forms of external stress. The time course of adaptation is of particular interest to those planning the schedules of athletes who intend to compete in mountainous regions; the advantages of full acclimatization must be nicely balanced against expense and other adverse aspects of prolonged residence in an abnormal environment.

Respiration

The "hunting" pattern of intermittent respiration is gradually lost, and after a period of three to six weeks at altitude, the sea level STPD ventilation can be maintained quite comfortably while sitting at rest.

The earliest biochemical change is a decrease in the buffering capacity of the cerebrospinal fluid; the bicarbonate content of this fluid is actively regulated by the choroid plexus, so that within a few hours of reaching altitude, the normal environment of the medullary CO_2 receptors is restored despite the lower arterial CO_2 tension. There may also be some decrease in the buffering capacity of the arterial blood, but this is a slower process, occurring over the course of several weeks.

On first arrival at altitude, the drive to the respiratory centres is derived largely from the carotid chemoreceptors. During the next few weeks, the importance of the medullary chemoreceptors is restored, and ultimately there is an enhanced responsiveness to CO_2 at a given oxygen tension. However, the increased discharge rate of the chemoreceptors does not disappear with more prolonged residence at altitude, and indeed at very high altitudes ventilation continues to be regulated by oxygen lack.

Pugh has estimated that the adaptation achieved by an increase of ventilation is most effective between the altitudes of nine and fifteen thousand ft. In this range, acclimatization may increase the alveolar oxygen pressure by 8–9 mmHg, equivalent to a three to four thousand foot decrease of altitude.

Although the respiratory adjustments are generally beneficial, the diminution of alkaline reserve reduces the capacity of the blood to transport carbon dioxide from the active tissues. Fortunately, this loss of buffering power is largely offset by an increase of haemoglobin level; haemoglobin is also a very important blood buffer (p. 143).

Pulmonary Diffusion

West and his colleagues have carried out measurements of pulmonary diffusing capacity quite close to the summit of Everest. While the membrane properties are unaltered by altitude acclimatization, there is a small increase in the overall diffusing capacity due to (a) an increase in the haemoglobin content of the blood and (b) a speeding of the reaction rate θ at low oxygen pressures (see p. 138).

Blood Transport

Increases in the red cell count and haemoglobin level are well-recognised adaptations to high altitude. There is undoubtedly a long-term stimulation of erythropoiesis, much as occurs in the patient with congenital heart disease and in the chronic heavy smoker. An increased formation of red cells can be demonstrated within two hours of arrival at altitude; however, new production rarely raises the count by more than 1% to 2% per day, and the total adjustment of 50% seen at nineteen thousand ft. would require at least a month to achieve. Increases found on the first day at altitude thus reflect largely the initial decrease of plasma volume. If the subject continues at altitude, the plasma volume remains reduced, but the total blood volume is gradually restored by an increase of red cell mass.

Initially, rather immature red cells may be released into the circulation. These are larger than normal, with a poor haemoglobin content. However, when adaptation is complete, the haemoglobin content of individual cells is restored to normal, and the cells also have a normal life span.

The increased haemogobin content of unit volume of blood increases λ (p. 48) and thus the potential transport of oxygen by unit volume of blood. This advantage is offset by an increase in blood viscosity, which becomes of practical significance at haemoglobin levels above 20 gm/100 ml. (Fig. 36). In some animals such as the llama, a shift of the oxygen dissociation curve also helps the process of adaptation; however, in man any changes in the oxygen-binding properties of haemoglobin are small and unimportant.

At rest and during moderate work the heart rate and cardiac output revert towards sea-level values as the ventilation and haemoglobin level increase. The maximum cardiac output is depressed less as the normal blood volume is restored, but the sea level maximum heart rate is not attained even after prolonged periods at high altitudes.

The resident at altitudes of more than eight to ten thousand feet has a high pulmonary arterial pressure (pulmonary hypertension) and there are associated anatomical changes, particularly an increase in the muscularity of the pulmonary arterioles. Grover and his colleagues regard the hypertension as a "useful" adaptation, since it increases blood flow through the poorly perfused apical region of the lungs (p. 100).

Tissue Adaptations

The study of tissue adaptations to altitude is still in its infancy; to date, there is evidence of mitochondrial enlargement, with adaptive changes in respiratory enzyme systems and increases in the myoglobin content of muscle fibres. High altitude natives also incur a smaller oxygen debt than partially acclimatized athletes working at the same intensity of submaximal effort; this suggests that muscle blood flow or capillarity is greater in the permanent resident at high altitude.

Loss of Acclimatization

The Kenyan endurance athletes had an excellent performance in Mexico City, and this immediately raises the possibility of improving human endurance by training above the altitude at which a competition is planned.

On return to sea level there is an immediate resting hyper-ventilation, since there is a deficiency of buffers within the cerebrospinal fluid. This could well cause an athlete to overbreathe during a competition, leading to an excessive consumption of oxygen by the respiratory muscles. However, the return of medullary and cerebrospinal bicarbonate concentrations to appropriate sea-level readings is completed within a few hours.

The other main adaptive change to altitude (the increased red cell count) is a little more persistent, but two thirds of the increase developed at eighteen to twenty thousand feet is lost with as little as seventeen days residence at sea level; both a decrease in the production of red cells and an increase in the rate of destruction seem to be involved.

Relatively few athletes have tested the effect of altitude training on sea level performance, but there is some evidence that a small bonus is obtained on the first few days after return from a mountain training camp.

The High-Altitude Native

The discussion to this point has been restricted largely to the adaptations that occur when sea-level natives are moved to high altitudes. Many early investigations were based on the comparison of sea-level and high altitude natives. Such studies suffer from the usual difficulty encountered in cross-sectional comparisons—are the observed differences an expression of genetic endowment, or a genuine adaptation to an adverse environment? Until recently, many of the high altitude natives have been drawn from rather distinctive ethnic groups, such as the Sherpas. On the other hand, some of the observed differences from sea-level natives, such as a high haemoglobin level, mirror the pattern of response seen in more satisfactory "longitudinal" experiments. The relative contribution of genes and environment to anatomical peculiarities (increased lung volume, greater alveolar size, increased pulmonary capillary bed and greater heart size) is more problematical. There is some evidence that the chemoreceptors of the high altitude native show a reduced sensitivity to both CO_2 and oxygen lack, but again the basis of this adaptation (genetic or environmental) has yet to be resolved.

Altitude and Performance

Mexico City

Physiologists engaged in many attempts at predicting the likely loss of performance in the 1968 Olympic Games. The final concensus was based partly on previous athletic contests in Mexico City and Johannesburg and partly on physiological considerations. It was forecast that because of diminished air resistance, new records might be set in short-distance running and in throwing (discuss and javelin); times for events of intermediate distance would be near the expected level, and because of the diminution in maximum oxygen intake, endurance events would be impeded by 7 percent to 8 percent. Recovery from shorter events might also take longer than under sea-level conditions. The first two predictions proved correct, but even in endurance events the apparent loss of performance was often no more than 1 percent to 2 percent; in assessing such figures, allowance should be made for the continuing progression of athletic records (p. 380). Furthermore, many of the successful competitors were either high altitude natives such as the Kenyans or had spent long periods of training and acclimatization at comparable altitudes. Modifications of both pace and ventilatory pattern are essential to success in endurance events at altitude, and many of the competitors undoubtedly learnt the necessary new techniques through their substantial period of training at mountain camps.

Mountaineers

Mountaineers have maintained for many years that they can climb almost as fast at twenty thousand feet as at ten thousand feet. The disbelief of physiologists has now been quelled by measurements of energy expediture during climbing; irrespective of altitude, the typical rate of oxygen consumption is 25–30 ml/kg min. However, at sea level, this represents no more than 50 percent of the climber's power, whereas at twenty thousand feet it amounts to 80 or even 90 percent of his maximum oxygen intake. The possible duration of individual bouts of climbing thus decreases progressively with altitude, and frequent rest pauses become ever more essential. Pugh noted that on the higher slopes of Everest, the climbers found it necessary to stop as often as every twelve paces.

Industry

The highest industrial operations in the world are to be found in the Chilean sulphur mines (19,000 feet). The need for adequate initial acclimatization of employees with provision of living accommodation at lower altitudes has already been stressed. As with the mountaineers, the normal working limit of 50 percent of aerobic power is readily exceeded, and care must be taken to ensure that suitable rest pauses are introduced into the work schedule.

Oxygen and Performance

Physiological Changes

Let us suppose that oxygen is supplied to a subject working at eighteen thousand feet (380 mmHg pressure). Time is allowed for elimination of nitrogen. Assuming that the alveolar partial pressure of water vapour is 47 mmHg and that the corresponding CO_2 pressure is 40 mmHg, then the alveolar oxygen pressure must substantially exceed the sea level value of 100 mmHg. As would be predicted from the normal response to oxygen breathing (p. 363), the STPD ventilation and the heart rate in submaximum exercise are reduced, and may indeed fall below the anticipated sea level readings breathing air. The maximum heart rate also returns towards its sea-level value, and the maximum aerobic power is largely restored.

Sea-level alveolar oxygen pressures can be attained or exceeded by the use of efficient oxygen equipment up to 33,000 ft. At higher altitudes, the total ambient pressure is so low that the alveolar oxygen pressure inevitably falls. A subject breathing pure oxygen at forty thousand feet is in the same situation of oxygen lack as a man breathing air at ten thousand feet. If still higher altitudes are to be explored, it is mandatory that the pressure of respired gas should be increased by using some form of pressure breathing equipment (p. 98). Vapourization of tissue fluid occurs at 65 to 70,000 feet (depending on the temperature of the exposed parts) and at yet higher altitudes a full pressure-suit must be worn.

Oxygen Supply

Oxygen may be supplied by increasing the general ambient pressure (as in most aircraft and space vehicles), or by provision of personal oxygen equipment.

In the cabin of a standard commercial aircraft, the pressure is raised by a blower system. Compression of the air tends to make it hot, and refrigeration may be needed, particularly during take-off and climb in tropical regions. Humidification prevents respiratory discomfort in the dry air of the stratosphere, but during rapid descent misting may dangerously reduce a pilot's vision. A minimum ventilation of 10 cu ft/min should be provided for each passenger.

In spacecraft, a closed-circuit system is used, with replenishment of oxygen as it is used. In such a system, care must be taken to avoid accumulation of CO_2 and toxic vapours emanating from either the spacecraft or the human body (for instance, the degradation of haemoglobin to carbon monoxide).

Personal oxygen equipment is designed to maintain the alveolar oxygen pressure at or near the ground level value; alveolar oxygen pressures of more than 300 mmHg are best avoided because of certain hazards of oxygen toxicity (p. 151). The ideal mask supplies oxygen to the subject without imposing a noticeable resistance to breathing (p. 153). During normal use, the inspiratory effort should not exceed a suction of more than 5 cm H_2O. The dead space should be small, and the equipment should meet both the anticipated steady rate of gas flow and any high frequency transients such as occur during speech; a pilot's oxygen mask is thus designed to accomodate a steady flow of 50–100 litre/min, with peaks of 125–250 litre/min.

The demands of the climber are even more exacting. The specifications of all components of the breathing system, including reducing valves, regulators, tubing, connectors, and face-piece valves should be tested against maximum likely flow requirements.

Other desirable properties of a personal oxygen system include a good facepiece seal (to avoid leakage) appropriate air channelling (to avoid freezing of valves), a drain for saliva and condensed expirate, and good acoustic properties (without resonance or chatter of the valves).

Because of the penalty imposed by the weight of a gas cylinder, the carriage of oxygen by the mountain-climber is of advantage only at extreme altitudes. However, the design of a light-weight and efficient oxygen system undoubtedly played a role in the final conquest of Everest.

Medical Problems of Air Travel

The Healthy Individual

The speed of air travel creates environmental problems even for the healthy individual through transition from hot to cold climates and vice-versa, swift ascents to mountainous regions, and disruption of normal diurnal rhythms. However, the cabin altitude itself (8000 feet or less) is well-tolerated by a healthy person.

On emerging from an aircraft, the traveller may be confronted by a host of unfamiliar and aggressive microorganisms, and appropriate vaccination is thus a necessary prelude to travel. The voyager and/or his aircraft may also carry disease to the host country, and to avoid major epidemics, WHO International Sanitary Regulations require stringent quarantine arrangements against smallpox, cholera, plague, yellow fever, typhus, and relapsing fever.

Minor Abnormalities

Motion Sickness. Motion sickness arises from an excessive stimulation of position receptors in the inner ear. Some aircraft passengers are unduly sensitive to light turbulence. The problem seems exaggerated by anxiety, hyperventilation, air-swallowing, head movements, and attempts to read fine print. Affected individuals are usually helped markedly if a compound of the hyoscine class is taken immediately prior to travel. If possible, they should select a seat over the wing, on the left-hand side of the aisle; this is near the centre of gravity of the aircraft, and has the added advantage that spinning ground is invisible when the aircraft makes a normal right-hand turn.

Gas Expansion. Problems may arise from expansion of gas pockets within the body (dysbarism). Expansion of abdominal gas can give rise to colicky stomach pains. However, there is little relationship between the quantity of gas in the intestines (as seen on X-Ray film) and the reported sensations; much seems to depend upon the sensitivity of the individual. The initial problem can be minimized by avoiding carbonated drinks and other likely sources of gas, and the pain is usually relieved by belching or rectal evacuation of gas.

Expansion of trapped air in the teeth can give rise to a painful toothache (aerodontalgia); the wise traveller obtains a dental inspection before commencing a major journey.

Expansion of air within a blocked paranasal sinus can cause intense pain. However, the offending plug of mucus is usually forced from the sinus entrance during ascent. The traveller should be encouraged to blow any expelled mucus from his nose to avoid problems on descent. If he is suffering from a recent upper respiratory infection, a combined antihistamine/decongestant tablet may be a helpful prelude to travel.

Blockage of the Eustachian tube is potentially the most serious form of dysbarism. During ascent, gas can escape freely from the middle ear to the nasopharynx unless the tube is blocked by mucus or inflammatory swelling. However, during descent the increasing external pressure tends to collapse the relatively weak cartilaginous supports of the tube; this tendency must be reversed by deliberate swallowing, pulling the tube open through the action of the salpopharyngeus muscle. The critical pressure differential for complete collapse of the Eustachian tube is no more than 50–60 mmHg; if ignored, collapse can be followed by acute pain, haemorrhage, the formation of exudate within the middle ear and rupture of the ear drum.

Preventive measures include a preliminary decongestion of the nasopharynx in patients with upper respiratory infections, the waking of all passengers during descent, encouraging swallowing by provision of food or candy (sweets), and (except in emergency) minimizing the rate of descent of the cabin relative to the external altitude.

Chronic Disease

The small reduction of oxygen pressure within the cabin may prove critical for patients with diseases affecting the oxygen transport system (for example, anaemia, angina, heart failure, and chronic respiratory disease). Where possible, the condition of such individuals should be improved by appropriate medical treatment, and the extent of dsability should be evaluated by appropriate function tests. Commercial aircraft will provide an oxygen supply if this seems necessary; international regulations require a five minute supply of oxygen for all passengers, and a continuous supply of oxygen for 10 percent of passengers.

The combination of reduced oxygen pressure and the excitement attending a journey often increases the systemic blood pressure, and a mild sedative may be helpful in correcting this. There is a risk of haemorrhage- if the sea-level pressure is already high (hypertension) or the blood vessels are weakened by peptic ulceration or acute leukaemia. The coronary-prone individual may also succumb to his disease while in flight. The negro with sickle-cell anaemia may develop a splenic infarct, and several deaths have arisen from this cause at altitudes of around eight thousand feet. In view of the substantial incidence of the sickle-cell abnormality in negroes (~15%), the blood of negroid passengers should ideally be tested for this condition.

Lack of oxygen often worsens the condition of patients with mental disease, and may provoke attacks of epilepsy. The aircrew should be warned of any serious mental abnormality in a passenger, and appropriate sedation should be given, together with avoidance of in-flight alcohol.

The alteration of diurnal rhythms, unusual meals, and air sickness may together disturb an otherwise well-adjusted diabetic. Such a patient should carry his own supply of insulin and sugar, and make no attempt to adjust his feeding schedule until after the flight has been completed.

Expansion of abdominal gas can threaten a peptic ulcer with perforation; it may also cause a hernia to become incarcerated or a colostomy to expel its contents. The likelihood of these contingencies is reduced by measures to control abdominal gas (see above). Expansion of a pneumothorax may embarass both the circulation and respiration; a patient should thus avoid air travel within one week of the refilling of a pnemothorax. Occasionally, expansion of an unsuspected and partially calcified tuberculous cavity may cause haemorrhage or the spread of infection.

Despite these many possible medical hazards, most patients withstand air travel remarkably well, and indeed if adequate facilities for treatment are not available locally, air evacuation to a major hospital may be the procedure of choice.

References

Goddard, R.F.: *The International Symposium on the Effects of Altitude on Physical Performance.* Athletic Institute, U.S.A., 1967.

Margaria, R.: *Exercise at Altitude.* Dordrecht, Netherlands, Excerpta Medica Foundation, 1967.

Jokl, E., and Jokl, P.: *Exercise and Altitude.* Basel, Karger, 1968.

Scano, A., and Venerando, A.: Studi salla acclimatazione degli atleti Italiani a città del Messico. Rome, Italian Olympic Committee, 1968.

Faulkner, J.A.: Maximum exercise at medium altitude. In *Frontiers of Fitness.* Springfield, Thomas, 1971.

McFarland, R.A.: *Human Factors in Air Transportation.* New York, McGraw Hill, 1953.

Armstrong, H.J.: *Aerospace Medicine.* Baltimore, Williams and Wilkins, 1961.

9

UNDERWATER ACTIVITY

The problems of exercise at increased ambient pressure are being encountered by an increasingly large proportion of the total population, in such activities as recreational diving, tunnelling through swampy land, building the foundations of river and estuary bridges, escaping from submarines, and exploiting the ocean bed. The hazards depend on the type of equipment used, the personality and experience of the user, and the nature of any external dangers. While small increments of pressure are relatively harmless in tunnelling operations, there is no "safe" minimum depth for the diver. Drowning can occur in a few inches of water, and lung rupture is theoretically possible following submersion to no more than four or five feet.

Types of Equipment

Breath-hold Diving

The simplest approach to underwater exploration is to use no equipment, but to hold one's breath throughout the dive. This method has been used for centuries by the oriental pearl divers, and is remarkably successful if only a short period of submersion is required. In 1968, Croft reached a depth of 240 feet using no equipment other than contact lenses and saline-filled goggles; he remained underwater for 148 seconds.

The Traditional Diver

The traditional diver has worn an armoured helmet, breast-plate and weighted suit. The system is supplied with air from a surface line, fed by a compressor with an emergency reservoir tank. The power of the compressor must be increased as greater depths are explored; for instance, if it is intended to accomodate a respiratory demand of 50 litre/min BTPS, an airflow of 100 litre/min will be required at thirty-three ft, 200 litre/min at one hundred feet and 300 litre/min 165 ft. The compressor can be replaced by a battery of compressed air cylinders, but care must then be taken to ensure an adequate total gas supply to cover all emergencies. The heavy equipment and surface line greatly restrict mobility, but traditional equipment of this type is still used quite successfully for static underwater tasks such as salvage and construction.

At very great depths, there are dangers of both oxygen poisoning and nitrogen narcosis; in consequence, the nitrogen content of air is replaced by helium. It would be impracticable to supply large quantities of such an expensive gas, to the diver,* and accordingly a partial recirculation of air is arranged, expired gas being directed to a CO_2 absorbing soda-lime canister carried on the back.

Surface Demand System

The diver is connected by a mouthpiece and neutrally buoyant hosepipe to a demand valve at the surface. Because the buoyancy of the man is less than when wearing a traditional diving suit, it is possible to replace the weighted boots with fins, and in consequence mobility is greatly improved. On the other hand, the light surface line is vulnerable to kinking and fracture. It is thus a wise precaution to carry a small self-contained underwater breathing apparatus for emergency use.

Self-contained Open-circuit System

This system is widely used for recreational purposes. Gas is supplied via a demand valve from compressed air cylinders carried on the back. Exhaled gas is vented into the water. The main disadvantage is the limited endurance of cylinders when they are used in an open-circuit fashion; this precludes adherence to any lengthy decompression schedule, as may be required in commercial diving. From the military point of view, it is also unwise to provide a potential adversary with a tell-tale trail of bubbles.

It is difficult for a diver to read cylinder gauges while swimming, and accordingly exhaustion of the system is signalled by a valve that imposes a resistance to breathing; this valve is tripped when three quarters of the cylinder contents have been used.

---

* In North America, helium costs about $10 for 150 cu ft (150 x 28 litres); in Europe, the gas is much more expensive.

Economy of gas usage may be achieved if the diver breathes through a "snorkel" when he is close to the water surface.

Self-contained Closed-circuit Systems

Self-contained closed-circuit breathing apparatus is of two main types—pendulum and recirculating systems (Fig. 61). With either form of equipment, nitrogen should be flushed from the lungs and blood prior to use, in order to avoid diluting the oxygen content of the system. Oxygen is supplied to a 7 litre bag at a fixed rate of about 1 litre/min and excess gas escapes from a blow-off valve adjusted to a suitable excess over water pressure (10–30 cm H_2O).

The pendulum system has the advantage of simplicity, with no valves to maintain, and because of the bidirectional flow

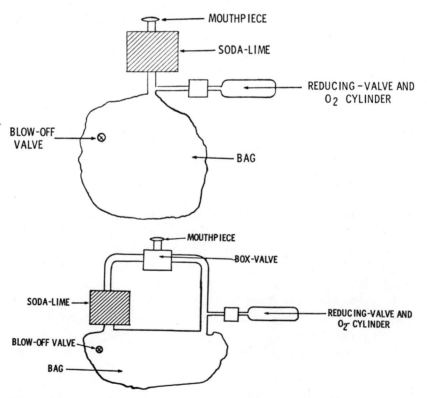

Figure 61. Self-contained closed-circuit underwater breathing systems. (*Top*) *Pendulum type.* (*Bottom*) *Recirculating system.*

the efficiency of CO_2 absorption is increased. On the other hand, there is inevitably a substantial dead space; this latter difficulty is avoided in the recirculating system.

The soda-lime canister holds about 1 kg of absorbent granules. This is sufficient to absorb 200 litres of carbon dioxide and it is thus exhausted in one to two hours, depending on the intensity of effort.

Because oxygen is used there is a risk of oxygen toxicity, and standard closed-circuit systems are not suitable for depths greater than twenty-five to thirty feet. The operating range can be extended by breathing mixtures of oxygen and nitrogen, so adjusted that the oxygen content of the bag does not fall below 20 percent even when the diver is developing an oxygen intake as large as 2 litre/min. At 140 feet, 40 percent oxygen is supplied at the increased flow rate of 8 litre/min and at 180 ft 32.5 percent oxygen is supplied at 13 litre/min. In the event that depth and duration of dive make this necessary, a decompression schedule is calculated as for an equivalent dive breathing air (p. 288).

Diving Clothing and Equipment

In warm and temperate waters, normal bathing trunks may provide adequate clothing, but a more formal diving suit provides both thermal insulation, and also protection against sharp objects such as coral and wreckage; if dark in colour it is reputed to discourage molestation by sharks.

A rubberized suit tends to trap air, and this can cause a subcutaneous "squeeze" (p. 276); at depth, compression of the air also largely destroys its insulating properties. Accordingly, it is useful to make provision for increasing suit inflation during a dive.

The "wet" suit is an alternative outfit. Since this is permeable to water, problems of a subcutaneous "squeeze" are avoided. Water is trapped beneath the suit and this tends to be warmed by the body, thus providing some thermal insulation. The main problems of a "wet" suit are loss of buoyancy, and discomfort when out of the water.

All equipment that is carried must be resistant to both water and external pressure. A reliable watch provides a check on cylinder endurance. A compass, depth gauge, and decompression sickness computer (Fig. 64) are other useful aids. Communication with the surface may be by radio and telephone, or by the simpler rope signals, message slates, and small explosive charges. Electrical equipment is safe while underwater, but a very dangerous short-circuit may occur on lifting equipment from the sea; regular checks of earthing and insulation must be maintained. Power tools are liable to propel the diver in a circle, and there is still a need to develop mechanical equipment that will exert minimal torque upon the operator.

The Caisson

When bridge-building, it is common to use a caisson. Compressed air is pumped into a rigid box to exclude water from a river or estuary while the foundations of a bridge are prepared (Fig. 62). Cement is also pumped into the caisson, and since the setting of

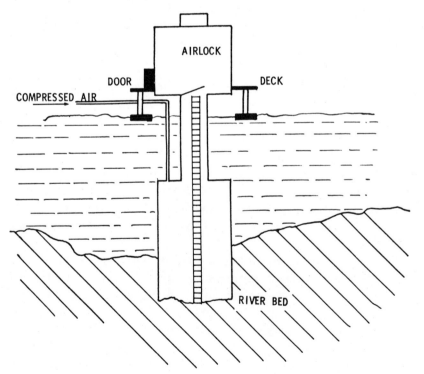

Figure 62. A simple caisson as used in bridge construction.

cement is an exothermal reaction, there is often a hot and humid environment at the working surface on the river bed. The pressure to which the builders are exposed depends on the depth of the river; in tidal waters, it may fluctuate by $\frac{1}{2}$ to 1 atmosphere over the course of a working day.

At the end of the shift, the workmen climb to a small lock at the top of the caisson, and are decompressed to normal ambient pressures. Within the lock, conditions are crowded, with a high CO_2 concentration, and a cold, clammy humidity. The men are impatient to leave, and often it is difficult to enforce prescribed rates of decompression.

The Tunnel

As in the caisson, pressure is needed to exclude water during construction; however, high pressures are required only at the immediate work-face, and finished sections of a tunnel can be held at an intermediate pressure. There is thus scope for a slow and progressive decompression to occur while the workers are walking from the work-face, showering and changing.

The Submarine

A submarine normally operates at sea-level pressures. However, in the event of damage, it must be flooded as a prelude to escape. Compression of gas leads to an undesirable concentration of atmospheric contaminants—particularly CO_2—and modern vessels thus contain a separate escape chamber with an independent supply of oxygen and nitrogen. The submariners must spend a substantial period at increased pressure, awaiting their turn to escape and the various physiological hazards of sustained high pressure (p. 277) may develop over this time.

If equipment such as the Davis escape apparatus is worn, the sailor can ascend relatively slowly, allowing time for decompression of inert gas. Normally, only a buoy is worn, and ascent is rapid (about 4 feet per second).

If the submarine is damaged in cold water, death from subsequent chilling is a serious possibility. The submariner is given an inflatable suit which provides some insulation, but he must use a nice judgment in balancing exhaustion of air within the escape compartment against the likely time of arrival of rescuing craft.

The Underwater Habitat. The need for extensive exploration of the continental shelf is leading to the design of underwater habitats. The aquanaut concerned is "saturated" with gas at an intermediate pressure (10–12 atmospheres), and makes periodic excursions to much greater depths. Typical schedules have ranged from two days at 432 feet to twenty-two days at 330 feet. By living at depth, the loss of working time through adherence to lengthy decompression schedules is much reduced. In designing living quarters, considerable thought must be devoted to prevention of fire. There have been several tragic conflagrations within high-pressure chambers, usually, traced to some minor source such as an electrical spark.

The Gill. Compartive physiologists have been fascinated by the possibility of developing a gill that would allow a man to derive oxygen from and excrete CO_2 freely into the surrounding water. Calculations to date suggest that survival would be technically possible, but that the necessary gill would be dangerously fragile and bulky, and would need exposure to a brisk stream of moving water.

Physiological Problems of Increasing Pressures

During a diving descent, there is a progressive and relatively rapid increase of ambient pressure. This produces many of the problems encountered during descent from altitude (baro-otitis, aerodontalgia, aerosinusitis, see p. 261) and may indeed compound difficulties of a recent air journey.* As with altitude exposure, the best approach seems to avoid deep diving during upper respiratory infections, and to keep the teeth in good condition.

If the breath is held during diving, either deliberately (breath-hold dive) or through inexperience (as in the use of self-contained underwater breathing equipment), the intrathoracic gas volume is compressed towards residual volume. Depending on the initial volume of gas in the lungs and the change of external pressure, the chest cage may be reduced to its minimum size without abolishing all the pressure differential between the water and lung gas. At the same time, the large capacity vessels of the legs are compressed, driving as much as a litre of blood into the lung vessels. The intravascular pressure rises and there is a tendency for the pulmonary vessels to rupture, with oedema

* For instance, one of the Canadian divers at the Edinburgh Commonwealth Games (1970) sustained a ruptured eardrum, and in her case there was reason to believe that the initial collapse of the eustachian tube developed on the flight from Canada.

formation and haemorrhage into the lungs. This syndrome is described as a "thoracic squeeze."

The same type of pressure differential may develop between other air pockets and blood vessels in the underlying skin. Thus, air may be trapped beneath rigid goggles, leading to conjunctival haemorrhage, bleeding into the eyelids, and even haemorrhage into the fat pocket behind the eyes (retro-orbital fossa). Air trapped beneath a tightly fitting waterproof immersion suit may cause haemorrhage into folds and ridges of skin over the trunk, while if the ears are covered, blood blisters may develop in the external auditory meatus and on the tympanic membrane.

There is a dramatic reduction of light intensity on passing beneath the water-surface, and divers can gain a substantial advantage from a preliminary period of dark adaption, wearing red goggles. The rod pigment rhodopsin (visual purple) is bleached by daylight, and a full resynthesis is required for "night" vision.

Physiological Problems of Maintained Pressure

If a man remains at increased ambient pressure for an extended period, problems arise from oxygen toxicity, inert gas narcosis, an increase in the work of breathing, retention of carbon dioxide, increased heat loss, and difficulty in communication.

Oxygen Toxicity

We have noted already (p. 151) that 100 percent oxygen has some toxicity if it is breathed for an extended period. Lung collapse occurs, due to pulmonary congestion, depression of the alveolar macrophages that normally form lung surfactant, oxidation of the unsaturated fatty acids used in surfactant production, and absorption of oxygen in occluded airways. There is also some retention of CO_2, pulmonary vasoconstriction, and an increase of pulmonary vascular permeability. These effects normally develop within twelve hours, and may occur in as short a time as six hours. Air compressed to more than 3 to 4 atmospheres contains a toxic pressure of oxygen, and if used for an extended period, it creates similar problems.

More severe toxic effects are encountered if 100 percent oxygen is breathed at high pressure. Initial symptoms include substernal distress, cough, nausea and pallor, with an increase of pulse rate and blood pressure. Laboratory evaluation shows a reduction in the vital capacity and a circumscription of the visual field. Changes of vital capacity provide a useful index of respiratory effects, while the visual changes reflect cerebral toxicity. If the initial signs and symptoms are ignored, the patient may develop convulsive seizures and/or a syncopal attack. At rest, two atmospheres of oxygen are tolerated for six hours, 3 atmospheres for three hours, and 4 atmospheres for some thirty minutes. However, these safety margins are greatly reduced by physical activity, and during exercise no more than thirty minutes can be tolerated at 3 atmospheres. The tolerance limit also seems less for the diver than for deliberate chamber exposures, and when swimming or diving with oxygen, a limit of one hour at a depth of no more than twenty-five feet is recommended.

> The cause of the cerebral changes is still debated. Carbon dioxide retention may play some role, since men who are acclimatized to CO_2 are more resistant to oxygen convulsions. A more important consideration is the inhibition of vital enzyme systems by either the high pressure of oxygen per se, or the associated "free radicals" that are produced. Possibly essential sulph-hydryl groups are oxidized. Vulnerable enzymes and metabolites include cytochrome c reductase, glutamic acid decarboxylase, GABA (gamma amino-butyric acid), and DPNH (diphenyl nitrohydrazine). GABA plays an important role in the normal functioning of the brain, and seizures are associated with low GABA levels. Further, GABA therapy protects against both lung damage and convulsions. It is thus tempting to assign the responsibility for oxygen toxicity to either a reduced formation of GABA (glutamic acid decarboxylase inhibition), or an enhanced breakdown of this metabolite. A further source of disturbed function may be the oxidation of structural lipids in the cell membranes. Removal of the adrenal and thyroid glands protect some animals against oxygen poisoning, but the mechanism remains obscure.

Inert Gas Narcosis

As early as 1835, Junod noted that when breathing compressed air "the functions of the brain are activated, imagination is lively, thoughts have peculiar charm, and in some persons symptoms of intoxication are present." Subsequent analysis of symptomatology has shown a similar chain of events to that encountered during exposure to hallucinogenic drugs. The highest functions of the brain including the capacity for self-criticism are inhibited, and a cheerful euphoria develops, often with an exaggeration of the normal personality. With very deep diving (300–400 feet), there may be a sense of impending black-out, manic or depressive states, and changes in sensory perception. There is also a marked dulling of mental ability, usually unappreciated by the individual. The state of the diver is potentially very dangerous, and if symptoms are ignored neuromuscular incoordination and loss of consciousness may occur. Recovery is rapid on decompression.

The depth at which functional loss is first seen depends upon the sensitivity of the test and the familiarity of the subjects with the evaluation procedure; loss of reasoning ability, reaction speed and manual dexterity is apparent in the first twelve minutes at one hundred feet (4 atmospheres); more prolonged exposures give difficulty with simple mental arithmetic and a decrease in the frequency at which a flickering light appears as a continuous source (flicker-fusion test).

> The basis of symptoms seems the increase in partial pressure of nitrogen in the respired gas. Other inert gases, such as xenon, argon, and krypton are even more narcotic and it is possible to draw a parallel between the lipid solubility of a given gas and its narcotic potency. This finding is reminiscent of the parallel between lipid solubility and potency of aliphatic anaesthetics. It suggests that inert gases behave essentially as anaesthetic agents, disturbing the conductance of cell membranes within the central nervous system. Details of the disturbance have yet to be agreed. Probably there is a solution of gas in the lipid phase of the membrane, and this may displace oxygen, leading to a type of histotoxic hypoxia. This in turn could cause a failure of the "sodium pump," with an alteration in the concentration of intracellular cations and a delay in the transfer of food materials from the supporting glia to the active nerve cells. Certainly, experimental studies show a sustained depression of neuronal transmission, with a depression of evoked potentials both at the lumbar synapses and also in the cerebral cortex.

At one time, accumulation of CO_2 and/or oxygen were thought to contribute significantly to the narcosis. Accumulation of carbon dioxide is a not uncommon problem in high pressure work.

The increased partial pressure of oxygen favours retention of carbon dioxide by the body, and this tendency is abetted by some restriction of external ventilation (secondary to both the increased density of respired gas and the resistance imposed by the water and breathing equipment). Defects of ventilatory pumps and/or inefficiency of CO_2 scrubbers may also impose an increasing inspired CO_2 concentration; whereas 0.25 percent CO_2 is unimportant at sea level, it becomes a very significant burden at three hundred feet. Certainly an excess of carbon dioxide could contribute to the depressed neural transmission, and there is some evidence that assisted ventilation diminishes the risk of narcosis. However, direct measurements of intracerebral gas pressures have failed to link inert gas toxicity with increases in either oxygen or carbon dioxide pressures.

It is technically possible to carry out diving operations to three hundred feet, breathing compressed air. However, because the average subject is not aware of the development of intoxication, very careful supervision is then required, and a less experienced team would do well to restrict themselves to a depth of one hundred feet or less. At greater depths, oxygen should be mixed with a relatively nontoxic gas such as hydrogen or helium. Hydrogen is unpopular because of the danger of explosions, and helium is commonly used. This has some advantages in terms of the work of breathing (see below), but unfortunately it also has a high thermal conductivity and thus leads to an increased heat loss in cold water. Bennett has studied the value of a number of drugs in preventing inert gas narcosis. The most promising are "Frenquel"-azacyclonal hydrochloride- and carbachol; however, further investigation is needed before these compounds can be recommended to divers.

Work of Breathing

Many factors conspire to increase the work of breathing at depth, until it imposes a significant limitation upon performance. The most important single consideration is the change in density of the respired gas. The turbulent component of airway resistance increases in proportion to $\sqrt{D}$, where D is the density of the breathing mixture. (p. 61). There is also an increase in the force required for convective acceleration of gas, as it passes from the lung spaces to the airways of narrower total cross section. In consequence, the pressure drop along the length of the airways is more rapid than at sea level, and the "equal pressure point" (Fig. 28) tends to be displaced peripherally, beyond the bronchi with cartilaginous supports. The diver thus has a low maximum expiratory flow rate while he is at depth and attempts at more vigorous expiration merely lead to collapse of the airway and "wasted" ventilatory effort. His remedies are twofold—to lengthen expiration at the expense of inspiration, thereby decreasing the expiratory pressure gradient, and to increase the mean chest volume, thereby strengthening the elastic forces resisting collapse.

Some ventilatory resistance is imposed by the viscosity of the water itself. In Snorkel-diving and other situations where the air pressure is less than the water pressure around the chest, the thoracic cage is compressed. The subject is forced to operate over an unfavourable part of his compliance curve (Fig. 29), and a much larger pressure is required to overcome elastic resistance; the airways are also narrowed and more liable to collapse, so that the viscous resistance to breathing is large. In other situations, the air pressure may exceed water pressure; the chest is then forced towards the inspiratory position. A small positive pressure may ease the work of breathing, but an excessive intrapulmonary pressure leads to an unnatural pattern of breathing with a forced expiration and relaxation during inspiration; the body responds by hyperventilation during rest and light activity.

All breathing equipment should have minimal resistance (p. 153). An external work-load that is well-tolerated at sea-level may become quite unbearable when the gas density is increased tenfold. The effect of more moderate external resistance depends on the location of the "equal pressure" point. If the diver has reached the maximum possible expiratory flow rate for a given gas density, and is "wasting" respiratory work in fruitless attempts to produce a greater flow, then a substantial external load may be accepted at little apparent cost to the work of breathing.

Accumulation of Carbon Dioxide

Even if a subject is not encumbered by breathing equipment, the increase in the work of breathing is sufficient to depress maximum voluntary ventilation; at one hundred feet, the M.V.V. is 50 percent of the sea-level value, and at four hundred to five hundred feet it is only 25 percent of the sea-level figure. The limits of sustained ventilation are poorly understood (p. 114), but it seems unlikely that an exercising diver breathing through valves, tubing and soda-lime canisters can develop more than 50 percent of his maximum voluntary ventilation over a fifteen minute period. Even assuming the diver is fortunate enough to have an M.V.V. of 200 litre/min he is thus restricted to an external ventilation of 25 litre/min BTPS when swimming at a depth of four hundred feet.

It is possible that the increased gas density worsens alveolar ventilation, both by slowing the diffusional exchange of alveolar and bronchial gas (p. 122), and also by enhancing inequality of ventilation. But even if alveolar ventilation remains as in exercise at sea level, it is no more than 80 percent of external ventilation, or 20 litre/min BTPS at four hundred feet.

> Let us suppose the diver is swimming at a speed of 1 knot per hour. His CO_2 production will approach 2 litre/min STPD and with an alveolar ventilation of 20 litre/min BTPS there is inevitably a pressure gradient of 86 mmHg between inspired and alveolar gas.[*]
> Let us further suppose that the dead space and other inefficiencies of the breathing equipment raise the inspired CO_2 concentration to 0.25% (18 mmHg at 10 atmospheres); the total alveolar CO_2 pressure then reaches the dangerously toxic level of 104 mmHg. It is hardly surprising that divers soon attain a tolerance to increased pressures of carbon dioxide, and that it is difficult to sustain vigorous work at extreme depths.

The problem of CO_2 retention is greatly reduced if all of the nitrogen and a part of the oxygen in the respired mixture are replaced by helium. The density of the inhaled gas is then reduced to a fifth of normal or less, and the turbulent resistance is reduced by at least $\sqrt{5}$; convective acceleration also demands less

[*] Irrespective of ambient pressure, $PA,{CO_2} = 863 \dfrac{\dot{V}E,{CO_2} \ (\text{litre/min STPD})}{\dot{V}A \ (\text{litre/min BTPS})}$

pressure, and the maximum expiratory flow rate is greatly improved. The main disadvantages of helium mixtures are a small increase in the viscous resistance to breathing and in increased body heat loss. By using a suitable mixture (at least 95% helium), a diver can sustain a CO_2 output of 2 litre/min at a depth of four hundred feet, and still keep the alveolar CO_2 tension within the relatively safe range of 50 to 60 mmHg.

The influence of increased oxygen pressures upon CO_2 retention has already been stressed (p. 151). A further complication in some habitual divers is an inadequate ventilatory response to exercise. This reflects partly a long-term change in the sensitivity of the respiratory centre, induced by repeated exposure to high partial pressures of CO_2, and partly a more immediate depression of the medulla by inert gas narcosis.

Other Physiological Problems

The convective conductance of heat increases with ambient pressure. This has implications for the ventilation of compressed air workings and for human thermoregulation. The thermal conductivity of helium is about six times that of air, and despite the effects of density and kinematic viscosity, it also has a greater convective conductance than air. Thus the insulating properties of "dry" diving suits are largely lost when the diver breathes helium mixtures at great depths. The thermally neutral temperature for water immersion is between 33° and 34°C, and these conditions are rarely met in diving. The temperature on the continental shelf is often around 10°C. During vigorous swimming, body heat production may be sufficient to prevent serious cooling, but during nominal rest periods added activity is often necessary to maintain body temperature. It is important to avoid shivering when using diving equipment, as this can lead to loss of control of the mouthpiece.

Clear speech is particularly vital to the success of team operations, since water visibility may not permit adequate hand signals. Unfortunately, the pressure of the water or gas on the cheeks, and of a helmet upon the jaw, coupled with the need to grip a mouthpiece or wear a resonant facemask all militate against intelligible speech. The problem is compounded by many sources of interference (the movement of clothing and equipment, the hissing of gas, and noise from shipping and marine life). The psychological tensions of diving further reduce the likelihood of either careful speech or careful listening. The use of helium adds a peculiar high-pitched resonance, at about 1.8 times the normal speech frequency. At sea level, the helium breather's voice sounds odd, but has a rather normal intelligibility (95–100%); at depths of more than one hundred feet, the loss of intelligibility seems worse in helium than in air, but the difference is difficult to document.

> Communication can be improved by the use of high fidelity microphones that will handle the high pitched speech. Others have proposed various methods of lowering the frequency of speech (such as recording the diver's voice and playing it back at half the recording speed, sampling of 50 percent of the tape, or lowering the frequency electronically by amplifying selected harmonics). Intelligibility is not improved by the use of filters, and surprisingly the low frequency sounds make a larger than normal contribution to communication. Perhaps the understanding of speech becomes unusually dependent on time cues provided by the low frequency sounds.

A diuresis commonly occurs on diving, and this can present problems if the subject is encased in a waterproof suit! The physiological mechanism seems an increase of central blood volume secondary to the increased external hydrostatic pressure; atrial stretch receptors are stimulated and inhibit secretion of the antidiuretic hormone of the pituitary gland.

Prolonged residence at depth imposes a substantial psychophysiological stress. Various measurements of this stress, such as the fall in eosinophil count and the excretion of 17-corticosteroids suggest that it reaches a maximum in three to five days. As in the arctic winter, so in diving exploration, there is a need for adaptation of the cerebral cortex to limited input of sensory information. Both the arctic adventurer and the diver are commonly afraid of becoming lost, and their happiness can be much increased by the use of simple direction markers.

The artificial atmosphere of an underwater habitat makes heavy demands upon air quality. Indeed, a small impurity such as carbon monoxide can have disastrous consequences even with simple compressed air diving. If several months of underwater residence are contemplated, then endurance may be limited by the need for CO_2 absorbent, which can fill much of the available space! Other vapours and fumes from body sources, cooking, machine lubricants and batteries can all accumulate in an alarming manner, and any material admitted to an underwater habitat must receive exhaustive screening for its potential toxicity.

Physiological Problems of Pressure Reduction

The main problem of ascent from diving or tunnelling operations is decompression sickness. If the ascent is too rapid, structural injury may occur in the lungs, and difficulty can also arise from expansion of abdominal gas as in ascent to altitude (p. 266).

Symptoms of Decompression Sickness

The symptoms of decompression sickness can develop after ascent from diving or during flight at cabin altitudes of more than 25,000 feet. There are slight differences in the clinical picture, since at altitude tissues that have become saturated with gas over a lifetime are decompressed, whereas in the diver, a relatively brief period is available to produce supersaturation. In the aviator, symptoms commonly arise in fatty tissues, and obesity predisposes to decompression sickness; in the diver, on the other hand, obesity is a less well-documented hazard, and lesions of the spinal cord and long bones are more common.

The release of gas bubbles during decompression was first noted by Boyle in the seventeenth Century. The clinical picture of decompression sickness was initially described in caisson workers by Pol and Watella (1854), and de Mericourt (1868) pointed out similar incidents in divers.

The most common complaint is the bends—a discomfort or pain in or near one of the large limb joints. This commences as a dull ache, during or for some hours after decompression. It may lead to clumsiness and weakness of the affected limb, and sometimes progresses to an unbearable pain with symptoms of secondary collapse (pallor, sweating, nausea, vomiting, and even loss of consciousness). The pain passes quickly on recompression, but if a second decompression is made within a few hours, there is often a recurrence at the same site. Residual stiffness and aching may persist for some days.

Skin lesions are more common in the aviator than the diver. There may be itching of the thigh, arms, and trunk, a mottled reddening of the skin (erythema) or a capillary (petechial) rash, and sometimes a patchy swelling of the subcutaneous tissue.

The *"Chokes"* is a more serious manifestation. This commences as a shortness of breath accompanied by a sense of oppression in the chest and a dry cough. The lungs feel overdistended, and there is a sense of suffocation. Respiration becomes rapid and shallow, with an "inspiratory catch," and there is sometimes a mottled cyanosis of the trunk. Collapse may follow.

Neurological symptoms are also a warning of dangerous sickness. In the aviator, the commonest neurological problem is a defect in part of the visual field—either a shimmering light or blindness. Often there is an accompanying migraine-like occipital headache. These symptoms persist for up to half an hour following recompression. In the diver, epileptiform attacks, temporary vertigo, and spastic paralysis of the legs have been described; however, their occurrence is rare, and the symptoms normally disappear if the patient is rapidly recompressed.

Collapse may be secondary to severely painful bends or other discomfort. It may also follow the chokes or neurological symptoms, and can arise as a primary phenomenon. The affected individual becomes pale, with a cold sweat on the extremities, a rapid and "thin" pulse, nausea, and syncope. Recovery occurs quickly upon recompression. More rarely, collapse may occur one to four hours after recompression; treatment is then more difficult, and occasionally death may result from circulatory or renal failure.

Bone necrosis is sometimes seen in divers or tunnellers some months after exposure. The areas particularly affected are the head and lower diaphysis of the long bones—the femur, tibia and humerus.

Pathology of Decompression Sickness

The essential pathology of decompression sickness is a supersaturation of the tissues with inert gas. When a certain excess pressure is developed relative to ambient air, bubbles form, intracellularly or extracellularly. Injury may be produced by disruption of tissues (intracellular bubbles) or by distortion (extracellular bubbles). Intravascular bubbles may occlude the circulation, and perivascular bubbles may cause arterial spasm.

Evidence for these statements includes (a) the preventive effect of a change in composition of respired gas (such as preliminary oxygen breathing by the aviator) (b) the prompt resolution of most symptoms by recompression, and (c) the preventive value of computers based on the theory of bubble formation.

Bubbles commonly develop in tissues such as periarticular fat, with a poor blood supply and a high nitrogen content. Symptoms may be precipitated or relieved by local factors such as exercise, heat and pressure. The relationship between bubble formation and symptoms is by no means linear, and a radiograph may disclose many bubbles within a joint or bursa despite the absence of symptoms.

The migraine-like attacks are thought due to a spasm of the cerebral vessels induced by perivascular bubbles.* The central nervous manifestations, including delayed shock, were once thought due to disruption of tissues by the gas bubbles, with either formation of fat emboli or release of toxic substances; however, the usual dramatic response to recompression suggests that the major responsibility again rests with bubble formation, probably intravascular emboli. Residual effects are probably attributable to irreversible changes in nervous tissue during the period of vascular occlusion, but fat emboli and anoxic damage to the pulmonary capillaries may contribute to the shock syndrome. The chokes are usually attributed to intravascular bubble formation, with occlusion of the pulmonary capillary bed.

Bubbles do not form immediately a tissue becomes supersaturated; as was recognized many years ago by Haldane and his colleagues, there is a critical ratio of tissue to ambient pressure, and if this is not exceeded then the diver is safe. Various authors have set this ratio at 1.75–2.25 to 1. The ratio is smallest for the most poorly perfused tissues, and may also be somewhat smaller for helium than for nitrogen.

The saturation of the tissues during a dive and the subsequent release of gas follows an exponential course. The exponent for

---

* In migraine visual disturbances may arise from spasm of the basilar artery.

any given tissue depends upon the ratio of local blood flow to the product of tissue volume and gas solubility (Fig. 63). In general, the times involved are quite lengthy. Equilibration is speeded by exercise, and because it has a lower solubility in fat, helium is eliminated from slowly decompressed tissues twice as rapidly as nitrogen. If a man breathes oxygen for five hours, he has still only eliminated 94 percent of body nitrogen. The times required for saturation of poorly perfused tissues are equally

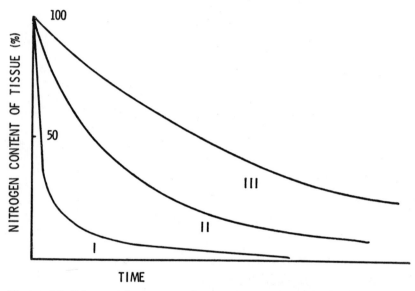

Figure 63. Schema of nitrogen elimination in a subject breathing pure oxygen. In tissue I, the ratio of blood flow to the product (tissue volume x N_2 solubility) is large, and elimination is rapid. In tissues II and III the ratio is smaller, and elimination is consequently much slower.

long, and a worker fails to reach the saturation point either in brief dives (10–30 min) or in the usual caisson shift (4 hours). The Canadian Navy has now developed a small pneumatic analogue computed (Fig. 64) that enables the diver to predict the gas content of different tissues, and thus the safety of further diving operations. The analogue represents the body by four small rigid compartments corresponding to the volume/ solubility product of different tissues. The apertures to individual compartments are suitably scaled to represent blood flow, and a gauge indicates the maximum pressure differential between ambient gas and any one of the four compartments. If this ratio exceeds 1.75 : 1, the diver halts his ascent until a safe pressure differential is indicated.

Once bubble-formation has occurred, the diver remains liable to a recurrence of decompression sickness in the affected region for several days. This is difficult to explain on normal curves of gas elimination, and it has been postulated that a bubble/tissue complex is formed with a very long half-time.

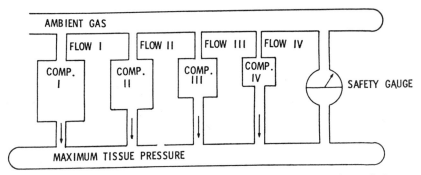

Figure 64. A pneumatic analogue used in monitoring the safety of diving operations. The four rigid compartments correspond to the volume/solubility products of different tissues, and the apertures are scaled to represent the corresponding regional blood flows.

Prevention of Decompression Sickness

Personnel Selection. Some individuals are more susceptible to decompression sickness than others, and the incidence of symptoms can thus be reduced by appropriate selection of personnel. Formal decompression tests are not necessarily helpful to the selection process, since susceptibility varies quite markedly from one occasion to another, and a highly paid diver or test-pilot may in any event fail to report symptoms for fear of losing his job; certainly, employment should not be restricted if a man develops minor bends, but a change of occupation may be desirable if more serious symptoms (chokes, migraine, or collapse) occur. The routine testing of aviators involves one hour's exposure to 25,000 feet (breathing oxygen), followed by one hour's exposure to 37,000 feet. The pattern of symptoms reported then includes bends (18%), collapse (impending and actual) 7%, chokes (0.4%) and neurological symptoms (0.4%).

Adjustment of breathing mixture. The aviator may be given preoxygenation (thus eliminating body nitrogen prior to ascent). Alternatively he may ascend slowly to a cabin altitude of 25,000 feet, eliminating nitrogen en route. The diver, particularly if operating from an underwater habitat, may change his gas mixture periodically, so that no foreign gas ever accumulates to a dangerous pressure, and he also may breathe oxygen during decompression.

Predisposing Factors. Exercise, heat, cold, oxygen lack, injury, infection, alcohol, recent previous exposure to inert gas, poor circulation (including ageing and lack of fitness) and obesity (in the aviator more than the diver) all increase the susceptibility to decompression sickness. Many of these factors are avoidable hazards to be noted in a preventive programme.

Acclimatization. There is some evidence that with repeated exposure to high pressures of foreign gas, the likelihood of decompression sickness is reduced. The physiological basis of such acclimatization is unknown.

Rate of ascent. Until recently, divers have relied upon a series of tables indicating the permissible rate of ascent according to depth and duration of exposure. The tables were originally devised for the British navy by Haldane, on the basis of experiments on goats. He found that if the "bends" developed in a major joint, a goat tended to hold the affected limb in a characteristic position, and on this rather tenuous basis he succeeded in drawing up an extensive series of diving tables that were used very successfully for many years.

Tables are still relevant to operations such as tunnelling, where the shift length and pressures are relatively constant. However, this type of approach is inefficient in free diving. Once a man has surfaced, he has no means of monitoring the subsequent behaviour of the tissues, and he is thus uncertain when it is safe for him to make a further descent. The possible frequency, duration, and depth of diving have been much extended by two recent developments—the Canadian navy analogue computer, and saturation diving (a technique where the worker eats and sleeps for several weeks at an intermediate but relatively high pressure).

Treatment of Decompression Sickness

Most forms of decompression sickness respond well to immediate recompression and a subsequent more gradual release of pressure. The administration of oxygen is generally recommended, although the beneficial effect of this gas upon nitrogen elimination is offset by an associated slowing of the circulation.

Many deep diving operations now include a pressure chamber for any necessary recompression therapy. Coastal bathing patrols might usefully locate the nearest facility of this type; in addition to military and commercial diving units, many large hospitals now have high pressure facilities.

Recompression does not lead to an immediate solution of the offending bubbles, but it does reduce their volume drastically—to 25 percent of the initial size at one hundred feet, and to 17 percent at 165 feet. This reduces the chance of permanent injury, particularly if there is compression or vascular occlusion within the central nervous system.

Any patient who complains of more than a simple attack of bends should be admitted to hospital, and observed for at least twenty-four hours. Delayed collapse is potentially very dangerous, and more than half of the first thirty reported cases were fatal. Medical treatment for shock and renal failure may be needed, including oxygen, intravenous fluids, cortisone, and dialysis.

Structural Injuries Arising From Gross Expansion of Gas

Trapped gas expands during decompression, and this can give rise to tissue injury, particularly in the lungs. The problem may occur during a diving ascent, a submarine escape, or the "explosive decompression" of an aircraft.

During submarine escape, no difficulty is likely unless the breath is held as the man ascends. If the glottis remains closed, the chest expands progressively to its inspiratory capacity, and a differential pressure then develops between lung gas on the one hand, and the water (and thus the circulatory system) on the other. Experiments on anaesthetized dogs suggest that the tissues will withstand a differential pressure of no more than 80 mmHg. If higher pressures are developed, the lung may rupture into the pleura (giving a pneumothorax), into the mediastinum (causing surgical emphysema), or into the pulmonary vessels (leading to air embolism). This last danger is the greatest, and depending upon the posture of the animal, and thus the intravascular distribution of gas bubbles, death from cerebral vascular occlusion is very likely.

The effective differential pressure can be reduced by applying external pressure to the chest, either by deliberate tensing of the respiratory muscles or by application of tight binders to the thorax. However, the most effective method of preventing injury is to teach the diver to exhale a constant stream of bubbles during ascent. This prevents laryngeal spasm, and at the same time reduces the gas content of the thorax. Submariners now undergo instruction in escape towers until they have mastered the appropriate technique. Formal escape apparatus such as the Davis equipment includes a valve that automatically releases gas from the breathing bag; however, accidents can still occur if the diver fails to exhale and indeed the number of mishaps is no less in escapes where apparatus has been worn.

Explosive decompression implies to the aviator a forced ascent at a rate of 5000 feet/min or greater. If an aircraft passenger is decompressed from sea level to an altitude of 40,000 feet, there must be a 7.6 fold expansion of gas within the lungs. However, the density of the gas is reduced, and for this reason there is normally little difficulty in carrying out what amounts to a forced expiration in the allotted time. Extremely rapid decompressions have been carried out on experimental animals. Dogs and rats have been "exploded" from eight thousand feet to 45,000 feet in 19 msec, and although there has been some haemorrhage in the ears, and partial collapse and haemorrhage into the lungs, there have been no fatalities. The extent of pathology has depended largely upon the patency of the airways. With even more rapid "explosions," the limiting factor becomes the capacity of the individual cells to alter in shape. Rats have been exploded from sea level to 65,000 feet in 12 m sec, and have sustained a variety of lesions, including emphysema-like changes in the lungs, congestion of the brain sinuses, rupture of the diaphragm, tearing of the kidneys, and myocardial damage from dilatation of the heart.

The rate of decompression has been relatively slow in most incidents affecting commercial aircraft; variables to be considered are the size of the hole relative to cabin volume, the power of emergency blowers, the pressure differential, and the ultimate liability of the passengers and crew to oxygen lack. The main hazard in the Comet disasters was thought to be the equivalent of a hurricane force wind (140 mph); this led to fracture of cabin furniture and secondary injury of passengers.

Other Problems of Underwater Activity

Selection for Diving Work

Many of the principles underlying selection of the diver have already been discussed. Since activity is to be vigorous and sustained, with an appropriate reserve of energy for emergencies, a good cardiorespiratory status is mandatory. The British Royal Navy sets an upper age limit of forty. Psychological stability is an important consideration, particularly if an emergency arises; some authors have suggested that those attracted to underwater activities often lack the stability of temperament necessary to both the diver and his partner.

Medical requirements are largely self-evident. The diver should be free of respiratory infection, and capable of venting his middle ear cavities. He should also have a normal musculoskeletal system, and be free of any condition adversely affected by severe exercise.

Energy Expenditure of the Swimmer

The energy consumption of any given swimmer is approximately proportional to his water speed (p. 538). An oxygen consumption of 1.5 litre/min is common at a speed of 1 knot per hour, and at higher velocities an individual may reach at least 90 percent of his maximum oxygen intake (p. 411). Lactate levels in maximum swimming are comparable with those in other forms of maximum effort but perhaps because of water pressure on the thorax, ventilation is somewhat smaller in the swimmer than in the runner.

Physiology of Breath-hold Diving

The danger of loss of consciousness during breath-hold diving has already been mentioned (p. 150). If the swimmer takes a

normal deep breath prior to a dive, several factors contribute
to the cessation of the breath-hold, including a rising CO_2 pressure in alveolar gas and arterial blood, a falling O_2 pressure and
a reduction of lung volume due to external water pressure, O_2
absorption, and displacement of blood from the limbs to the
thorax. When the breaking point is reached, the swimmer surfaces. The reduction of external pressure leads to an expansion
of the lungs and a rapid drop in alveolar pressures of O_2 and
CO_2. Nevertheless, the O_2 pressure does not drop low enough
to cause loss of consciousness, unless the duration of the breath-
hold has been deliberately extended by preliminary hyperventilation.

The commercial pearl diver of Japan, the Ama, shows a number of physiological adaptations over the course of the working
season, including an increase of vital capacity and forced expiratory volume, and a decreased ventilatory response to inhaled CO_2. Nevertheless, O_2 and CO_2 pressures at the breaking
point of a breath-hold dive remain much as in normal individuals
with little experience of diving.

Marine Injuries

The nature and risk of marine injuries varies with the local
ecology. In general, the hazards are greater in warm than in
cool water.

Injuries from coral may give rise to an urticarial reaction.
Stings from jellyfish, sea nettles, and Portugese man o'war cause
intense local pain, and in sensitive individuals they may give
rise to systemic reactions, including anaphylactic shock. One
particularly dangerous variety is the "Sea Wasp" (Chiropsal-
mus), found in North Australia and the Indian Ocean; this can
kill a man in as little as three minutes. First-aid treatment consists in removing as much of the tentacles as possible with a
cloth-covered hand, washing the affected area with water or
ammonia, and local application of antihistamine creams. If there
is a more general reaction, the physician may administer oral
antihistamines, and systemic and topical adrenocortical hormones.

Attacks from whales and sharks are rare unless the creatures are provoked by the swimmer. Nevertheless, both can cause dangerous bruising, and a shark bite may lead to a massive and fatal haemorrhage. It is thus prudent to regard any shark over four feet in length as dangerous, and to remain still until it has moved away. Antiriot chemicals such as "mace" are sometimes used as shark repellants. A bather may occasionally tread on a stingray. This leaves a sizeable ragged wound which must be cleaned and sutured, and the injected toxin may give a more general systemic reaction, requiring the usual medical treatment for shock.

Concussion is a fairly common hazard, both from diving into rocks or wrecks, and ascending into overhead obstructions such as boats or piers. Seaweed and other marine plants may enmesh the diver, preventing swimming.

The extent of these various dangers is much reduced by a watchful colleague. No one should dive or swim alone.

Infections

In warm weather, swimming and wading pools, shallow rivers and lakes, and associated changing rooms can all transmit infections to the swimmer.

Often, the infection is of a minor nature. Upper respiratory viruses are transmitted from the anterior nares to the water, the macerated skin of the external ear readily transmits and receives bacterial infections (otitis externa), and the wet floor of changing rooms serves to transfer fungal infections (athlete's foot). Adequate chlorination of the water, preliminary showering, inspection of bathers for overt infection, avoidance of overcrowding, and proper drainage of changing areas all reduce the frequency of such incidents. Occasional episodes have involved the transmission of more serious systemic infections such as typhoid fever and anterior poliomyelitis; particular watch must be kept for faecal contamination when bathing is permitted in shallow rivers and lakes.

Drowning

Drowning continues to take a heavy toll of life in many nations.

The physiological processes involved have now received extensive study. Initially, inhaled water irritates the bronchial tree and may give rise to both bronchospasm and breath-holding. However, with continued submersion, breathing returns, and the lungs become inundated with substantial quantities of both water and vomit. This leads in turn to hypoxia, hypercapnia and acidosis, with the usual chain of events seen in impaired gas exchange (a rise of blood pressure, a slowing of the heart, the development of arrhythmias, a fall of blood pressure, hyperpnoea, and terminal gasping).

The immediate picture is modified somewhat by the composition of the water. In fresh-water, the osmotic pressure of the inhaled fluid is less than that of the blood; water is thus drawn into the blood stream, leading to a fall of plasma sodium ion concentration. There is also some increase of plasma potassium, now attributed to tissue hypoxia rather than rupture of red cells. In salt water drowning, these processes are reversed; fluid is drawn from the blood into the lungs, with a rise of plasma sodium and a general haemoconcentration. The likelihood of ventricular fibrillation is increased by a drop in plasma sodium concentration, so that arrhythmias are more likely in fresh than in salt water. Indeed, mice survive the filling of their lungs with buffered saline for as long as eighteen hours, providing that oxygen is supplied under high pressure. For this reason, some authorities have recommended that bathing pools should be filled with saline.

In man, drowning differs somewhat from that seen in experimental animals. There are less changes of blood composition, the liability to ventricular fibrillation is greater than in some small mammals, and there is more likelihood of secondary problems such as "shock" and pulmonary oedema. As many as 25 percent of clinical cases of "near-drowning" later succumb to secondary complications.

The immediate first-aid treatment of a drowning person should consist of removal to a place of safety, with rapid application of artificial respiration by an accepted technique (p. 157). Obvious debris should be removed from the mouth and throat, but time should not be wasted in fruitless attempts to drain water from the lungs. Bronchospasm and a decrease of lung compliance make necessary the use of quite high ventilatory pressures. If the pulse has stopped, cardiac massage (p. 78) or defibrillation (p. 77) will be needed. A suitably trained first-aid worker can carry out adequate cardiac massage until more formal medical treatment can be instituted.

Blood samples may be drawn to test for disturbances of electrolyte balance, and appropriate remedial infusions can be given. However, current clinical opinion attaches more importance to the acid/base status of the victim than to sodium and potassium balance; infusions of bicarbonate may thus prove useful. Pulmonary oedema seems a reaction to the irritant contents of swimming pool water. Antibiotics may be helpful in preventing secondary infections and at this stage administration of plasma may be needed to maintain the circulating blood volume. Bronchospasm may be sufficiently intense to require treatment with bronchodilators. It should be emphasized that once the victim has reached hospital, there is usually little difference between fresh water and salt water drowning, and careful treatment of either type of casualty is essential to subsequent survival.

References

Duffner, G.J., and Lanphier, E.H.: Medicine and science in sport diving. In Johnson, W.R. (Ed.): *Science and Medicine of Exercise and Sports.* New York, Harper, 1960.

Miles, S.: *Underwater Medicine.* London, Staples Press, 1962.

Lambertsen, C.J.: *Underwater Physiology.* Baltimore, Williams and Wilkins, 1967.

Bennett, P.B.: *The Aetiology of Compressed Air Intoxication and Inert Gas Narcosis.* Oxford, Pergamon, 1966.

Bennett, P.B., and Elliott, D.H.: *The Physiology and Medicine of Diving and Compressed Air Work.* London, Baillière Tindall and Cassell, 1969.

10

HOT AND COLD CLIMATES

Mechanisms of Heat Exchange

The Homiothermic Condition

Reptiles, insects and various "lower" forms of animal life are *poikilothermic*—their body temperature varies almost directly with that of the external environment. In contrast, birds and mammals are *homiothermic*, maintaining a practically constant body temperature in the face of wide variations in their thermal environment. Advantages and disadvantages of the homiothermic condition have already been discussed briefly (p. x).

Although many people regard the human body temperature as maintaining a constant value of 98.6°F, this reading is no more than the average resting oral temperature. The rectal temperature is commonly 0.5°F higher, and both oral and rectal temperatures show a diurnal variation of about 1°F. The diurnal change is probably related to parallel variations in the level of arousal, and hence changes of muscle tone induced through the γ loop mechanism (p. 173). If a man is engaged on shift work, the normal rhythm of both temperature and arousal is reversed, high temperatures being recorded at the end of the night rather than at the end of the day. Women show a significant variation of body temperature with the oestrus cycle; there is a slight fall at the time of menstruation, and a rise of almost 1°F coincident with ovulation. Much larger changes of temperature are induced by exercise, fever, and heat exposure. The highest temperature compatible with full recovery of cerebral function is about 107°F, although in patients with fatal hyperpyrexia terminal readings as high as 110°F have been recorded. Only limited chilling is compatible with safety; recovery from accidental cold exposure is likely if the body temperature does not fall below 90°F.

Despite the limited range of permissible body temperatures, man has a very varied rate of heat production. Under basal conditions, the heat of metabolism is about 1.1–1.2 kcal/min (1 kcal is the energy required to raise 1 kg of water through 1°C). During maximum effort, an athlete may increase his energy expenditure to 30 kcal/min; even supposing that 25 percent of this energy is converted to useful work, the remaining 22.5 kcal/min must appear as heat. A delicate adjustment of the heat exchange between a man and his immediate environment is thus essential to meet the normal range of human activity; the exchange proceeds continually by several routes—conduction, radiation, convection and evaporation.

Conduction

Conduction implies the transfer of heat to and from the skin by direct contact, without the interposition of air. Normally, it accounts for only a small component of the total heat transfer, due to the insulation provided by clothing. However, appreciable quantities of heat may be conducted to the body when a man walks barefoot on hot sand or when he sits on an overheated car seat wearing only light clothing; conversely, a combination of conduction and convection lead to quite rapid heat loss on immersion in cold water.

Radiation

Radiation implies the transfer of heat as a wave motion. All objects radiate energy, at a rate dependent on the nature of their surface and the absolute temperature. However, it is convenient to distinguish the low temperature radiation of terrestrial objects (~300°K, 20–50°C) from high temperature solar radiation. Low temperature radiation has a relatively long (infra-red) wavelength, and most surfaces have a large emissivity at these wavelengths; this means that they emit and absorb radiation much as a black surface, with little reflection. Whether heat is gained or lost from an object depends simply on its absolute temperature and its geometric relationship to surrounding surfaces. Thus, when a man is sitting indoors under temperate conditions, the wall temperature is lower than that of his skin and overlying clothing, and the body loses heat by radiation. Conversely, in a tropical climate, wall temperature often exceeds skin temperature and the body then gains heat from the walls of the building.

Radiant heat gain reaches a maximum when a man steps out of the shadows into the direct path of the sun's rays. Owing to the very high temperature of the sun, outward radiation from the man to the sun can be neglected. The wavelengths of solar radiation are shorter than for the terrestrial radiator, and for this reason appreciable amounts of energy are reflected from the skin and from light coloured clothing.

The thermal load imposed upon a human subject can be expressed as the *mean radiant temperature,* measured by a radiometer or a thermometer enclosed in a black globe. In the latter case, allowance must be made for air temperature and air movement (corrected effective temperature, p. 305). The globe thermometer may overestimate the stress in sunlight, since it absorbs nearly all of the incident radiation, and presents a larger relative surface to the sun than does a standing man. The globe can be painted a suitable shade of gray to adjust for an individual's skin reflectance and postural effects; the modified globe still functions as a "black" surface with respect to the lower frequency radiations from terrestrial objects.

Convection

Convection implies the forced transfer of heat induced by movement of gas or fluid. In the context of human heat exchange, there are three main barriers to convection—the subcutaneous fat, clothing, and a film of stationary air or water in immediate contact with the clothing. The rate of heat transfer thus depends on the temperature gradient across each of these impedances, the thermal conductivity of the convected matter, and the total convective flow across the barrier.

In the case of subcutaneous fat, the thickness of the barrier and the thermal conductivity of the blood are relatively fixed quantities, and heat transfer varies according to the temperature gradient from the core of the body to the skin surface and the rate of skin blood flow.

Heat loss at the surface of the skin or clothing is increased by wind or water movement, running and swimming; since the "stationary" film of air or water is disturbed, convective currents across the film are increased thereby. Heat loss is also increased if the normal ambient air is replaced by a gas such as helium, with a high thermal conductivity (p. 283). At high altitudes, the number of molecules of gas per unit volume of the "stationary" film is less, and the impedance to heat transfer is thus increased. Conversely, the number of molecules per unit volume of gas is increased at depth, and this compounds the problem of maintaining body temperature in the diver.

Evaporation

Evaporation of 1g of water requires about 0.58 kcal of energy (the latent heat of vaporisation). The body normally loses heat through diffusion of water vapour across the skin surface (insensible perspiration) and the membranes of the respiratory tract. In an exercising subject, there is also a substantial evaporation of sweat and any externally applied water. In order to lose heat, sweat must be not only secreted but also evaporated. Light clothing may thus be helpful in a hot climate, providing an extended wick-like surface from which evaporation can occur, while at the same time conserving sweat that might otherwise have accumulated as a useless pool on the floor.

The rate of evaporation depends on the gradient of water vapour pressure across the film of stationary air surrounding the skin and on the thickness of this stationary film. An increase of atmospheric pressure impedes the movement of water vapour molecules, and the converse is true of low ambient pressures.

The evaporative loss from the lungs depends on the BTPS ventilation, the dryness of the atmosphere, and the barometric pressure. When men are working hard in the dry air of high mountains, the loss may amount to as much as five to seven pints per day (p. 240); this is a substantial load in terms of both heat loss (1300–1800 kcal) and fluid replacement.

The Influence of Clothing on Heat Transfer

The main function of clothing is to impose an additional impedance to heat loss, supplementing the "stationary" air film in contact with the skin. Insulation is achieved largely by virtue

of air trapped in the clothing, and is independent of the type
of fibre used.* The efficiency of clothing was originally rated
in arbitrary *"clo" units*. One clo provides sufficient insulation for
the indefinite comfort of a man sitting in a room heated to
21°C, with an air movement of twenty feet per minute, and a
relative humidity of less than 50 percent. This corresponds quite
closely with normal British domestic life, from which we may
deduce that the indoor clothing popular in Britain provides
1 clo of insulation. The corresponding thickness of clothing is
about a quarter of an inch.

> More recently, garments have been evaluated in physical terms,
> and rated in terms of the temperature difference required to produce
> unit flow of heat. 1 clo is equal to an insulation of 0.18°C m² hr/
> kcal. The insulating properties of clothing may be useful not only
> in the cold, but also in a hot environment, protecting an individual
> against heat gain by radiation and convection. A loosely fitting
> porous garment is most appropriate for the latter purpose. At one
> time it was thought that brain damage could result from a direct
> penetration of the skull by radiant energy; this seems the basis of
> the picturesque helmet and spine pads of the colonial tropical uni-
> form. Unfortunately, there is no evidence that such helmets serve
> more than a tourist attracting function.

Clothing may present an appreciable barrier to the transfer
of water vapour from the skin surface to the atmosphere. Fibres
that will "wet" transfer sweat fairly readily, and conserve fluid
that would otherwise drip from the body; on the other hand,
closely woven nylon garments offer an almost insuperable barrier, and nylon clothing has contributed appreciably to heat-
related incidents during football games in the southern United
States.

The Concept of Heat Balance

The Equations of Heat Balance

The body reaches a state of equilibrium with its environment
when metabolic heat production (M) is balanced by the

---

* However, a high wind penetrates loosely woven material, displacing the
trapped air and destroying insulation. Clothing for arctic conditions should
therefore include an outer windproof layer.

algebraic sum of heat transferred by convection (C), radiation (R), conduction (K) and evaporation of water (E)

$$M = E \pm C \pm R \pm K$$

Equilibrium may not be reached for several hours following a change in environmental conditions, and during the period of adjustment heat may be either lost from or stored within the body. The average specific heat of the body tissues is about 0.83 (that is, 0.83 kcal of energy are needed to raise 1 kg of tissue through 1° C). Thus, if we denote heat storage by S, we may rewrite our equation of heat balance as:

$$M - S = E \pm C \pm R \pm K$$

The situation may be complicated by a change of body mass due to sweating; in absolute terms, the thermal capacity of the body is reduced, although this does not necessarily disturb the equilibrium as defined by our equations. During exercise, useful external work W is also performed. The equation then reads:

$$M - S - W = E \pm C \pm R \pm K$$

The Assessment of Heat Balance

In order to draw up a heat balance sheet, it is necessary to assign values to our various constants. The metabolic heat production (M) is readily calculated from the overall oxygen consumption and the respiratory quotient (p. 558); for many purposes it is sufficient to assume that an oxygen intake of 1 litre/min measured under STPD conditions, is equivalent to a heat production of 5 kcal/min. The external work (W) may also be determined for many forms of exercise (p. 20). The greatest problem is presented by heat storage (S). Where can the change of body temperature be measured? Virtually all possible body apertures have been used to test core temperature; unsuspecting subjects have had thermometers or thermocouples thrust into the mouth, oesophagus, rectum, bladder, ear drum, and stomach. Unfortunately, all possible techniques are open to a number of criticisms (p. 425).

In order to calculate changes in heat storage, it is necessary to take account of both core and skin temperatures; the equation commonly used is:

$$S = 0.83W \left[(0.65 Tr_1 + 0.35\ Ts_1) - (0.65\ Tr_2 + 0.35\ Ts_2) \right]$$

where W is the body weight, Tr_1 and Tr_2 are the initial and final rectal temperatures, and Ts_1 and Ts_2 are the initial and final skin temperatures. The skin temperature itself must be a suitably weighted average of readings obtained from many body sites; Newburgh has suggested the following weightings: head—7 percent, arms—14 percent, hands—5 percent, trunk—35 percent, thighs—19 percent, legs—13 percent, and feet—7 percent.

The main route of heat loss during exercise in either a temperate or a warm climate is evaporation. The sweat loss can be calculated quite simply by weighing the subject, and correcting for the intake of food and fluids and the voiding of urine and faeces. Providing that all sweat is evaporated, the change in body weight is proportional to the evaporative heat loss. It is very difficult to obtain accurate figures for conduction, convection and radiation, but an overall impression of the stress imposed by a given climate can be obtained from the various indices of effective temperature discussed below.

The Assessment of Climate

Air Temperature. The air temperature is measured by a standard mercury thermometer, shielded from any large source of radiant energy.

Relative Humidity. The simplest method of measuring relative humidity is a sling psychrometer. The bulb of a mercury thermometer is surrounded by moistened gauze and whirled through the air to evaporate the water and obtain the wet bulb temperature. If the air temperature is also known, the relative humidity and absolute water vapour pressure can then be obtained from tables. In more sophisticated psychrometers, air is drawn over the moistened thermometer bulb by a small electric motor. Continuously recording psychrometers are commonly based on wet and dry junction thermocouples, but sometimes use the simpler expedient of a fibre that changes length with humidity.

Air Movement. The speed of air movement is conveniently recorded by a hot-wire anemometer. Convection and evaporation both increase with air speed.

Radiant Temperature. The use of a black or grey globe thermometer to assess the mean radiant temperature has been discussed above.

Effective Temperature. The severity of the thermal stress imposed by various combinations of relative humidity, wind speed, and radiant energy is conveniently expressed as a single index, the "effective temperature." This scale is based on the subjective comparison of various environments, and it refers to an equivalent temperature for still air saturated with water vapour (Fig. 65). The original nomograms for the calculation of effective temperature ignored the problem of radiant energy, but an appropriate allowance can be made for radiation if the globe temperature is measured in place of the dry bulb tem-

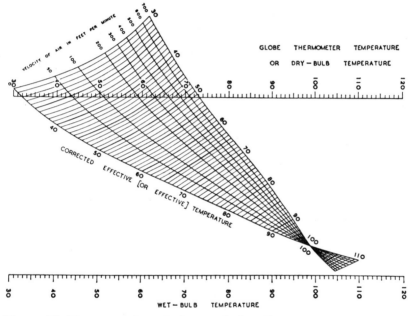

Figure 65. Nomogram for calculation of the effective temperature (men stripped to the waist and performing moderate activity). Copyright American Society of Heating, Refrigerating and Air Conditioning Engineers. Reprinted by permission from ASHRAE Handbook of Fundamentals, 1967.

perature (Fig. 65). The reading thus obtained is described as the "*corrected effective temperature.*" The subjective assessments used in creating the effective temperature scale were made on men stripped to the waist and performing moderate work. A rather different ("normal") scale is used when subjects are wearing indoor clothing, and some further modification is desirable when very vigorous exercise is to be performed.

The WBGT Index

An alternative and rather simpler method of synthesizing wet bulb, dry bulb and globe thermometer readings was proposed by Minard. He developed the wet bulb globe temperature index (WBGT) as follows:

For men outdoors　　WBGT = 0.7 (WBT) + 0.2 (GT) + 0.1 (DBT)

For men indoors　　WBGT = 0.7 (WBT) + 0.3 (DBT)

where WBT, GT, and DBT are the wet bulb, globe, and dry bulb temperatures respectively. The index was designed initially for the United States Marine Corps, and it refers to men carrying out normal duties while wearing standard United States combat uniforms; if violent athletic practice is contemplated, or impermeable clothing is worn, the limits suggested may thus impose an excessive heat stress.

Minard recommended that caution should be observed if the index surpassed 82, that the activity of unacclimatized men should be restricted at an index of 85, that all except fully acclimatized individuals should limit their effort at an index of 88, and that outdoor activity should be replaced by lectures and demonstrations when the index exceeded 90.

A Comfortable Environment

The environment is comfortable when a man is neither gaining nor losing heat. The ideal temperature thus depends on the extent of activity that is contemplated, the amount of clothing to be worn, and any acclimatization of the individual to a hot or a cold environment. The sedentary office worker commonly prefers a temperature of 70° to 75°F, while a range of 65° to 70°F is more comfortable in a factory requiring moderate activity.

A water temperature of 90° to 92°F is comfortable for a completely inactive person, but 75° to 80°F is a reasonable temperature for a swimming pool where vigorous activity is anticipated (higher temperatures are also undesirable in a pool, since they favour more rapid bacterial growth).

Mechanisms of Thermal Regulation

Thermal Regulation in a Comfortable Environment

The resting metabolic heat is partially dissipated through insensible water loss; evaporation through the skin is not less than 0.5 litre/day, and losses from the respiratory tract add a further 0.3 litre/day. The minimum evaporation is thus about 0.5 ml/min, corresponding to about a half of the resting heat production. The residual heat loss occurs by radiation and convection, and is adjusted through changes in skin temperature. If the environmental temperature falls, heat losses by radiation and convection initially increase, and there is thus a slight immediate fall of temperature at the body surface. The increased thermal gradient from the core to the skin in turn tends to increase heat loss, but an appropriate reduction of skin blood flow rapidly reduces heat transport to its previous level. Equilibrium is now restored at the expense of a lower skin temperature, and possibly a small reduction of core temperature.

Conversely, if activity is increased, there is a tendency for core temperature to rise. Skin blood flow is then increased, and because both flow and thermal gradient are greater than normal, more heat is transported to the body surface. In consequence, the skin temperature rises and heat loss by radiation and convection is inevitably increased. However, the major basis of adjustment to physical activity is through an increase in sweat production (Figs. 66 and 67). At equilibrium, the core temperature is raised by an amount proportional to the relative intensity of exercise. Thus, Saltin and his colleagues found an oesophageal temperature of 37.3°C in subjects exercising at 25 percent of aerobic power, with readings of 38.0°C and 38.5°C at 50 percent and 75 percent of aerobic power respectively. Rectal temperatures were about 0.1°C higher than the oesophageal readings, and muscle temperatures were 0.6° to 0.8°C higher still. These findings imply that a physically fit individual with a large aerobic power can sustain a given rate of working with a lesser rise of body temperature than a man who is unfit. It is unlikely that there are great differences of radiant or convective heat loss

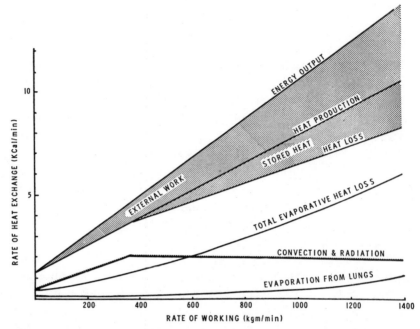

Figure 66. The several routes of heat transfer during physical activity in a temperate climate (based on data of Nielsen).

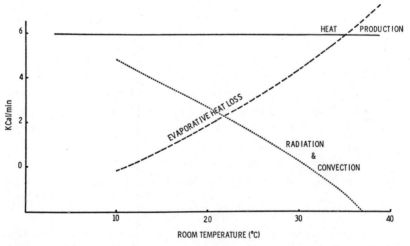

Figure 67. The influence of room temperature upon the relative proportion of the total heat loss dissipated by evaporation. Nude subject, exercising at a load of 900 kgm/min. Based on data of Nielsen (1938).

between fit and unfit subjects, and we may thus presume that the well-trained individual sweats more at a given absolute rate of working. This presumption is borne out when the rate of sweat loss is measured by weighing. Although the body temperature of the athlete is lower during moderate effort, he also has a surprising tolerance for very high core temperatures during prolonged and exhausting effort. Pugh has observed rectal temperatures of 41°C and more in marathon runners competing at an environmental temperature of 23°C.

> Both sweating and skin blood flow are regulated primarily by centres in the hypothalamus; the anterior hypothalamus responds to the temperature of the perfusing blood, and is most active when body temperature is rising. The posterior hypothalamus contains a coordinating centre for cutaneous temperature receptors, and is most active when body temperature is falling. Zotterman has identified specific cutaneous receptors for cold and heat. The cold fibres reach a peak discharge at a skin temperature of 25° to 30°C, and their activity rapidly ceases at higher temperatures. The "warm" fibres commence to discharge at 25° to 30°C, and reach a maximum activity at about 40°C; above 45°C, their activity also ceases, but the cold fibres may show a "paradoxical" discharge (accounting for the phenomenon of shivering on entering a hot bath). Both types of fibre adapt rapidly. This is best appreciated on jumping into a cool lake; the cold receptors initially make a brisk protest, but soon the water feels quite pleasant. Efferent fibres pass to the cutaneous blood vessels and the sweat glands; cold also increases the discharge of motor fibres (leading to shivering) and (particularly in smaller animals) stimulates metabolism through an increased output of thyrotropic and adrenotropic hormones from the pituitary gland.

The normal "setting" of the thermoregulatory mechanism corresponds to a hypothalamic temperature of 37°C (98.6°F). Cooling of the skin stimulates the cold receptors, raising this setting and bringing cold conserving mechanisms into play. Conversely, heating of the skin lowers the setting. Both exercise and bacterial "pyrogens" raise the temperature to which regulation occurs.

Sweating seems influenced by both skin and hypothalamic temperatures (Fig. 68). It may in turn influence the blood supply to the skin, through local cooling and the associated secretion of a bradykinin-like vasodilator substance.

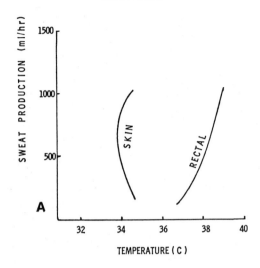

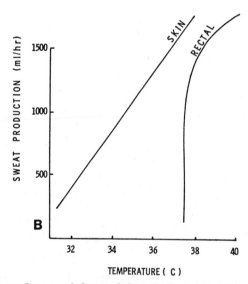

Figure 68. The influence of skin and deep body temperature on sweat rate. Based on data of Robinson. (a) Varying rate of working; (b) Constant rate of working, but varying environmental conditions. Based on material in *Physiology of Heat Regulation and the Science of Clothing*, Division of Medical Sciences, National Academy of Sciences—National Research Council, Washington, D.C., 1957. By permission of author and publishers (Saunders).

Thermal Regulation in Warm Conditions

Whether a clothed man is active or not, under warm conditions (>80°F) his thermal regulation is dependent largely upon evaporation of sweat. The internal impedance to heat transfer is also minimised by a massive dilatation of the blood vessels supplying the skin. This involves both a release of constrictor tone in the sympathetically innervated vessels of the hands and feet, and an active dilatation of vessels in the trunk and proximal parts of the limb. As much as a quarter of the cardiac output may be diverted to the skin in near maximum exercise; this in effect acts as an arteriovenous shunt, and it limits the maximum attainable arterio-venous oxygen difference (p. 96).

During the first few minutes of vigorous activity in the heat, the maximum oxygen intake does not differ from that found under more temperate conditions. However, the pulse rate is substantially greater at a given submaximal effort, and the stroke volume is correspondingly reduced. The diversion of blood away from visceral organs (p. 97) is also greater under hot conditions.

The maximum rate of sweat production (1–2 litres per hour) is sufficiently large that activity is normally limited by the ability to evaporate sweat rather than by the ability to produce it (Table IV). Providing the added burden of radiant heating is avoided, the hot dry climate of a desert is tolerated much better than the hot wet climate of a jungle region. The rate of evaporation of sweat normally depends on (a) the skin temperature, (b) the absolute water vapour pressure in ambient air, and (c) the rate of air movement; however, until the skin is completely wetted, the area of the sweat film is the controlling factor.

TABLE IV

EXPECTED WEIGHT LOSS OF 90 KG ATHLETE DURING NINETY MINUTE GAME UNDER CONDITIONS SPECIFIED

Temperature (°F)	Relative Humidity			
	40%	40%–60%	60%–80%	80%–100%
100	2.7	3.1	3.3	3.5
90	2.3	2.6	2.8	3.1
80	1.8	2.2	2.4	2.6
70	1.4	1.7	1.9	2.2
60	0.3	0.5	0.7	0.9

If the evaporative heat loss is insufficient for equilibrium, skin and core temperatures rise; the rate of evaporation of sweat is increased thereby, but at the same time the rate of sweating is markedly increasing (Fig. 68). Unfortunately, much of the added sweat is lost without evaporation; Kerslake has calculated that sweat starts to drip from the skin when the overall production is one third of the maximum evaporative capacity. Sweating is particularly inefficient if parts of the body are excessively clothed; the skin temperature rises rapidly in these regions, and leads to a local overactivity of the sweat glands.

Individuals vary widely in their ability to produce sweat. If a standard exercise/heat stress is applied, then a man acclimatized to a hot environment sweats earlier and in greater quantities than a person who is accustomed to more temperate conditions (p. 319). Trained individuals sweat less than the untrained at a given absolute workload, but it is probable that they sweat more if pushed to maximum effort; certainly, there is a considerable interaction between physical training and heat acclimatization (p. 320).

If exercise or heat exposure is prolonged, there is a gradual decline of sweat production. This occurs even if body fluids are well-maintained. It is thought to reflect a blockage of the sweat ducts secondary to maceration of the skin, and it occurs most readily if excessive clothing is worn or the conditions are unduly humid.

Sweat contains 15–20 mE of sodium ions per litre; thus, considerable quantities of salt are lost from the body during a period of heavy sweating. Such deficiencies must be made good in order to avoid disturbances secondary to changes in the concentration of sodium ions. The iron loss (1.5–2.0 mg/litre of sweat) has been suggested as a factor contributing to anemia in some athletes.

The intensity of thermal stress imposed by a given combination of environment, clothing, and activity is commonly summarised as a *predicted 4-hour sweat rate*. This is obtained from a rather complex nomogram (Fig. 69). The *basic 4-hour sweat rate* is obtained by joining the dry bulb and appropriate wet-bulb scales, and noting the intercept on the corresponding B-4 SR scale (Fig. 69). The

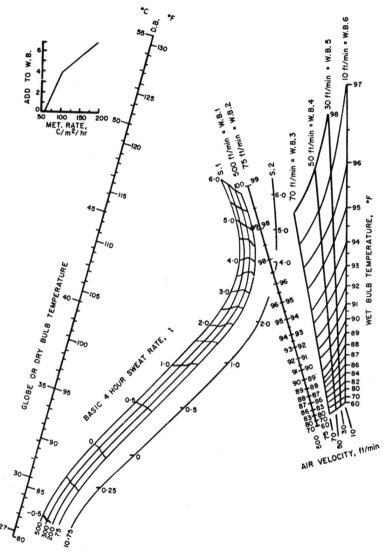

Figure 69. A nomogram for prediction of the 4-hour sweat rate (Smith, as redrawn by Kerslake). From: A textbook of Aviation Physiology, by permission of the author; British Crown Copyright.

point of entry to the wet bulb scale of the nomogram is increased (Δ_t) in the following circumstances:

(a) if the globe temperature (G_t) exceeds the dry bulb temperature (D_t): $\Delta_t = 0.4 \ (G_t - D_t)$

(b) if the metabolic rate is greater than 0.9 Kcal/min/n^2; Δ_t is as shown on the insert

(c) if the clothing has an insulation greater than shorts; (for example, Δ_t for overalls $= 1°C$).

The predicted four hour sweat rate is only equal to the B4SR if the men under study are sitting in shorts. If they are wearing overalls, the figure must be increased by 0.25 litres, and if they are undertaking any form of physical activity, the B4SR rises by an amount proportional to the metabolic rate (M, kCal/min/m^2):

$$P4SR = B4SR + 0.84 \ (M - 0.9)$$

The nomogram can be used to obtain an approximate figure for unevaporated sweat. The chart is entered at the lowest possible wet bulb reading, and the calculations are repeated; the difference between this figure and the actual P4SR represents unevaporated sweat.

Tolerance of Brief Heating

Leithead and Lind have carried out detailed studies of this question, with reference to the very high temperatures encountered in fires and other emergencies. The limit is usually set by a man's capacity to withstand thermal pain; in dry air, 120°C is tolerated for ten minutes, and 200°C for two minutes.

Tolerance of Prolonged Heating

The tolerance of prolonged activity may be set by an excessive rise of body temperature, an "exhaustion" of the sweat glands, a failure of fluid replenishment, or a combination of these problems.

Leithead and Lind have suggested that a P4SR of 4.5 litres represents a safe limit of thermal stress for young men, and that in view of the poorer heat tolerance of older people, the limit should be reduced to 3 litres for those aged forty-five and over. Further restrictions are required if the stress is to be sustained for an eight hour shift rather than a four hour period. Blockley has found that in more acute exposures a heat storage of 50 kcal/m^2 leads to appreciable discomfort, and a burden of 80 kcal/m^2 is usually associated with some impairment of consciousness; given a specific heat of 0.83, this is equivalent to a 2.5°C rise of body temperature. Blockley's experiments were measured in minutes, and the somewhat greater temperatures tolerated by the marathon runner are reached over much longer periods.

In the industrial setting, the loads tolerated by a worker of average fitness are relatively light—180 kcal/hr at 30°C, 300 kcal/hr at 28°C, and 420 kcal/hr at 26°C. Failure of adaptation is shown by the progressive rise of both pulse rate and body temperature over the working day. Wyndham suggests that working conditions are easy if the rectal temperature does not rise above 38°C, but that the combined heat and work stress is excessive if the rectal temperature reaches 39.2°C. Often, the optimum working conditions can be restored quite simply. Factories can be constructed without windows or with reflecting surfaces, and in some cases can be built underground. Ventilation can be improved, with dehydration and refrigeration of the circulating air. Local radiant surfaces can be enclosed by appropriate shielding. Where these remedies are inadequate, much can be gained from a preliminary training and heat acclimatization of the workers. Thus, Wyndham and his colleagues carry out a series of climatic chamber exposures on all recruits to the Johannesburg mines. Not only are the men prepared thereby for hard physical work under adverse conditions, but it is possible to eliminate from the labour force those recruits who are unduly susceptible to heat stress. Other possible approaches include the introduction of rest pauses, and a reduction in the average intensity of activity. Since the working limit is often set by accumulation of heat, some theoretical advantage is gained from an initial chilling of the body. However, in view of the effects of warm-up on performance (p. 190), this approach is unlikely to commend itself either to the worker or the athlete. If the total environment cannot be brought within the limits of human tolerance, then the worker must be provided with an appropriate micro-climate—a piped-supply of refrigerated air distributed over the body surface by a suitable system of ducts.

In the athletic setting, the maintenance of fluid balance is very important, particularly in prolonged events (Table IV). If dehydration occurs, the stored heat becomes distributed through a smaller total mass, and the body temperature inevitably rises. Snellen has estimated an increase of 0.3–0.5°C per kilogram of dehydration, so that in events such as marathon running (where 4–5 litres of dehydration can occur), it is hardly surprising that temperatures of 40–41°C are encountered under temperate conditions. Unfortunately, many distance athletes cherish the belief that fluid replacement impairs performance. Wyndham comments that it is dangerous to deplete body weight by more than 3 percent, and he criticises the international rule that forbade drinking of water in the first ten miles of a marathon race as "criminal folly in warm weather." Certainly, many athletes lose more than 3 percent of body weight during summer contests (Table IV). One recent study of the Ohio State University football team showed an *average* weight loss of almost 3 kg during September practice games.

When calculating fluid requirements, account should be taken of the hydration of glycogen (approximately 2.7 ml per gm) and the water liberated by combustion (about 0.6 ml per gm). If body glycogen stores are exhausted, some 1650 ml of water is produced; this is adequate to dissipate more than half of the associated heat production. Perhaps because water of hydration is lost when exercise is performed, much of the total weight loss is intracellular, whereas when a man is resting in a hot climate fluid is lost largely from the plasma.

Although the aerobic power is unchanged by a sweat loss amounting to 5 percent of body weight, the tolerance for prolonged work is reduced. The explanation may be that because the initial blood volume is reduced, the body is less well-equipped to withstand the progressive exudation of fluid that accompanies physical activity (p. 102). This view is supported by the reduced tolerance of a dehydrated person for the upright position (on tilting, there is an early increase of heart rate and greater than normal liability to fainting). The resistance of the physically trained individual to dehydration is also in keeping with such a hypothesis; training increases both total and central blood volume. Alternatively, intracellular dehydration may influence the tolerance of the muscle towards accumulation of metabolites, or even disturb the chemical processes of contraction. Some authors have found a small ($<10\%$) decrease of maximum isometric strength after dehydration, and it may also be significant that endurance is affected more by exercise (intracellular dehydration) than by heat (extracellular dehydration).

The athlete's voluntary intake of fluids often fails to match his rate of dehydration, even if fears of performance impairment by drinking are resolved. It is thus important to carry out regular intake of fluid (e.g. 100 ml–200 ml several times per hour). If repeated bouts of activity are undertaken, the loss of sodium and potassium ions must also be made good. At one time it was common to provide salt tablets (5–15 gm per day), but these may cause gastric irritation, and can pass straight through the intestines without absorption. Proprietary drinks that contain suitable concentrations of sodium and potassium ions are now available.* Alternatively, enteric-coated salt capsules may be given.

In addition to the loss of physiological endurance, an uncomfortably hot environment leads to a progressive deterioration of mental performance. This can be demonstrated objectively by standard psychomotor and vigilance tests (p. 220). The threshold temperature for a decrement of performance depends upon the acclimatization of the subject, and the sensitivity of the test used. A well-acclimatized man may tolerate a temperature of 30°C, whereas someone who is unaccustomed to heat may show a loss of psychomotor skills at 25°C.

The deterioration of function is less obvious in well-motivated than in uncooperative subjects; The observed changes are probably a reaction to the minor discomforts encountered. However, if physical work is performed, a reduction of cerebral blood flow may contribute to the terminal decrement in score.

Thermal Regulation in Cold Conditions

Less problem is presented by cold than by heat, since modern wind-proof clothing and portable housing protect even arctic expeditions from all except the most extreme environments. The immediate response to cold is a vigorous general constriction of the cutaneous blood vessels. This can be induced by directing a jet of cold air upon a relatively small area of skin. However cold the environment, a certain minimum blood flow is needed to meet the metabolic requirements of the subcutaneous tissues, and this could lead to an excessive flow of heat from the core to the periphery. A second adaptive mechanism

* For instance, "Sportade," a preparation containing potassium bicarbonate, sodium chloride, vitamin C, sugar, dextrose, citric acid, and various flavouring agents.

is thus provided through a constriction of the superficial veins; blood returning from the limbs is diverted from these superficial vessels to the venae comitantes that overlie the main arteries. In consequence, the blood is cooled by the venous return almost immediately upon entering the limb. Heat exchange mechanisms of this type are particularly well-developed in arctic animals such as the whale.

An excessively cold environment may provoke a "paradoxical" dilatation of the skin vessels. This can alternate with periods of intense vasoconstriction (a "hunting" reaction), leading to a severe heat loss. It is blamed on a paralysis of the arteriovenous anastomoses by the extreme cold.

Vasoconstriction holds heat losses by radiation, convection, and conduction to a minimum. However, a certain evaporative loss cannot be avoided; insensible perspiration continues at the skin surface and the respiratory loss also persists, although under extreme conditions the quantity of water vapour expired is diminished by the decrease of air temperature. Some sweating also continues, particularly on the palms and soles of the feet, and in the axillae; this secretion is increased by anxiety or excitement.

If body temperature continues to fall, metabolic heat production is increased through shivering (an increase in tone of the voluntary muscles), an increased secretion of thyroid hormone, adrenaline, and adrenocorticoids, and voluntary modifications of activity. Eskimos on long arctic voyages frequently find it necessary to beach their boats and run vigorously to restore body temperature. In some animals, piloerection provides a final mechanism of adaptation; contraction of small muscles attached to the fur leads to a useful increase of trapped air and thus thermal impedance.

Tolerance of body cooling is quite limited. Discomfort and a deterioration of psychomotor performance occur when the body has lost some 40 kcal/m² of heat. Tasks requiring fine coordinated movements are particularly affected, due to the impaired function of both cutaneous receptors and muscle propriocepters. The maximum safe loss of heat is about 80 kcal/m². A deterioration of cerebration is apparent at a rectal temperature of 35°C

(95°F) and heat regulation fails at about 32°C (90°F); lower temperatures have been attained during surgically controlled hypothermia, but the risks of cardiac arrest and/or fibrillation are unacceptable outside of the operating theatre.

Excessive local cooling gives rise to frostbite if the blood supply to an area of skin is sufficiently reduced to permit tissue destruction by freezing. Owing to the substantial osmotic pressure of tissue fluid, freezing occurs at −1° rather than 0°C.

Tolerance of arctic conditions is greatly influenced by the prevailing wind-speed and by the activity of the subject. An inactive man wearing garments that provide a total insulation of 4 Clo may lose 80 kcal/m² of heat with two to three hours exposure to a temperature of 40°C. However, a deliberate energy expenditure of 2 kcal/min may be sufficient to counteract heat loss and establish an equilibrium with this environment.

Adipose tissue has a low metabolic rate, and thus requires a limited blood flow. Individuals with a substantial layer of subcutaneous fat fare better than thinner subjects when exposed to extreme cold. This, together with greater buoyancy, gives the fat individual a substantial advantage in long-distance swimming events.

Acclimatization

General Features of Acclimatization

When an individual is repeatedly exposed to a physiological stress, acclimatization tends to occur; a fully acclimatized person can function normally despite the unusual environment to which he is exposed. The extent and rate of acclimatization is influenced more by the intensity than by the frequency or duration of the applied stress. On removal from the adverse environment, acclimatization is gradually lost.

Heat Acclimatization

The primary feature of heat acclimatization seems an earlier and a greater production of sweat. This is not always appreciated by the subject, partly because the increased output is largely evaporated, and partly because the distribution of sweat production changes, relatively more being secreted by the trunk and proximal parts of the limb. The increased sweat secretion lowers the temperature of the skin surface, and in consequence a greater quantity of heat is carried from the core to the skin per unit of blood flow. If heat dissipation was inadequate prior to acclimatization, then adaptation may be associated with a greater blood flow to the skin, particularly over the upper half of the body. On the other hand if equilibrium was possible prior to acclimatization, the steady-state condition is sustained with a smaller cutaneous blood flow, thereby permitting better perfusion of the viscera and active muscles. These changes, together with some increase in the tone of the capacity vessels of the legs and possibly an increase of blood volume are sufficient to account for a lower pulse rate at any given work load.

The excretion of salt in the urine and sweat diminishes with acclimatization. Robinson has argued that this is secondary to sodium ion depletion, and does not occur if an adequate salt intake is maintained. Other authors have suggested that repeated heat exposure increases secretion of the hormone aldosterone, leading to a retention of sodium ions and an increased loss of potassium ions.

Relatively long-term adaptations to heat have been described. In some species (but perhaps not in man) the secretion of thyroid hormone is reduced, with a consequent reduction of basal metabolism. The movement vocabulary is modified, and unnecessary exuberant activity is avoided. The exposed individual learns to avoid intense heat—he walks in the shade and avoids the hot tar-mac. Finally, there is some habituation to the sensations encountered in a hot climate, so that a given disturbance of physiological function can be endured with a minimum psychological reaction.

There are many points of similarity between the response to cardiorespiratory training and heat acclimatization. Individuals who are in good physical condition make a good adaptation to a warm climate, while the elderly and obese respond more poorly. Adaptation to heat is temporarily impaired by overindulgence in alcohol or lack of sleep. Cardiorespiratory training partially prepares a man for the heat, and the reverse is also true. Nevertheless, if hard physical work is to be undertaken in the heat, maximum acclimatization can only be attained through a combination of physical activity and heat exposure.

The changes associated with acclimatization take place in an exponential manner. Much of the total adaptation occurs within the first three days of exposure, and changes are largely completed within two weeks. On leaving a tropical area, the adaptations persist for several weeks, and they can be restored at an accelerated speed should the individual return to tropical conditions.

In terms of the practical preparation of either servicemen or athletes for activity overseas, it should be stressed that the full range of adaptation cannot be achieved through a series of heat exposures in a laboratory environmental chamber. Features of the tropical environment such as an unfamiliar pattern of life and a range of new microorganisms are inevitably encountered for the first time when the tropical zone is reached.

Cold Acclimatization

It is much more difficult to demonstrate convincing physiological adaptations to a cold environment. While the general level of skin blood flow is reduced in an attempt to conserve heat, there may be an increase in the blood flow to the exposed extremities, restoring the dexterity of the hands, and permitting skilled work to be carried out once again. However, it is difficult to measure the precise extent of such changes, because blood flow remains relatively small, and the precision of plethysmography (p. 93) is inevitably restricted by shivering.

Some animals show an increased basal metabolic rate on prolonged exposure to cold. However, it is less certain whether man has the capacity to make this response. The greater resting metabolism of arctic peoples such as the Eskimo may reflect rather the specific dynamic action of their traditional high fat diet.

If careful records of subjective comfort and of shivering are maintained, it can certainly be shown that acclimatized individuals feel more comfortable and shiver less. However, their body temperature is often lower than that of unacclimatized men exposed to the same stress, and much of the apparent adaptation may be no more than habituation to a variety of unpleasant sensations.

With prolonged residence in the cold, a more forceful pattern of movement is adopted, and various tricks of organization of house, clothing and outdoor movement minimize the cold stress to which the individual is exposed.

Extreme cooling of the hand is a particular problem in the fishing industry. LeBlanc has shown that with repeated immersion in ice-cold water, the extremities undergo a considerable degree of local acclimatization. The normal intense vasoconstriction is suppressed, and the hand remains warm and nimble enough to perform precise work. Raynaud's phenomenon (p. 96) is the converse situation—an excessive sensitivity of the digital blood vessels to cold.

The Pathology of Extreme Climates

Heat Syncope

Perhaps the commonest reaction to an excessive combination of effort and thermal stress is heat syncope. The venous return to the heart is inadequate, and the blood pressure falls, triggering a vasovagal attack, with a slow pulse rate and muscular vasodilatation. The problem is commonly initiated by a decrease of central blood volume, due to (a) fluid loss in the sweat (water exhaustion), (b) excessive pooling of blood in the relaxed peripheral veins, and (c) increased exudation of fluid (heat oedema of the dependent parts). A competition between the circulatory needs of muscle and skin may also contribute to the fall of blood pressure. The situation is rapidly restored by (a) lying down with the legs elevated, (b) tepid sponging, and (c) oral administration of fluids.

Mild Heat Exhaustion

Mild heat exhaustion is a lesser degree of circulatory inadequacy frequently encountered in industry. The symptoms include fatigue and irritability particularly at the end of the working day, together with a deterioration of mechanical efficiency. The affected individual becomes accident prone, and there is a reduction in both his own production and that of other workers with whom he interacts. Vernon found 50 percent more mining accidents when the temperature exceeded 80°F; interestingly enough, the increase was in minor rather than fatal accidents. The productivity was also reduced, being only 74 percent of that in the cooler and better ventilated areas of the mine. Suitable methods for minimizing heat exhaustion have been discussed elsewhere (p. 315).

If ignored, exhaustion may progress to a chronic neurotic reaction (*"heat neurasthenia"*), with loss of energy, initiative, and interest, and complaints of "dizziness" and "black-outs." The picture is not dissimilar to the effort neurasthenia seen in more temperate climates, and recovery is usually rapid on removal from the hot environment. Before dismissing complaints as heat neurasthenia, it is important to exclude more serious causes of exhaustion such as salt or sweat deficiency.

Heat Stroke

Heat stroke is a dangerous and potentially irreversible failure of the heat regulating mechanisms. Although relatively uncommon, the mortality is high. It is most likely in an obese, unfit and unacclimatized person who is forced to exercise hard in a hot environment. A warning sign is a rectal temperature higher than 104°F (40°C). A progressive rise of body temperature is compounded by dehydration, a diminishing secretion of sweat (*anhidrotic heat exhausion*), and a diminished blood flow to the skin. The combination of rising body temperature and an inadequate blood flow to the brain may cause cerebral irritability, hallucinations, coma, and irreversible cerebral damage. A combination of visceral vasoconstriction and a failing circulation may also damage the kidneys (with a suppression of urine formation) and the adrenal cortex (heat shock). The immediate treatment consists in cooling the patient by tepid sponging; a physician may also administer intravenous fluids and hydrocortisone preparations to counteract the circulatory failure.

A number of athletes have died of heat stroke. Contributory factors include the wearing of clothing that is impermeable to sweat (p. 98), a deliberate restriction of skin blood flow through the illegal administration of drugs of the amphetamine class (p. 50) and the deliberate restriction of water intake (p. 316).

Heat Cramps

The normal loss of salt (sodium chloride) from the body is no more than 12 gm per day. However, a man who is sweating hard can lose as much as 20 gm of salt per hour, and unless this loss is replaced, the body pool of some 175 gm is soon depleted. The usual physiological manifestation of salt depletion is a liability to painful muscular cramps ("Stoker's cramp"). The symptom is most common on first arrival in a tropical climate, partly because adaptive changes in the salt content of the sweat and urine are incomplete, and partly because the newcomer has not yet acquired the habit of deliberately supplementing his salt intake. Salt depletion in turn exacerbates dehydration, since the body endeavours to restore the osmotic pressure of the blood by excreting water. *Salt deficiency exhaustion* often presents as a general chronic weakness, and it must be carefully distinguished from heat neurasthenia. Sometimes symptoms may be more acute, with marked weight loss, constipation, a scanty urine, headache, and (if dehydration is advanced) nausea and vomiting, sunken eyes, an inelastic skin, and circulatory failure. Once vomiting is established, chloride loss is increased, and the condition can be fatal. However, all symptoms are corrected rapidly on restoration of a normal plasma composition.

Heat Rash

There are several forms of heat rash. "Prickly heat" is so named on account of the intense prickling sensation which occurs. A papillary rash and vesicles appear from three days to several months after commencing work in a hot and humid environment; the condition is seen especially on the elbows and forearms, the waist, axillae, and behind the knees. The pathological basis seems a blockage of the sweat ducts secondary to excessive sweating, as discussed above, but in long-standing cases the situation may be complicated by secondary infection. Other skin conditions, particularly fungal infections, flourish under hot conditions. Occasionally, skin reactions may be sufficiently severe that it becomes unwise for the individual to work in a hot environment.

Sunburn

Sunburn may occur in any climate if the individual is exposed to an excess of ultraviolet radiation. However, it is particularly serious in tropical areas, since the body loses vasomotor control over the affected parts, and sweating also ceases in these regions of the skin.

Cold Exposure

Survival in cold water is quite brief. A lightly clothed man does not survive for more than one hour at 5°C, or fifteen minutes at 0°C; the critical factor is a wetting of the clothing with loss of insulating properties, and many hours of survival can be achieved through the simple expedient of wearing a light but waterproof plastic outergarment when boating in cold weather. The course of heat loss depends on body build. Swimming may help a fat man to maintain his body temperature, but the heat loss of a thin man is accelerated if a relative water movement is induced by vigorous swimming. The minimum water temperature compatible with maintenance of heat balance is surprisingly high (about 68°F, 20°C).

Stimulation of cutaneous cold receptors may be very intense, giving rise to reflex hyperventilation, breathlessness, and an inability to control respiration. Occasionally, cardiac arrest or fibrillation may be induced by the shock of immersion. Slowing of muscular contraction, malfunction of sensory receptors, and a progressive deterioration of cerebral function all compound the difficulty of the swimmer. The effort required for propulsion is also increased, due to an appreciable rise in water viscosity (1.8 centipoise at 0°C, compared with 1.0 centipoise at 20°C).

Repeated exposure to cold water, as in the Korean diving women, gives a similar pattern of acclimatization to that discussed for exposure to cold air.

Cold Air. Pugh has recently drawn attention to a number of deaths occurring in English hill walkers under relatively mild conditions (atmospheric temperature greater than 10°C); the problem seems to have been caused by a combination of high wind speeds, limited shelter, and loss of insulation due to soaking of the clothing by mist and rain.

During such activity, the fittest members of a party are often able to maintain heat balance by a deliberate increase in their rate of walking, but those in poorer cardiorespiratory condition are unable to sustain the necessary effort. Exhaustion of the weaker climbers occurs after about five hours, with postural hypotension, ketonuria, and mental changes. The effects of cold are compounded by the incipient exhaustion, and the risk of injury is increased. In the event of immobilization through injury, body temperature falls rapidly.

Treatment of a patient following cold exposure is difficult, and many die. Complications include respiratory depression, metabolic acidosis, circulatory failure, and renal failure; cardiac fibrillation may also develop. The usual plan of treatment includes fairly rapid rewarming, assistance to ventilation including the administration of oxygen, and injection of hydrocortisone to counteract circulatory failure.

References

Burch, G.E., and DePasquale, N.P.: *Hot Climates, Man and his Heart.* Springfield, Thomas, 1962.

Leithead, C.S., and Lind, A.R.: *Heat Stress and Heat Disorders.* London, Cassell, 1964.

Kerslake, D. McK.: The effects of thermal stress on the human body. In: Gillies, J.A. (Ed.): *A Textbook of Aviation Psysiology.* Oxford, Pergamon, 1965.

Edholm, O.G., and Bacharach, A.L.: *The Physiology of Human Survival.* London, Academic Press, 1965.

Polk, G.E.: *Introduction to Environmental Physiology.* Philadelphia, Lea & Febiger, 1966.

Adolph, E.F.: *Physiology of Man in the Desert* New York, Interscience, 1947.

Dill, D.B.: *Handbook of Physiology.* Section 4. Adaptation to the environment. Baltimore, Williams & Wilkins, 1964.

Lee, D.H.K., and Minard, D.: *Physiology, Environment and Man.* New York, Academic Press, 1970.

11

DRUGS

Tobacco

An Overview of Cigarettes and Society

The use of tobacco by man is not a recent development. North American Indians have smoked the pipe of peace for many centuries, and in Western Europe also the tobacco habit has a history of at least four hundred years, going back to the time of Sir Walter Raleigh. However, the twentieth century has seen an important change in tobacco usage. Previous generations were content to chew tobacco, inhale snuff, and smoke pipes and cigars, and although these pursuits incurred the wrath of the British monarch James I, there were apparently no major ill-effects on the community. Now, the cigarette predominates, and unfortunately it cannot be extended the same clear bill of health.

Cigarette manufacturing machines were first developed about 1870, and world production has increased progressively ever since; thus the annual output of United States factories was 4 billion (4×10^9) in 1900, and is now about 580 billion. The attractions of the cigarette relative to other forms of tobacco include low unit cost, mildness (permitting inhalation of the smoke and thus rapid absorption of nicotine), the short time required for smoking, and relative inoffensiveness to others.

While the total production of cigarettes is still increasing, this now reflects an increasing world population rather than a greater per capita demand. Again taking figures for the United States, where the current situation is well documented, a peak production of 4345 cigarettes per adult per year was reached in 1963, and the provisional 1968 figure (4195) is marginally lower (Fig. 70). It would be gratifying if the halting of the per-capita increase could be attributed to publicity linking cigarette consumption and ill-health. Massive documentation such as the United States Surgeon General's report of 1964 apparently had a small ($<5\%$) effect on cigarette sales that persisted for about a year. Dramatic increases in the taxation of cigarettes in the United Kingdom had a similar short-lived effect. However, little of the "curve flattening" seen to date

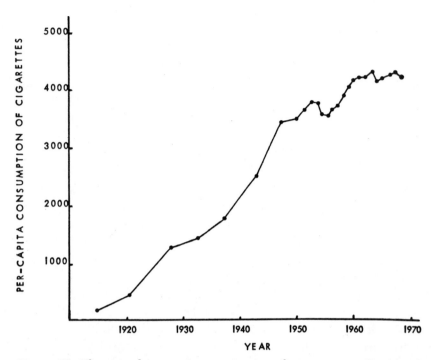

Figure 70. The annual per-capita consumption of cigarettes in the United States (adults 18 years of age and over; based on data of United States Department of Health, Education, and Welfare, Public Health Service, Health Services, and Mental Health Administration).

can be related to health publicity or taxation; it simply reflects the fact that almost all of the population have now been exposed to the temptations of the cigarette industry since adolescence. It has been quite acceptable for a man to smoke cigarettes for at least fifty years, and public smoking by women has also been widely accepted for thirty or forty years.

The future of the cigarette industry is problematical. At the present time, the number of young people taking up smoking is decreasing, and some older adults are also abandoning the habit. Such is the pressure of conformity in western society that if the proportion of smokers were to fall below 40 percent of the population, then the habit might disappear quite rapidly; on the other hand, if marijuana cigarettes were legalised, then consumption might show a further upward curve.

Characteristics of the Smoker

At the present time, about a half of the United States male population are regular cigarette smokers, and about a third of the women also smoke regularly. Some 19 percent of the men and six percent of the women have successfully abandoned the habit.

Cigarette smoking is characteristic of the poor man with limited education and intelligence. Fifty-five percent of men earning $3000 dollars or less smoke, compared with 44 percent in those earning $10,000 dollars or more. Men with less than five years education have a 53 percent chance of being a smoker, while men with thirteen or more years of education have only a 41 percent chance. Perhaps because of greater social pressures, the reverse pattern is seen in women (Fig. 71). Smoking is also associated with city life; 51 percent of metropolitan men and 36 percent of metropolitan women smoke, compared with 45 percent of farm men and 16 percent of farm women.

The greatest percentage of smokers is found between the ages of twenty-five and forty-five; in women, particularly, there is an appreciable deficit of smokers over the age of fifty-five.

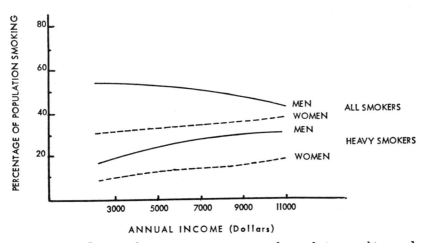

Figure 71. Influence of income on percentage of population smoking and percentage of heavy smokers (> 20 cigarettes per day). Based on data from the United States Department of Health, Education and Welfare, Public Health Service, Health Services, and Mental Health Administration.

This deficit will probably disappear as the present twenty-five to forty-five year age group becomes older (Fig. 72).

In both sexes, the most common personal estimate of consumption is from ten to twenty cigarettes per day. Most people apparently underestimate their consumption, and if production is related to population, then the true average for the United States is between nineteen and twenty cigarettes per day. This confirms the suspicion that consumption is regulated largely by the size of the cigarette package, and it explains the interest of the industry in longer

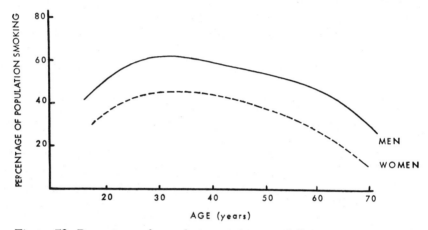

Figure 72. Percentage of population smoking at different ages. Based on data from the United States Department of Health, Education and Welfare, Public Health Service, Health Services, and Mental Health Administration.

cigarettes, twenty-five-packs, and "weekender" cartons that incorporate four packs to be consumed in less than three days. Income has some influence on consumption (Fig. 71); the heavy smokers (> pack per day) are more common in the $10,000 dollar income group (male 29%, female 16%) than in those with a $3000 dollar income (male 18%, female 9%). Former smokers are more common among the wealthy and the intelligent.

Cigarette Smoking and Health

As early as the 1930s scientists began to suspect that cigarette smoking might be one factor responsible for the rising incidence of lung cancer. In the United States, less than three thousand persons died of this condition in 1930, but by 1965 the number was approximately fifty thousand. Exhaustive research over the past decade has established beyond reasonable doubt (Table V) that cigarette consumption is associated not only with cancer of the lung, but with a wide range of other diseases leading to both disability and premature death. The liability to both disability and death is increased in proportion to the number of cigarettes consumed, and decreases progressively from the day when the cigarette habit is abandoned. It

TABLE V

NINE CRITERIA THAT SHOULD BE MET IF THE ASSOCIATION BETWEEN A HABIT (SUCH AS CIGARETTE SMOKING) AND THE SUBSEQUENT INCIDENCE OF DISEASE IS TO BE REGARDED AS CAUSAL RATHER THAN CASUAL

(modified from Bradford Hill)

1. *Strength.* The association is a strong one; for instance, the relative risk of lung cancer is high in the presence of cigarette smoking, but low in its absence.

2. *Consistency.* The association has been reported by many investigators studying different populations in different countries and using different techniques.

3. *Specificity.* The association between the suspect diseases and cigarette smoking is relatively specific: however, there are other confounding features (constitution, income, intelligence, health consciousness) which distinguish the smoker from the nonsmoker.

4. *Temporality.* Ideally, a person with a suspect disease should always have an antecedent history of smoking. Unfortunately, a proportion of patients developing such conditions as lung cancer, chronic bronchitis and atherosclerotic heart disease give no such history. Thus this criterion of a causal association is not fully satisfied.

5. *Biological gradient.* There is good evidence of a graded dose-response relationship for both disability and death, whether "dose" is expressed in terms of the number of cigarettes smoked, the total years of smoking, or the estimated depth of inhalation.

6. *Plausibility.* There are now a number of reasonable mechanisms whereby cigarette smoking could cause disease—thus the association makes "biological sense."

7. *Coherence.* The hypothesis provides a coherent explanation of the data; smoking and the diseases in question show concomitant variation, and the hypothesis is consistent with other known facts about cigarette smoking.

8. *Experimental verification.* If animals such as dogs are made to smoke, tumours develop; if man stops smoking, the incidence of disease and disability falls.

9. *Analogy.* It is well recognized that some of the constituents of cigarette smoke can induce carcinogenic changes in animal cells under suitable experimental conditions.

is thus difficult to infer that the cigarette smoker has some constitutional weakness which increases his susceptibility to the diseases of concern. One bastion of the cigarette industry has been the lower incidence of cigarette-related diseases in women; however, there are now several reasonable and well-documented explanations of this: (a) women have been smoking for a shorter average period than men, (b) they are less likely to inhale deeply, (c) they take fewer puffs per cigarette, and (d) they throw cigarettes away while they are still relatively long, for fear of staining their fingers (both the temperature of combustion and the degree of filtration of the smoke are influenced markedly by the length of the cigarette).

The majority of diseases to be discussed are peculiarly related to cigarette smoking. This seems mainly because cigarette smoke is mild enough to inhale. Determined individuals who inhale deeply on cigars or pipes are rewarded by an equal range of ailments.

The precise toxic materials in cigarette smoke are still open to discussion. A number of potentially carcinogenic tars are produced during combustion. Some authors have considered traces of radioactive polonium an important constituent of the smoke. Carbon monoxide has been suggested as a major factor in producing ischaemic vascular disease. The dust particles themselves can cause bronchospasm and possibly increased secretion of bronchial mucus. Finally, ciliary paralysis is caused by various toxic constituents of the smoke, and this in turn may lead to a retention of naturally occurring air pollutants.

Diseases currently regarded as related to smoking include cancer of the lungs, larynx, mouth, lip, oesophagus, bladder and urinary tract, chronic bronchitis and emphysema, various forms of ischaemic vascular disease, cirrhosis of the liver, and gastric ulcer.

The largest effect on death rate occurs in what many regard as the most productive years of life (45–64). In men of this age, the likelihood of death is almost doubled in the cigarette smoker, and in women also, mortality is increased by 30 percent (Table VI). Men show a doubling of deaths from all forms of cancer, with an eight-fold increase in the risk of a fatal lung cancer. The chances of a circulatory death are also doubled. In women, the likelihood of death from lung cancer is twice as great in those who smoke and the risks of a circulatory death are also increased 60 percent. In older people, the adverse effects of cigarettes are a little less dramatic, but over the age range sixty-five to seventy-nine years, smoking still increases the male death rate by 40 percent, and the female rate by 23 percent.

The effects of cigarette smoking are even more dramatic when broken down in terms of the number of cigarettes consumed and the estimated depth of inhalation. On average, a twenty-

TABLE VI

DEATH RATE PER 100,000 OF POPULATION—SMOKERS (S)
VERSUS NONSMOKERS (NS)

(Based on data of United States Department of Health, Education and Welfare,
Public Health Service, Health Services, and Mental Health Administration.)

	Age 45–64				*Age 65–79*			
	MEN		*WOMEN*		*MEN*		*WOMEN*	
	S	NS	S	NS	S	NS	S	NS
All Causes	1729	708	584	453	5196	3642	2867	2331
All Cancer	267	127	201	197	973	555	572	518
Lung Cancer	87	11	15	7	262	23	30	17
All Diseases of Heart and Circulation	802	422	256	161	3238	2471	1831	1434
Ischaemic Heart Disease	615	304	148	83	2159	1586	1029	803
Violence, Accidents and Suicide	72	60	32	23	129	116	64	51

five-year-old man smoking two or more packs of cigarettes per day shortens his life by eight years (Fig. 73).

Until recently, lung cancer has provided the main focus of public interest in the cigarette controversy. However, in terms of human misery and economic loss the excess of chest and

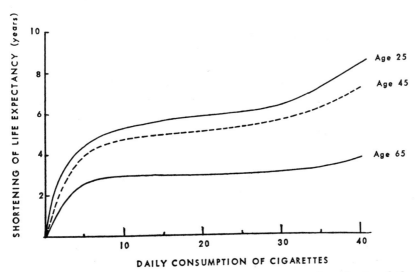

Figure 73. The shortening of life expectancy associated with the daily consumption of cigarettes. Based on data of United States Department of Health, Education and Welfare, Public Health Service, Health Services, and Mental Health Administration.

atherosclerotic disease in the smokers is of much greater importance, because the percentage of those at risk who develop the disease is much larger than in the case of lung cancer. The practical effects of chronic illness can be assessed in terms of days absence from work, days of bed disability and days when physical activity is restricted by illness. On any one of these criteria a man who is a typical heavy smoker (2 packs or more per day) has twice as much disability as a nonsmoker.

Economics of Smoking

The production of cigarette tobaccos makes a major contribution to the economy of many rural areas, particularly North Carolina and Kentucky in the United States, and Western Ontario in Canada. Tobacco farming has largely defied attempts at mechanisation and it thus provides employment for a substantial population in the poorer areas of North America. The cigarette factories, also, provide direct employment for some 36,000 citizens of North Carolina, Kentucky, and Virginia. The corporations concerned are currently diversifying their interests, and some have taken the word "tobacco" from their name.

Some $300,000,000 per year is spent on the advertising of cigarettes in the United States. Until the recent ban on radio and television presentations, two thirds of this expenditure was for television time. This figure gives some measure of the investment that would be needed to produce an alteration of public attitudes. Cigarette manufacturers have been by far the heaviest purchasers of television time.

Cigarettes are a popular basis of taxation in many nations. In 1968, the United State federal and state revenues derived from tobacco products amounted to a total of $4 billion. This was 1.4 percent of federal income, and 2 percent to 16 percent of state income. While politicians would be reluctant to sacrifice financial support of this order, a number of calculations have now shown quite conclusively that the costs of the cigarette to the economy in terms of premature death, disability and hospital care far exceed any taxation that is collected.

Public Attitudes to Smoking

Despite overwhelming scientific proof of the effects of smoking on health, the populace at large has been reluctant to accept this evidence. Surveys have shown that a substantial minority of the general public are still unaware of the dangers of cigarette smoking, and many of the remainder cherish a belief that it is only excessive smoking that is harmful. The definition of excessive smoking is usually a figure slightly greater than the individual's daily consumption. However, the recent switch from regular to filter-tipped cigarettes suggest that many people are increasingly suspicious that there may be something harmful to them in cigarette smoke. This is borne out by the results of a recent questionnaire circulated in the small town of Lindsay, Ontario. More than 80 percent of the adult and high school population knew that smoking was in some way injurious to health. Some 67 percent knew of the specific risk of lung cancer, but the other potential harmful effects were uniformly unrecognised. The knowledge of the community was only marginally improved by a massive smoking and health educational programme. Interestingly enough, the majority of the adults in this community derived their health information from newspapers, rather than the television and radio programmes. For the students, as might be anticipated, television was the most important medium. Neither adults nor students apparently paid much attention to a large numbers of health leaflets circulated in the community, and the campaign had little impact on the cigarette consumption of the average smoker in the area.

The cigarette habit is commonly acquired at the age of twelve or thirteen, and any programme of education would thus be most effective if carried out at a relatively early age. The example of parents is most important, and where one or both parents smoke, the children are very likely to follow their example. Addiction is relatively rapid once regular and open smoking is possible. A boy or girl who is smoking five cigarettes a day at the age of seventeen will commonly have progressed to twenty cigarettes a day at the age of eighteen. Addiction takes three main forms. The *physiological addict* encounters disturbances of the sympathetic nervous system when cigarettes are withdrawn. The *psychological addict* has emotional symptoms such as tenseness and irritability if cigarettes are denied. The third type of addict is the *habitual smoker;* in his case, smoking has become a conditioned reflex response to many environmental situations. The physiological addict is the most easily cured, while the habitual smoker is the most difficult type of person to treat.

About 20 percent of those who decide to stop smoking are successful in their resolve. The proportion can be increased to 30 to 40 percent through various types of clinic and group support, and in one recent British survey some 40 percent of physicians had themselves succeeded in breaking the habit. The physicians were asked how difficult they had found it to stop; 33 percent of the unsuccessful and 17 percent of the successful "quitters" found it "very difficult," while 35 percent of the unsuccessful and 53 percent of the successful had found it "quite easy." About half of the successful quitters found their difficulty lasted for less than six months, but some (14%) were still tempted by cigarettes for as long as two to five years. The times when the need for a cigarette was felt most acutely included social gatherings (73%), periods of stress (25%), and after or on missing meals (13%). Those who were unsuccessful in quitting the habit more frequently reported a desire when under stress (61%) and when writing or reading (41%). Of the exsmokers, 81 percent noted advantages in giving up smoking, and only 31 percent reported any disadvantages; however, advantages and disadvantages were evenly balanced by those who failed to abandon the habit. Advantages claimed included a reduction in coughing and upper respiratory disease, a cleaner mouth, improved appetite, smell, and taste, more energy, and the saving of money, bother and mess. Disadvantages included an increase of weight, and an increase of irritability (the latter being reported mainly by those who were unsuccessful.)

The reasons for deciding to stop smoking included current minor ailments, future dangers to health, and expense. Even among the physicians who were successful quitters, current symptoms provided more motivation (67%) than future concern (50%); among the general population, future health concerned only 24 percent of the quitters, and 11 percent of those who were unsuccessful in abandoning the habit. Expense was an important consideration in this sample, since the tobacco duty in Britain is high; 27 percent of continuing smokers and 42 percent of exsmokers were influenced by the cost of cigarettes.

Physiological Effects of Smoking

Overall Endurance. Present knowledge of the harmful effects of smoking is such that experiments where nonsmokers are persuaded to smoke no longer seem justified. Information must thus be derived from scientifically less satisfactory approaches such as comparing smokers and nonsmokers, or evaluating the changes that accompany voluntary cessation of smoking.

The endurance time in an all-out run is apparently diminished by the smoking of one or two cigarettes, and in one comparison recently reported from Edmonton nonsmokers were able to continue with a progressive treadmill test for 16.5 minutes, compared with 13.2 minutes in smokers of the same age.

Circulatory Effects. Many of the immediate circulatory effects of smoking are attributed to absorption of nicotine; the average person retains about 1 mg for each cigarette that he smokes. Most textbooks suggest that absorption occurs "in the lungs," but in fact nicotine is freely miscible with water. Thus if inhalation occurs, much of the nicotine is absorbed via the bronchial circulation, and even if an attempt is made to hold the smoke within the mouth, absorption will still occur via the copious circulation of the tongue. The route of absorption of nicotine has some bearing on hypotheses regarding its mode of action on the heart and circulation. Burns and his associates have suggested that nicotine stimulates the release of noradrenaline at the sympathetic nerve endings, while Comroe has postulated a direct action on the chemo-sensitive tissues of the carotid bodies. If, as the present author suspects, absorption occurs in the upper part of the respiratory tract, the material passes via the bronchial circulation to the superior vena cava, and thus reaches the cardiac pacemaker in the wall of the right atrium. Any change of heart rate would then be likely to reflect liberation of noradrenaline at the pacemaker. On the other hand, if absorption occurs in the lungs, the nicotine is carried in relatively high concentrations to the left side of the heart, and thus reaches the carotid body in sufficiently high concentrations to act as postulated by Comroe.

A substantial part of the variation in *resting pulse rate* is due to time since the last cigarette. Some authors suggest that smoking can increase the heart rate by as much as 15 to 20 beats/min. However, the effect is relatively short lived; much of the increase passes in fifteen to forty-five minutes, and a stable pulse rate is reached with two to three hours of abstinence. The smoking of one or more cigarettes leads to a parallel increase in the pulse response to a given level of submaximal effort. However, the maximum heart rate and the maximum cardiac output are apparently unchanged by smoking.

The resting *blood flow to the skin* is reduced following smoking, and the tendency to cutaneous vasoconstriction persists in moderate exercise; perhaps for this reason, subjects who have smoked immediately prior to effort complain they sweat earlier and in greater quantities than when they are abstaining from cigarettes. The restriction of skin flow can have a beneficial influence on performance of the muscles; unfortunately, this occurs at the expense of impaired heat regulation. There is also a rise of systemic blood pressure, and this together with the tachycardia results in an increase of the cardiac workload both at rest and during moderate effort. Although the increased blood pressure may give some increase of coronary blood flow, a relative oxygen lack usually develops in the heart muscle, and occasionally this may be severe enough to cause electrocardiographic changes such as depression of the ST segment.

The immediate resting *muscle flow* is increased by smoking. On the other hand, some authors have found a larger postexercise oxygen debt in smokers than in nonsmokers. The oxygen debt remains unchanged if one or more cigarettes are smoked immediately prior to exercise, and it seems unlikely that the difference of debt between smokers and nonsmokers is a direct pharmacological response to nicotine. It may reflect partly the influence of carbon monoxide on oxygen transport, and partly a deterioration of the limb vasculature in the chronic smoker.

One particularly undesirable consequence of smoking is an increase in the irritability of the heart muscle; this is due in part to the increased release of noradrenaline, and in part to the relative myocardial hypoxia discussed above. Excessive exertion is more likely to induce ventricular fibrillation in a heavy smoker than in a nonsmoker, and perhaps for this reason the beneficial effects of deliberate exercise are less marked in the smoker (Table VII).

Carbon Monoxide. Cigarette smoke contains up to 4 percent carbon monoxide. This gas combines with haemoglobin more strongly than does oxygen. The ratio of affinities (usually designated M) varies somewhat from individual to individual, and in any given person it is also influenced by blood pH; the usually quoted range is 195–245 : 1.

TABLE VII

THE INFLUENCE OF SMOKING HABITS AND OF PHYSICAL ACTIVITY*
UPON TOTAL MORTALITY† OF ADULT MEN; DATA EXPRESSED AS
RATIO TO MORTALITY OF SEDENTARY GROUP
(based on data of Hammond)

Activity Level*	Nonsmokers	Heavy Smokers (>20 cigarettes/day)
Sedentary	1.00	1.00
Light Activity	0.69	0.95
Moderate Activity	0.58	0.75
Heavy Activity	0.57	0.70

* Total of occupational and leisure activity.
† Hammond estimated 47% was due to ischaemic heart disease.

The blood of a typical smoker contains 5% carboxyhaemoglobin; if he stops smoking, the level drops exponetially to a figure of about 1% carboxyhaemoglobin. The half-time of this process is a little under four hours. The carboxyhaemoglobin reading provides a useful and simple test of adherence to a smoking withdrawal programme. It is also an early physiological benefit that can be demonstrated to patients who may wish to see a tangible reward following abstinence from cigarettes.

Some authors have claimed a quantitative relationship between carboxyhaemoglobin levels and the number of cigarettes smoked. We have not been impressed with this, and suspect that other factors such as the number and depth of the puffs taken and the temperature of combustion of the cigarette have a more important bearing on the carboxyhaemoglobin reading.

If 5 percent of the haemoglobin is in the carboxy form, one might anticipate a corresponding limitation of oxygen conductance. In practice, there is little evidence of this except in acute smoking experiments. The faster heart rate provides one immediate compensatory mechanism, both at rest and during moderate work. The chronic smoker also develops a polycythaemia that helps to maintain his maximum oxygen intake; if he stops smoking, the potential gain of aerobic power from the dissociation of carboxyhaemoglobin is soon wiped out by a reduction in the red cell count and an increase of body weight. The polycythaemia of a heavy smoker rarely reaches the level at which a marked increase of blood viscosity occurs (Fig. 36) but it does increase the coagulability of the blood, and thus the liability to coronary infarction.

A second effect of substantial blood concentrations of carbon monoxide is to displace the haemoglobin dissociation curve (Fig. 39) to the left. This makes it more difficult for the tissues to extract their quota of oxygen, and may also lead to anoxia of the vessel walls, thereby initiating degenerative disease.

Some 10 percent of the carbon monoxide retained within the body combines with myoglobin. The pigment thus inactivated can no longer serve as an oxygen store, and there are obvious repercussions in terms of restricted anerobic "capacity" and power (p. 396), with a lowered tolerance for interval work (p. 449). The rate of clearance of carbon monoxide from myoglobin is much slower than its clearance from haemoglobin.

> Employees in tunnels and parking towers, and opponents of urban expressways and airports often quote with alarm the high concentrations of carbon monoxide in their immediate environment. No one would deny that a reduction of exhaust fumes would improve the quality of urban life. However, it seems a little illogical to become excited about an atmospheric carbon monoxide concentration of perhaps twenty parts per million while cheerfully inhaling cigarette smoke with a CO concentration of forty thousand parts per million. Certainly at least three quarters of the carboxyhaemoglobin of the typical metropolitan agitator could be eliminated by the simple expedient of ceasing to smoke for a few hours.

Respiratory Tract

The immediate response of the airways to cigarette smoke is a brisk bronchospasm. Nadel and his associates found that fifteen puffs on a cigarette were sufficient to cause a 31 percent decrease in the conductance of the airways. This began within a minute, and lasted rather more than half an hour. It was thought a direct reaction to dust particles in the smoke, and was independent of the nicotine content of the cigarettes.

Tobacco smoke particles are very fine (about 0.25μ), and for this reason the majority are carried to the finest air passages. These make a relatively small contribution to the overall airway resistance (p. 127), and the reported 31 percent decrease in overall conductance thus signifies a major narrowing of the smallest bronchioles. Spasm of the small airways has a marked effect on gas distribution, and the expected impairment with exposure to cigarette smoke has been demonstrated convincingly by such techniques as helium mixing curves (p. 119).

The 31 percent decrease of airway conductance is rarely appreciated by a resting subject, but in near-maximum effort, breathing is noticeably more difficult immediately following the smoking of one or more cigarettes. There is also a measurable increase in the oxygen cost of breathing; 10 percent rather than 5 percent of the available maximum oxygen intake is diverted to the chest muscles, and this is probably one of the main factors that reduce the endurance performance of the chronic smoker.

The bronchial cilia are briefly stimulated by cigarette smoke, but then show a more prolonged phase of depressed activity, lasting for thirty to forty minutes. The mucosa lining the bronchi swells with repeated exposure to cigarette smoke, and there is an increased production of mucus by the goblet cells. These changes further increase airway resistance, and lead to a retention of both bacteria and potentially carcinogenic tars.

Aerobic Power. The present author found negligible changes of predicted aerobic power when subjects were tested immediately before and one year after ceasing to smoke; indeed, when results were expressed per unit of body weight there was a slight deterioration in the final readings. These observations should perhaps be repeated with direct measurement of maximum oxygen intake (p. 411), but since smoking tends to *increase* the pulse response to submaximum effort, it is unlikely that direct measurement would establish a more "favourable" conclusion than use of the prediction procedure.

Body Composition. It is widely accepted that body weight increases when a person ceases to smoke. In our subjects, reexamined after an interval of one year, there was a gain of some 5 kg in those who were successful in abandoning the habit and smaller gains (~1 kg) in those who were unsuccessful but did reduce their cigarette consumption. Few of the patients reported any change in habitual activity, and there were substantial associated changes of skinfold thickness (6mm and 1–2mm, respectively in the two groups). The weight gain was thus due to an increase of body fat. Others have suggested problems of fat accumulation are less marked if observations are extended over a longer period. However, the need to restrict food intake remains greater in the nonsmoker than in the continuing smoker. Possible reasons for the increase in appetite on ceasing to smoke include a recovery in the senses of taste and smell, the adoption of alternative forms of indulgence (sweets and alcohol), and the previous action of nicotine in sustaining blood sugar levels between meals.

The disastrous rise of weight encountered by some patients has a profound negative influence on a smoking withdrawal programme. It emphasizes the importance of a total approach to improvement of health; a smoking withdrawal clinic should offer advice not only on smoking but also on diet and habitual activity.

Smoking and the Athlete. Some 15 to 20 percent of top athletes smoke while they are in training, but few are heavy smokers. In assessing these figures, we should note that not all athletic events call for endurance. It is rare to find a smoker among distance runners, swimmers, cyclists or cross-country skiers; apparently, performers in these events have found by experience that smoking is harmful to their competitive status.

Once training has been renounced, the smoking habits of the exathlete do not differ greatly from those of the general public. One study at Michigan State University showed 69 percent of exathletes and 60 percent of their sedentary classmates were smoking regularly. Any excess of smokers among the exathletes is probably attributable to their more extroverted personalities.

Alcohol

Alcohol and Society

The consumption of "alcohol" (ethanol) has many social connotations, but the influence of moderate doses on physical performance is slight. We shall thus discuss the question quite briefly, referring mainly to North American statistics. The apparent consumption of alcohol in the United States reached a peak of 2.5 gallons per adult per year in the decade 1901–1910, when the drive for prohibition was gathering force. In 1935, consumption had dropped to 1.2 gallons per adult per year, and since World War II usage has been relatively stable at two gallons per adult per year. Beer first became popular in the United States at the turn of the present century, and has since progressively replaced spirits as a beverage.

There are striking national differences in apparent alcohol consumption. Thus France consumes three times as much per capita as the United States, while the Scandinavian countries consume only about half as much. It may be helpful to translate the statistics cited into beverage usage. Over the last twenty years, about 40 percent of the United State population have consistently described themselves as abstainers, and perhaps a half of the remaining 60 percent use alcohol only occasionally. Thus the typical regular drinker is taking six to seven gallons of alcohol or twelve to fourteen gallons of spirits per year (4–5 oz per day). The percentage who are alcoholics is hard to determine. Jellinek has suggested that if the type of beverage and the nutritional status of a community are known, then the number of alcoholics can be estimated by multiplying the number of deaths from liver cirrhosis by a constant (4 for the U.S.). On this basis, there are currently more than five million alcoholics in the United States (4% of all adults); the number has increased roughly in proportion to the population over the last twenty years, and men have consistently outnumbered women by a factor of five or six to one.

As with smoking, the percentage of the population using alcohol is higher in men (76% in both U.S. and Canadian surveys) than in women (56% of U.S. women, 64% of Canadian women). There is also a smaller percentage of alcohol users over the age of fifty. As might be anticipated, there are more abstainers of Protestant than of Catholic or Jewish background. Alcohol consumption is also more common in the prosperous and well-educated (70%) than in the poor with little education (62%). In both the United States and Canada, the percentage of alcohol users is much higher in the big cities than in farming areas.

The personal use of alcohol commonly commences in the home at twelve or thirteen years of age, and about 50 percent of high school youth are taking some alcohol fairly regularly. Users are more common if one or both parents also drink; boys outnumber girls, and both extremes of the socioeconomic scale are overrepresented among the habitual drinkers. Alcohol is seen as a social beverage, rather than as a drug, and its use is associated with adult role playing in social occasions, celebrations and times of stress.

As with the sale of cigarettes, the use of alcohol has a considerable impact upon the economy. In recent years, some 3 percent of personal expenditures in the United States have been for alcoholic beverages, and the industry has given direct employment to more than 400,000 people through the production and sale of alcoholic beverages. A substantial part of federal (4.3%), state (5.9%) and local (0.4%) revenues is derived from the sales of alcohol. Advocates of abstinence have argued that the sum collected does not match the loss to the economy from problem-drinkers. Casual observation suggests this view is probably correct; however, reliable statistics have yet to be obtained. Total advertising expenditures in the United States have exceeded $200 million per year. The distribution of funds has differed from that of the cigarette manufacturers; more is spent on newspapers and magazines, and less on television time. These differences seem in part a reflection of self-regulation imposed by the distilled spirits manufacturers.

Alcoholism is currently one of the major clinical problems in industry. This is so despite the fact that a preponderance of alcoholics are either selfemployed (field salesmen and operators of small businesses) or are unable to obtain more than casual employment. Estimates of alcoholism in major industries range from 2 to 6 percent, depending in part upon the proportion of men in the labour force. Problem drinkers have about 2.5 times as many days absence from work as controls, and they are absent nearly three times as often. The young drinker has an increased liability to accidents "on the job," but beyond the age of forty he apparently learns various protective techniques and then has a similar accident experience to his more temperate colleagues. Where suitable treatment programmes have been established, 80 percent of problem drinkers have improved sufficiently to be retained in their place of employment. If treatment is unsuccessful, productivity becomes further limited by a variety of physical ailments, including cirrhosis of the liver, pancreatitis, polyneuritis, myocardial degeneration, and disturbances of the central nervous system. Many of these disorders are related to a limited intake of quality proteins and vitamins; the alcoholic meets his overall caloric requirements (Table I) and exhausts his budget before he leaves the beverage room.

The two main reasons currently advanced for abstinence are the impossibility of predicting who will become an alcoholic, and (perhaps more important) the incontravertible association between consumption of alcohol and road-traffic accidents. Many nations now impose a legal "ceiling" on the blood alcohol level of the drinking driver, testing either blood specimens or exhaled breath. Despite earnest pleas by defence counsel, the "breathalyser" is now established as an adequate technique for police use; the standard deviation of the blood alcohol estimated in this way is about 7 mg/100 ml. In Canada and in Britain the blood alcohol content of a person in charge of a motor vehicle must be less than 80 mg/100 ml; in Norway and Sweden the limit is 60 mg/100 ml, and in other countries it ranges from 30 to 150 mg/100 ml.

The relationship between alcohol consumption and blood level is influenced by the speed of drinking, the form of beverage, the accompanying food intake, body size, and habitual use of alcohol. Some 90 percent of the alcohol absorbed is ultimately metabolized to CO_2 and water; the blood is cleared at a relatively fixed rate of 10–20 mg/100 ml/hour, depending on the concentration of the enzyme alcohol dehydrogenase in the liver. Under average circumstances, four single whiskies or two pints of beer will produce a reading of 80 mg/100 ml.

The currently accepted legal standards represent a minimum in terms of public protection. As many as 10 percent of a population may show clinical intoxication (unsteady gait, slurred speech, and irresponsible behaviour) with blood levels of 10–50 mg/100 ml, and two thirds of the population are obviously intoxicated with blood levels of 100–150 mg/100 ml. Furthermore, if careful psychomotor tests are carried out (p. 220), there is no threshold dose of alcohol below which human performance remains completely unimpaired. The effects of a given blood level vary with personality. In general, extroverts show a larger deterioration of performance than introverts. Extroverts refuse to acknowledge their problem and drive at the same speed, but with greatly diminished accuracy. Introverts, on the other hand, strive to compensate for the effects of alcohol; they may drive slowly and cautiously, or attempt to prove their efficiency by fast but not very accurate driving. Another important aspect of personality is the liability to distraction by external stress or tension. There is an optimum level of cortical arousal for skilled performance (p. 198), and if this is exceeded, performance deteriorates. Some types of personality are normally near their optimum, but others may be excessively aroused by anxiety or other stimuli. In an overly anxious person, the deterioration of motor function induced by alcohol may be partially offset by a less intense and thus more favourable level of arousal.

Alcohol and Physical Performance

There is little question that doses of alcohol that impair either physical health or the sense of social responsibility have an adverse effect on physical performance. Large doses of alcohol can lead to an acute myopathy; the muscles become tender or aching and on biopsy show degeneration of the fibres. There is an associated myoglobinuria, and the rise of blood lactate levels following exhausting work is less than normal. Possibly, glycogen stores within the muscle are depleted when calories are supplied by alcohol rather than carbohydrate. The affected muscles usually recover after the drinking bout is over, but if the insult is repeated, a chronic myopathy may develop. Large doses of alcohol also lead to impaired function in a proportion of patients, even in the absence of overt alcoholism or cirrhosis of the liver; there may be evidence of heart failure, atrial or ventricular arrhythmias, and a variety of electrocardiographic abnormalities. In a proportion of patients, the myocardial degeneration has a dietetic basis, and recovery follows administration of vitamin supplements, but in others an acute fall of the blood magnesium level with an associated loss of intracellular potassium ions seems responsible.

Laboratory tests of the response to more moderate doses of alcohol all show an impairment of performance. The earliest acute manifestation is a deterioration in the higher functions of the brain, with an impairment of judgment and self-control, and a slowing of reaction times. Vision is also measurably impaired with blood concentrations of 40–80 mg/100 ml, and a hearing loss develops at concentrations between 100 and 150 mg/100 ml. A variety of measures such as arm steadiness, body sway, maintenance of equilibrium when walking, handwriting and more complicated psychomotor tests (p. 220) all demonstrate increased clumsiness of the voluntary muscles. In some individuals, motor function deteriorates when the blood alcohol is only 30 mg/100 ml, and all patients show a loss of motor performance at 100 mg/100 ml.

When observations are extended from the laboratory to real life situations, in most instances a loss of performance can still be demonstrated. However, there are specific exceptions. In industries that require heavy work but little skill, immediate productivity may be increased if drinking is allowed "on the job." The explanation seems that workers are then less conscious of fatigue. In some individuals, the maximum isometric force is also increased by moderate doses of alcohol; here, a lesser central inhibition of impulse traffic to the skeletal muscles may be responsible (see p. 199). Finally, as with a tense car driver, the competitive performance of some athletes may be impaired by excessive cortical arousal; in such individuals, the mild sedative action of alcohol can have a beneficial effect on performance. (Two pistol-shooters in the Mexico City Olympics were disqualified for alleged use of alcohol as a sedative).

Other responses to moderate doses of alcohol include cutaneous vasodilatation, an increase of resting pulse rate and sometimes of resting blood pressure, an increase in the acidity of gastric juice and a marked diuresis. The cutaneous vasodilatation gives a sensation of warmth to the skin, but heat loss is actually increased, particularly in a cold environment. Although the blood pressure may rise immediately following ingestion of alcohol, the long term response is a slight fall, particularly if the initial readings are increased by tension and anxiety. The diuresis is due in part to the large volume of fluid commonly ingested with the alcohol, but there is also a pharmacological inhibition of the release of antidiuretic hormone from the pituitary gland.

The circulatory effects of alcohol persists during moderate exercise. Cutaneous blood flow is greater than would otherwise be anticipated for a given work load; in consequence the pulse rate is faster, and the mean arteriovenous oxygen difference is smaller than in a completely sober individual. The muscle blood flow is unchanged or reduced, and because of the increased clumsiness of movement the oxygen cost of activity is increased. Dilatation of the skin vessels is a normal response to near-maximum effort, and thus it is hardly surprising that substantial doses of alcohol have no effect on maximum heart rate, stroke volume, arteriovenous oxygen difference, or maximum oxygen intake.

A deterioration of sprint performance might be anticipated from the effect of alcohol upon reaction time. A deterioration of endurance would likewise be anticipated from increased clumsiness. Some authors have reported up to 10 percent loss of performance following quite moderate doses of alcohol, while others have found no change with blood alcohol levels of 100 mg/100 ml. It is difficult to undertake controlled experiments with a substance that is so readily recognised, and there are probably wide individual differences in response. In some athletes, the greater confidence engendered by alcohol may compensate rather fully for any loss of skill and slowing of bodily reactions.

Alcohol and Fitness

Small doses of alcohol have little effect on fitness. In a tense and overanxious individual, alcohol may have a mild therapeutic effect. However, it seems undesirable to suggest that a patient treat his problems with alcohol; any tensions may equally be relieved by physical activity, with greater safety and benefit to health.

Alcohol consumption is commonly linked with obesity, and this may be due in part to the sedative nature of the drug. A second reason is the high calorie content (7 kcal/gm). The average drinker in North America takes at least 15 percent of his total calories in the form of alcohol, and there must be a proportionate reduction in the intake of normal nutrients if obesity is to be avoided (Table I).

Many athletes avoid the use of alcohol while in training, but exathletes are more likely to drink than their sedentary colleagues. As with exathletes and smoking, this is attributable mainly to differences of personality between the two populations.

Other "Social" Drugs

Drug Addiction

Many of the drugs considered in this section are important because of (a) their increasing usage by the younger generation, and (b) their marked tendency to cause addiction. An expert committee of the World Health Organization has defined addiction as follows:

> Drug addiction is a state of periodic or chronic intoxication detrimental to the individual and to society, produced by the repeated consumption of drug (natural or synthetic). Its characteristics include: (1) an overpowering desire or need (compulsion) to. continue taking the drug and to obtain it by any means; (2) a tendency to increase the dose; (3) a psychic (psychological) and sometimes a physical dependence on the effects of the drug.

A drug habit, as opposed to addiction, is associated with (a) a desire but not a compulsion for the drug, (b) little tendency for an increase of dose, (c) psychic but not physiological dependence, and (d) a detrimental effect on the individual rather than on society.

Some drugs such as the opiates and cocaine are rapidly addictive in all individuals. In others, the personality of the user seems a significant variable; thus with alcohol, some people are able to take small doses for many years without signs of addiction, but in others both psychic and physical dependence develop quite rapidly. Usage of many of the drugs to be discussed is a recent phenomenon, and for this reason evidence whether physical dependence can develop is often inadequate.

The "possession"* of many of the drugs described is currently a federal offence in both Canada and the United States. Those convicted may gain a permanent criminal record.

---

* The legal definition of possession includes (a) knowingly having a drug in the possession of another person, (b) storing it in any place, and (c) consenting to the possession of a drug by another member of a group.

Marijuana

Marijuana ("grass," "pot," "tea") consists of the dried mature flowering tops and upper leaves of the hemp plant (cannabis sativa). It is greenish brown in colour and is normally crushed to a peppery consistency; pieces of plant stem and seeds may persist among the particles thus produced. It is usually smoked in rather thin cigarettes ("joints") which have a characteristic odour (like burning hay or rope); however, it can also be brewed as a form of tea, or incorporated into food such as cakes. The main active ingredients are a group of tetrahydrocannabinols.

Hashish ("hash") is a brownish black resinous material exuded from the tops of the hemp plant. It is sold in blocks that have a soap-like texture, and the user normally puts a flake on the tip of a glowing cigarette. However, it can also be smoked in special pipes or consumed in foods. Hashish contains a high concentration of cannabinoids, and it is about five times as potent as marijuana.

Since the possession of any form of cannabis is a federal offence, it is difficult to obtain precise statistics on usage. One study in Toronto showed 6.7 percent of high school students had used the drug at least once in a six-month period; other estimates range as high as 13 percent. There are no figures on adult usage, but the general consensus is that the incidence is less than in teenagers.

The short-term effects of the drug are mainly psychological, and depend on the personality of the user, the environment, and the dose that is taken. In general, the inexperienced user has fewer symptoms than the habitual "pot-head". Small doses increase talkativeness and self-confidence, tiredness vanishes, and there is a sense of exhilaration and unusual perceptiveness. Larger doses give perceptual distortions and hallucinations; time passes more slowly and colours become more vivid. Physiological effects have been studied less fully, but there is some evidence of impaired muscular coordination, a slowing of reaction time, vasodilatation, and an increase in the resting heart rate. In one widely quoted but rather limited study of motorists, performance impairment was less than with alcohol, but many of the changes observed were similar in type. The effects of the drug last for several hours, and there may be subsequent lethargy and sleepiness, persisting to the following day.

A small proportion of users show panic and other adverse psychological reactions; panic seems most likely in the inexperienced. The long-term physical effects are unknown. Apart from the irritant properties of the smoke, the main risks seem a progression to "hard" drugs as a consequence of contact with "pushers," and the development of a psychological dependence on cannabis so that the individual becomes unable to face a normally perceived world.

Solvents

A variety of solvents are used as "social" drugs by teenagers. The compounds involved include polystyrene cements ("airplane glue"), nail-polish remover, lighter and cleaning fluids, gasoline and antifreeze. Addiction to hospital anaesthetics is an older but well-recognised problem. The active ingredients vary with the solvent, but include hexane, cyclohexane, benzene, naphtha, acetone, ethylacetate, carbon tetrachloride and toluene. All are lipid soluble volatile hydrocarbons.

The fumes are commonly inhaled from a soaked cloth or a closed bag, but in some instances the liquid solvent has been mixed with a beverage. The closed bag technique has led to a number of deaths from suffocation. Fatal explosions have also occurred from associated smoking. The odour of the solvent is persistent, and can usually be detected in the breath or on the clothing of the user. The typical "glue-sniffer" is about fourteen-years-old, and is more likely to be a boy than a girl. Antisocial personalities, the adventurous, and those from an adverse environment are largely represented, but in some areas as many as 5 percent of high school students are implicated.

The main effects of the solvents are upon the central nervous system, and depending on dosage the clinical picture ranges from mild intoxication or elation to confusion, slurring of speech, impairment of muscular coordination, distortion of perception, delusions of superior strength, and visual and auditory hallucinations. The user becomes drowsy, and eventually unconscious. Effects persist for five minutes to half an hour, depending on the saturation of body fat that has been reached. Physiological effects are not well-documented, but include local irritation of the nose and eyes. Performance is presumably affected much as by other intoxicants.

The main complications of solvent sniffing are psychological dependence on the drug, and dangerous behaviour while intoxicated. The body becomes biochemically habituated to the solvent used, so that increasingly large doses are required to achieve the desired level of intoxication. Withdrawal symptoms including restlessness, anxiety and irritability have been described, but it is not yet definitely established whether physical dependence can develop. It is suspected that frequent glue sniffing damages the mucous lining of the mouth and nose, the kidneys, liver, bone marrow, and chromosomes, but again this has yet to be proven.

Lysergic Acid Diethylamide

LSD, "acid" is a synthetic indole with psychedelic effects; it is about four thousand times as potent as the naturally occurring products mescaline and psilocybin. As a powder, it is white, odourless and tasteless; it can be taken either as a tablet or by impregnation of sugar cubes or blotting paper, and is occasionally given by injection. The average dose is 100–200 μg, and symptoms appear some thirty minutes after oral ingestion.

As with marijuana, possession of the drug is illegal, and little is known of the percentage of users. It is thought that most are under the age of thirty; some take the drug as an escape from anxiety and psychological pain, while others claim to seek increased self-awareness and understanding of life through the hallucinations that are induced.

The length of an individual "trip" varies from two to ten hours, depending on both the user and the dose. Although sensory distortions (intensified colours, distorted shapes and sizes, and apparent abnormalities of movement, time and space) are the most commonly reported effects, there are also a substantial range of physiological changes including tremors, numbness and tingling of the skin, weakness, increases of resting heart rate, systemic blood pressure and deep body temperature, hyperventilation, flushing of the face, sweating, papillary dilatation and an intolerance of bright lights. Many of these disturbances could affect physical performance, but details are not known.

It is widely agreed that LSD is a dangerous drug. Anxiety or panic during a "trip" can lead to suicide, homicide, and various forms of antisocial behaviour. In a proportion of users, particularly those who initially have an unstable personality, chronic anxiety and a variety of psychoses may develop. There are also reports of irreversible brain damage and the development of chromosome abnormalities among regular users.

DOM (STP, 2:5 dimethoxy-4 methyl-amphetamine) is a synthetic stimulant related to mescaline and amphetamine. It is about fifty times as potent as LSD.

DMT (dimethyltryptamine) is a component of hallucinogenic snuffs used by South American Indians. It is inactive by mouth and is thus smoked or taken as a snuff. Intoxication has a rapid onset, and panic is thus more likely than with LSD; however, the effects lack persistency, passing in thirty to forty-five minutes.

Mescaline ("mesc," "big chief") can be prepared from a Mexican cactus, but most users prefer a synthetic preparation, taking it in orange juice or cocoa to mask its unpleasant flavour. Kaleidoscopic visions are followed by a deep sleep that persists for up to ten hours after ingestion. Synthetic mescalines are intermediate in potency between LSD and DOM, and are reputed to induce particularly tranquil psychedelic experiences.

Psilocybin (4 hydroxy-dimethyltryptamine) can be extracted from a Mexican mushroom, and was once used by native tribes for religious purposes. The "high" induced by this drug is said to be less intense but more persistent than that produced by LSD.

Amphetamines ("Speed," "Dexedrine," "Benzedrine")

The amphetamines have been used medically for a number of years to treat mild depression and excessive appetite. They have also been valued as a means of preventing sleep, particularly by long-distance truck drivers and students "cramming" for examinations. More recently, large quantities of legally manufactured amphetamines have been shipped to Mexico, where they have found their way onto the black market. Substantial amounts are also prepared by backyard chemists. Trafficking is illegal, but "possession" is permitted by law.

The amphetamines may be taken ("dropped") as tablets (initially 10–20 mg, but increasing progressively to 1 gm or more as habituation occurs), sniffed in powder form, or injected intravenously (to "crank" or to "shoot"). They are chemically related to adrenaline, and effects are produced on both the sympathetic and the central nervous systems.

Oral ingestion gives increased confidence, loss of fatigue, and suppression of appetite. Concentration appears to be increased and users believe (often mistakenly) that their work has improved. Larger doses cause a restless excitement and subsequent sleeplessness; the user may thus oscillate increasingly violently between overdosage of "speed" and barbiturates.

Large intravenous doses give a sudden ecstasy (a "rush" or "total body orgasm") with strong emotions ranging from warmth and sociability to anger and fear. Other possible psychological effects include a sense of power or superiority, anxiety, irritability and hallucinations. The dose must be repeated every few hours to maintain a "high". Once the blood concentration falls, there is a rapid "crash"—a prolonged sleep, followed by depression.

Physiological effects of the amphetamines include a number of circulatory changes (constriction of cutaneous arterioles and superficial veins, with an increase of resting heart rate and systemic blood pressure); these changes could theoretically increase maximum oxygen intake. However, the cutaneous vasodilation of maximum effort is needed for heat elimination and the illegal use of dexedrine pills could thus expose an athlete to a dangerous level of heat stress. Some authors have found little improvement in physical performance following administration of amphetamines; however, critics of these experiments suggest that the drugs were given too close to a contest or in inadequate dosage. Smith and Beecher have reported a 1 percent improvement in times for one hundred to two hundred yard swimming events, and a 4 percent improvement in weight throwing in experiments where "benzedrine" was given two to three hours prior to the assessment of performance. While these gains are small (and still disputed), they would be hard to match by legal methods of additional training. Endurance is presumably modified partly by the elevation of mood, and partly through an increase of central blood volume. Any increase of strength is probably due to a release of cortical inhibition.

Large doses of amphetamines can produce palpitations and cardiac arrhythmias even while the subject is resting. The danger of ventricular fibrillation during exercise is almost certainly increased by the use of these drugs. Other physiological responses include dryness of the mouth, sweating, diarrhoea, blurring of vision, dizziness, and tremor. The last phenomenon is an indication of lesser damping of the γ loop system (p. 173).

The use of amphetamines carries many dangers. The athlete may be so euphoric that he ignores the usual warnings of fatigue and seriously overstress a muscle. Aggressiveness, delusions and hallucinations can lead to antisocial behaviour, and serious impairment of skilled performance such as driving; amphetamines may further change a sleepy drunk into a dangerously wide-awake drunk. The intravenous administration of any drug through poorly sterilized needles leads to epidemics of serum hepatitis, with the risk of permanent liver damage. Large intravenous doses of the amphetamines may produce a dramatic rise of systemic blood pressure, with risks of cerebral haemorrhage and cardiac failure. Frequent use of the amphetamines is also said to cause skin troubles, ulcers, pneumonia and convulsions in addition to the nutritional problems associated with suppression of appetite.

It is uncertain whether physical dependence can develop, but the possibility of this is suggested by (a) increasing tolerance of the drug and (b) reports of physical withdrawal reactions with depression, sleeplessness, and difficulty in micturition. Psychological dependence is common, particularly in those who take the drug intravenously.

Caffeine

Caffeine, theophylline and theobromine are three chemically related stimulants of the central nervous system. Caffeine is present in tea, coffee and cola. Theophylline is also present in tea, while theobromine is present in cocoa, chocolate and cola. All tend to be precipitated by addition of milk or cream to a beverage. A typical cup of coffee contains about 150 mg of caffeine; tea is usually less potent (depending on dilution), and cola drinks contain about 50 mg. These figures are all less than the usual pharmacological doses (0.2–1.0 gm).

The general actions of the three compounds are similar. Stimulation of the higher centres of the brain gives a quickening of thought, and a lessening of fatigue and drowsiness; with larger doses there may be difficulty in holding attention, restlessness, and insomnia. Effects upon the central nervous system are most marked following ingestion of caffeine. The stimulants are also ergogenic. The capacity for physical exertion is increased— soldiers can march further, with fewer "drop-outs", and in the laboratory 20 to 30 percent more work can be performed on a bicycle ergometer. The greater effort tolerance may be due mainly to a stimulation of higher centres, although large doses of caffeine can cause an increase of both cardiac stroke volume and aerobic power, together with a greater irritability of the myocardium. Ergographic measurements show an increase of muscular force, but coordination and recently acquired motor skills deteriorate. Large doses of the drugs cause tremor and convulsions. Some of these effects are attributable to a direct pharmacological irritation of the muscle; strength and extensibility are both increased. Theobromine has the greatest action in this direction. However, removal of central inhibition and a lessening of the sense of fatigue are also important, and caffeine is the most potent drug in this respect.

Theophylline acts primarily as a coronary vasodilator and diuretic; it thus has rather little influence on performance unless effort is limited by oxygen lack within the heart muscle.

Compounds of the caffeine class are undoubtedly taken by many endurance athletes, particularly long-distance cyclists. Providing intake is restricted to the drinking of normal beverages, there would seem no great objection to this, or indeed any easy basis of prevention. An excessive intake of coffee can cause indigestion and cardiac arrhythmias; there is even some development of dependence, with somnolence and irritability for a few days following withdrawal of the drug. Further, the regular consumption of five or more cups of coffee per day is associated with an appreciable (30%) increase of morbidity from coronary heart disease, possibly due to the increased irritability of the myocardium (see also p. 76). However, other factors may well be involved. Caffeine ingestion leads to a significant increase of serum free fatty acid levels, particularly if the drug is administered as a beverage without sugar; there are also statistical associations between the frequent drinking of coffee and both a high serum cholesterol and a large intake of sucrose.

Cocaine *("Charlie," "Coke," "Girl," "Snow")*

Cocaine is an alkaloid obtained from the leaves of the coca tree; natives of Peru and Bolivia have been addicted to the chewing of coca leaves for many centuries. Addicts in North America take either a snuff or intravenous injections.

In addition to its local anaesthetic properties, cocaine induces a general stimulation of the central nervous system. The action on the hypothalamus is particularly marked, and the results thus resemble peripheral stimulation of the adrenergic nerves. The pulse and respiration rates are increased, the systemic blood pressure rises, and the blood sugar and body temperature are increased.

Stimulation of the higher centres of the brain leads to excitement, garrulousness, and extreme restlessness. Intravenous injection gives an ecstatic sensation of physical and mental power, with increased activity, and absence of fatigue and hunger; this last for fifteen minutes or less. With repeated dosage, there is also an increase of deep tendon reflexes, tremor, spasm of muscles, and occasionally convulsions—the sensitivity of the γ loop system (p. 173) has been increased. Eventually, a toxic psychosis and paranoid delusions may develop.

The South American natives believe the coca leaf enables them to perform unusual feats of endurance. Laboratory experiments have suggested moderate doses of cocaine can postpone fatigue and increase the endurance of cyclists. However, the drug should never be used for this purpose, since addiction is extremely rapid.

Morphine *("M")*

Opium juice is derived from the unripe pod of the oriental poppy. It contains a number of alkaloids, of which the most important are morphine (10%) and narcotine (6%). Opium smoking extends back throughout recorded history, but present-day addicts more commonly use synthetically prepared morphine and its diacetyl derivative heroin. Morphine is given by injection, while heroin is smoked, taken as snuff, or injected subcutaneously. The extent of addiction in North America can be judged from the fact that in New York City the commonest cause of death between the ages of eighteen and thirty-five is an overdose of heroin; the New York area now boasts nearly one thousand deaths per year from heroin poisoning, or about one per one hundred and fifty adult man-years.

The main action of the opiates is a general depression of the central nervous system. Euphoria and facilitation of the imagination are the attractions noted by addicts. The reticular formation is depressed, and in consequence spinal reflexes are less active. The pulse and respiration are also slowed, and larger doses give sleep and coma.

Addiction is both rapid and difficult to treat, and while initially small quantities of the opiate are taken, eventually the craving is only satisfied by enormous doses, bought by crime or "pushing" the drug to other victims. The addict can sometimes be identified by a scarring of his arms, due to secondary infection at the sites of injection, and the diagnosis can be verified by paper chromatographic analysis of urine specimens.

Athletes and Drugs

"Doping"

"Doping" may be defined as an attempt to influence the outcome of an athletic competition by administration of drugs not required for the medical treatment of the individual. It is a cause for disqualification in most major competitions, including those sponsored by the International Olympic Association, the Amateur Athletic Union, and the International Amateur Athletic Federation. However, it is often difficult to draw the dividing line between "doping" and permissible forms of treatment. Performance may be improved by the use of sedatives such as barbiturates which ensure a sound night's sleep prior to a competition. Likewise, a tranquillizer may be prescribed for the control of pregame tension. A cocaine derivative may be injected into a joint to permit activity following a minor sprain and this may have not only local but also general effects. Finally, an athlete may habitually enjoy strong coffee or frequent cola drinks.

It is almost impossible to draw up a definition of doping that will cover all possible circumstances, and much must be left to the integrity and sportsmanship of the athlete and his attending physician. Perhaps the most tempting substances for the athlete to use are caffeine and the amphetamines. One is a constituent of natural beverages, and the other is closely related to the naturally occurring noradrenaline; thus, even if the policing of athletes by saliva, blood, or urine testing is thought desirable, it is technically quite difficult to obtain valid information. The sensible athlete polices himself. Fatigue is a warning to the body that the limit of performance—physiological or psychological—has been reached, and an individual who suppresses this warning system by the use of central nervous stimulants does so at his peril. Not only is there a danger of overstressing the body, but the drugs proposed as ergogenic aids are habit forming, with dangerous side effects.

Other Potential Ergogenic Aids

During exhausting work, the pH of the venous blood may drop as low at 7.0, and there is a consistent accumulation of lactate both in the active muscles and in the blood stream. The metabolically engendered acidosis could well contribute to the sensation of fatigue, and there has thus been an interest in extending performance by administration of buffers.

The compounds tested have usually been sodium and potassium salts such as bicarbonate or citrate. The initial response to an excess of such "alkali" is an increase of blood pH, with some decrease of ventilation (line AB of Fig. 74); the body then tends to restore blood pH by a further reduction in ventilation with retention of CO_2 (line BC). Changes within the cerebrospinal fluid proceed in the opposite direction; the pH falls with the initial hypoventilation (line AB), but within a few hours the bicarbonate levels in the cerebrospinal fluid have been increased, and a normal pH is restored (line BC).

The sequence of physiological events is rather complex, and the effects of alkalies upon performance undoubtedly depend on the time at which they are administered. Dennig has claimed substantial increases of endurance in moderately trained subjects following ingestion of a mixture of citrates and bicarbonates. Treatment started two days prior to testing and ceased five hours before assessment; this schedule permitted adjustment of buffer systems throughout the body. Others who have given "alkalies" to highly trained subjects nearer the time of competition have found no improvement of performance. Certainly, not all the effects of alkali are beneficial. The initial increase of blood pH

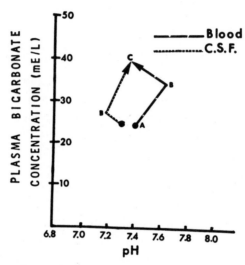

Figure 74. The effects of administering an "alkali." Initially, there is an increase of blood pH with some decrease of ventilation (AB). Later, pH is restored by a further fall of ventilation (BC). Changes within the cerebrospinal fluid proceed in the opposite direction.

causes a displacement of the oxygen dissociation curve to the left (making tissue oxygen extraction more difficult), and the subsequent increase of bicarbonate levels in the cerebrospinal fluid lowers the sensitivity of the respiratory centre to metabolically produced carbon dioxide.

If further research confirms the beneficial effects of early and sustained bicarbonate therapy, then interest will undoubtedly be directed to organic buffers such as THAM (tris-hydroxy-methyl amino-methane), which are less readily eliminated from the body.

It would be impossible to legislate against administration of sodium bicarbonate, since it is widely distributed in normal body fluids. On the other hand, athletes should be warned of possible adverse effects of excessive doses, including flatulence and purging. Further, in view of the ability of the body to regulate buffering capacity, it is questionable whether interference with normal regulation is advantageous; it seems likely that if an individual trains hard, he will already have developed an optimum adjustment of his tissue buffers. This indeed is one of the suggested advantages of accumulating lactic acid by prolonged-interval training. Organic buffers have no role in normal medical treatment, and their administration to athletes should definitely be regarded as doping.

Androgenic Hormones. Contestants in events such as discus throwing report a widespread illegal use of androgenic hormones, and some even maintain it is impossible to reach "world class" without the use of such compounds.

The naturally occurring testosterone is secreted by the interstitial cells of the testes from the time of puberty, and it plays some role in the adolescent strength spurt (p. 371). In certain synthetic derivatives of testosterone (for example, norethandrolone and oxandrolone) the masculinising effects have been eliminated, leaving simply a growth potentiating effect.

There is some evidence that compounds of this class are useful in treating the muscular wasting of older men, particularly following surgery. However, the rationale of administering androgenic hormones to young and normally virile men is obscure, and there is no objective evidence that performance is improved thereby. While the androgens can stimulate hypertrophy of wasted muscles, in a well-trained athlete the muscle fibres have already reached the maximum diameter compatible with continued oxygenation (p. 102). Further, the anabolic compounds have well-recognised and very dangerous side effects, including the possibility of kidney and liver damage and (in the adolescent) the premature closure of bone epiphyses.

Ergogenic Foods. Gelatin contains glycine, one of the three amino acids used in the synthesis of creatine; perhaps because of this, it was at one time thought that gelatin had an ergogenic effect. In fact, careful studies have failed to show this, and it is now appreciated that glycine is not an "essential" amino acid; it can be synthesized by amination of glucose residues.

Aspartate is another food material for which ergogenic properties have been claimed. Again it is difficult to see why ingestion of this particular compound should help an athlete. It can be formed by amination of oxaloacetic acid, part of the normal Krebs metabolic cycle, and the current concensus is that it has no effect on human performance.

In prolonged events, where muscle stores of glycogen become exhausted, performance is improved by administration of small quantities of sweet drinks (monosaccharides such as glucose, or disaccharides such as sucrose). Absorption takes about 30 minutes. Sugars are unlikely to have any physiological effect on the outcome of brief events.

Various vitamins have their advocates, but there is no objective evidence that any improve performance, at least in young, healthy and adequately nourished individuals. Indeed, an excessive intake of vitamins can be dangerous. Overdosage with vitamin A leads to swellings over the long bones, while an excess of vitamin D leads to osteoporosis, with potentially fatal calcification of the heart, blood vessels, lungs, and renal tissues.

Ultraviolet Irradiation. There have been claims that regular exposure to artificial ultraviolet irradiation improved physical performance. The main action of ultraviolet light is to increase the natural synthesis of Vitamin D_3 from the inactive sterol 7-dehydrocholesterol normally found in the skin. Thus, providing diet is adequate, it seems likely that any change of performance has a psychological rather than a physiological origin.

A second response to sunlight is a negative ionization of the air; this is brought about by cosmic irradiation, and can be produced experimentally by suitable equipment. Various extravagant claims have been made for negatively ionized air, including stimulation of ciliary activity in the trachea, increased secretion of adrenal glucocorticoids, an increase in the CO_2 content of the plasma, and dramatic improvements of static and dynamic work tolerance. The possible basis of such changes is far from clear, and more recent work suggests that negative ions have no great physiological role. The question should perhaps be resolved finally, since it has recently been reported that the converse of sunlight (air pollution) restricts athletic performance (p. 369). Track times were found to be correlated with concentrations of "oxidant" smog in Los Angeles, however, various mechanisms other than altered ionization could be responsible for the impaired performance, including decreased cortical arousal and motivation in adverse weather, chest and eye discomfort, an increase of airway resistance and thus the work of breathing and even an associated accumulation of carbon monoxide in the atmosphere.

Oxygen. It is generally agreed that the breathing of increased concentrations of oxygen has a beneficial effect on physical performance (p. 151). Bannister and Balke have both found that 66% oxygen increased treadmill endurance more than 100% oxygen. The mechanisms of action probably include a reduction in the work of breathing, an increase in the quantity of oxygen carried in physical solution in the blood, and a smaller accumulation of lactate in the tissues. The benefits of breathing oxygen are most obvious when oxygenation of the blood is impaired (for instance, in mountaineers, and patients with chronic cardio-respiratory disease); in these special cases, the use of portable oxygen equipment can materially extend performance. The lesser benefits obtained from 100% oxygen reflect a progressive accumulation of CO_2 in the brain, due to reduced ventilation, cerebral vasoconstriction, and a reduced buffering capacity of the fully oxygenated blood.

The use of oxygen before and after exercise has popularity in some sports, particularly professional football in the United States. Inhalation of oxygen immediately prior to brief events such as a one hundred yard swim gives some improvement of performance. Certain authors dismiss the benefit as purely psychological, but an evaluation of body oxygen stores (p. 152) suggests that a true physiological improvement can be obtained from several preliminary minutes of oxygen inhalation. There are also marginal physiological advantages to the use of oxygen during the recovery period (p. 152).

Hypnosis. Ikai and Steinhaus have suggested that strength is normally limited not by the maximum force that can be exerted by muscles, but rather by centrally acquired inhibitions. They were able to improve the recorded strength by 7 percent to 27 percent, using a variety of Pavlovian techniques of disinhibition, such as the firing of a pistol two to 10 seconds prior to activity, a shout at the time of contraction, hypnosis, and administration of amphetamines. The influence of such procedures is most marked in a suggestible individual, particularly if he has been warned frequently of the dangers of overexertion. If the inhibitions can be resolved, then an individual of this type may well show both an improved exercise tolerance and a greater acceptance of a strenuous training regime. However, it is less certain how beneficial such techniques are to healthy and normally active people with no fears of physical activity.

Glossary

The terminology of the drug user is sufficiently bizarre that a brief glossary may be helpful in understanding what the addict says; it is not suggested that the scientist himself should make a "phoney" incursion into the "Hippie" subculture. Many of the words listed have been collected by Dr. Bewley, a consulting psychiatrist in London, England.

Acid—LSD

African woodbine—marijuana

Bang—sensation after intravenous injection of drug

Benny—benzedrine

Black Bomber; Black and Tan; Black and White—amphetamine capsules

Block—hashish resin

Blocked—under influence of drug

Blow—smoke various forms of cannabis; masturbate; break with personal reality

Blue—amphetamine compound and other blue tablets. Policeman.

Boy—heroin

Bread—money

Brought down—depression following drug elation

Bugged—sores or abscesses resulting from subcutaneous injections

Bullet—a capsule

Bummer—unpleasant drug experience

Burn—take someone else's narcotic; smoke marijuana; purchase ineffective drug

Burned out—recovered from drug dependence

Business—apparatus for injection

Bust—arrest

Buzz—drug induced exhilaration

C—cocaine

Candyman—cocaine dealer

Caps—capsules of heroin

Charas(h)—black Indian cannabis

Charge—cannabis

Charlie—cocaine

Christmas tree—drinamyl spansules
Chuck—eat excessively during withdrawal from narcotics
Coke—cocaine
Cold turkey—stop taking narcotics suddenly
Come down—lose drug-induced exhilaration
Cook up—prepare injection
Cop—purchase or acquire
Corporation cocktail—coal gas bubbled through milk
Crank up—inject a narcotic
Croaker—physician who provides narcotics to addicts
Crutch—a split match used to smoke a marijuana cigarette completely
Cunt—area of vein for injection
Cut—adulterate drugs
D—detective
Deal—small amount of cannabis
Deck—injection (especially of heroin)
Derry—derelict house
Dex—dexamphetamine sulphate tablets
Ditch—cubital fossa (used for injection)
Drag—marijuana cigarette
Drop—inject
Drying out—slow withdrawal from narcotics or alcohol
Double blue—amphetamine/barbiturates
Dominoes—durophet spansules
Down—sedative, tranquillizer
Fix—injection of narcotic drug
Flash—effect of cocaine
Freak—hallucinate
Freddy—ephedrine tablet
Gage—cannabis
Get through—obtain drugs
Girl—cocaine
Goof—to spoil injection of narcotic/or give oneself away to police
Goof balls—barbiturates
Grass—cannabis
Green and blacks—librium capsules
Guide—person familiar with drug and relatively sober while others take it for the first time
Gun—syringe
H—heroin
Habit—addiction to drug/or dose commonly taken
Hash—hashish (cannabis)
Herb—cannabis
High—euphoria
Horrors—acute psychosis/or withdrawal symptoms

Horse—heroin
Hung-up—unable to get drugs, depressed
Hypo—addict (from hypodermic)
Jack—heroin tablet
Jack up—inject a narcotic
Jimmy—injection of narcotic
Job—batch of drugs
Joint—marijuana cigarette
Jolly beans—benzedrine
Joy pop—subcutaneous injection of drug
Juice—alcohol
Junkie—addict to narcotics
Lamb (chop)—injection of narcotic
LBJ—mixture of LSD, belladonna and strychnine
Load—stock of illegal drugs
M—morphine
Machine—syringe
Main-line—intravenous injection
Man—authority, police
Mary Jane—marijuana
Meth—methedrine
Minstrel—amphetamine
M—morphine
Mud—crude opium
O—opium
Paranatural—derealisation, depersonalisation or dissociation induced
    by drugs
Peace pill—mescaline, cocaine and LSD
Pellet—tablet
Per—prescription
Phy—Physeptone
Pipe—large vein
Point—needle
Pop—inject
Pot—marijuana
Purple heart—drinanyl
Push—sell narcotics
Rangoon—natural cannabis
Red biddy—methylated or surgical spirits
Reefer—marijuana cigarette
Roach—end of marijuana cigarette
Rope—marijuana
Sausage—marijuana
Scene—group of users, or place of drug usage
Score (v)—to obtain drugs/or get heroin in excess of requirement

Scratch—search for drugs
Script—prescription
Shirash—cannabis
Shit—heroin
Shmee—heroin; amphetamines
Shoot up—inject intravenously
Sick—symptoms of opiate withdrawal
Sleepers—barbiturates
Snort—take drug by sniffing
Snow—cocaine
Speedball—combination of cocaine, heroin and other opiates
Spike—hypodermic needle
Spliff—marijuana cigarette
Stick—marijuana cigarette
Straight—ordinary cigarette; person who rejects drug sub-culture
Strung out—feeling ill from lack of narcotics
Stuff—cannabis
Sugar—LSD
Sweets—amphetamines
Tampi—cannabis
Taste—small amount of drug giving just perceptible symptoms
Tea—marijuana
Tom (mix)—injection of narcotic
Turn-on—smoke a marijuana cigarette/or give nonaddict his first shot
Turn over—to rob
Uncle—police or informer
Weed—marijuana
Wired—addicted
Works—syringe, spoon, etc.
Wrap up—brown paper packet containing cannabis
Zen—LSD

References

U.S. Public Health Service: Smoking and health. *Report of the Advisory Committee to the Surgeon General of the Public Health Service.* Washington, D.C., 1964.

U.S. Public Health Service: The health consequences of smoking. *A Public Health Service Review.* Washington, D.C., 1967.

Terry, L.L.: *World Conference on Smoking and Health.* American Cancer Society, 1967.

Wynder, E.L., and Hoffmann, D.: *Tobacco and Tobacco Smoke.* New York, Academic Press, 1967.

Rode, A.: Acute and chronic effects of smoking on fitness. M.Sc. Thesis, University of Toronto, Toronto, Ont.

World Health Organization: Alcohol and alcoholism. *WHO Tech Rep 94,* WHO, Geneva, Switzerland, 1955.

Fox, B.H., and Fox, J.H.: *Alcohol and Traffic Safety.* U.S.P.H.S. Publication, *1043,* 1963.

Plaut, T.F.A.: *Alcohol Problems—a Report to the Nation.* New York, Oxford University Press, 1967.

Pittman, D.J.: *Alcoholism.* New York, Harper and Row, 1967.

Block, M.A.: *Alcoholism. Its Facets and Phases.* London, Oxford University Press, 1965.

Blum, R.H.: *Society and Drugs.* San Francisco, Jossey-Bass, 1969.

Blum, R. H.: *Students and Drugs.* San Francisco, Jossey-Bass, 1969.

Barber, B.: *Drugs and Society.* New York, Russell Sage Foundation, 1967.

McKennell, A.C., and Thomas, R.K.: Adults and adolescents smoking habits and attitudes. U.K. Ministry of Health, 1967.

Schwartz, J.L.: *Psychosocial Factors in Cigarette Smoking and Cessation.* Institute for Health Research, 301 Benvenue, Berkeley, Calif., 1968.

12

AIR POLLUTION

Knowledge of the effects of air pollutants upon human performance is in its infancy. However, the topic is of considerable current interest, and merits at least brief discussion.

There seems little question that high concentrations of the products of coal combustion (soot, sulphur dioxide, and—in the presence of oxidizing catalysts—sulphur trioxide) are physically harmful, particularly to young children, the aged and patients with chronic chest disease. Possibly there is some contribution also from a cold and foggy climate, and in the England of the 1950's (before smoke abatement laws had improved the environment) several thousand deaths seemed attributable to acute episodes of air pollution.

High concentrations of inert dust particles (such as may be found in a coal mine) induce measurable spasm of the bronchi. High concentrations of sulphur dioxide (greater than 5 parts per million) have a similar effect, although tolerance can apparently develop; certainly, workers in oil refineries may be exposed to as much as 30 ppm for many years without ill effects. Both dust and SO_2 increase the work of breathing, thereby inevitably reducing physical performance. Other gases, such as SO_3 and NO_2 are more toxic, and if inhaled in sufficient concentrations may induce pulmonary oedema; subclinical doses presumably have the effect of impairing gas exchange in the lungs, although this has not been well-documented.

Recent observations from California have suggested a negative correlation between the concentration of air pollutants and performance in running events. The usual Californian "smog" is rather different in chemical composition from a London fog, containing a higher concentration of both carbon monoxide and oxidants. Physiological reactions to oxidants, apart from a smarting and watering of the eyes are remarkably few, and it may be that the loss of performance noted is purely a subjective reaction to exercise in an unpleasant environment. It is also possible that some associated change, such as an alteration in the temperature or humidity of the atmosphere may be influencing performance. However, the smog does contain appreciable amounts of SO_2, ozone, and carbon monoxide, all of which could have a physical effect upon performance.

Carbon monoxide is currently receiving much attention from environmental engineers. On busy highways, concentrations can be 30 to 40 ppm, and where vehicles are idling under bridges and viaducts concentrations of 100 ppm may be seen. The physiological effects of carbon monoxide have been reviewed in the section on smoking, since this is the major factor causing accumulation of carbon monoxide within the body. Nevertheless, recent studies have shown that even the nonsmoker suffers some decrement of performance due to carbon monoxide, particularly if his home is in an urban environment and he drives in heavy traffic.

The changes demonstrated have been in the reaction time and other tests of psychomotor function; although the disturbances have been slight, they could affect the outcome of either a near traffic accident or a closely-contested short distance athletic event. The physiological mechanism is probably a cerebral oxygen lack secondary to displacement of the oxygen dissociation curve by the carbon monoxide.

What attitude should the science graduate adopt towards air contaminants? The several fatal episodes of acute pollution emphasize that in many large cities the concentration of pollutants can (under adverse weather conditions) approach the limit compatible with continued health. There is also a substantial suspicion that chronic exposure to the urban atmosphere operates synergically with cigarette smoking to increase the risks of lung cancer.

There are thus good medical reasons to press steadily (although not hysterically) for cleaner air. But on the basis of present evidence, the main emphasis of any drive against air or water pollution should rest not on health or performance, but on the possibility of an improved quality of life. Much has been achieved in London over the past ten years, and to see a clear sun shining over the River Thames, as fish play in the sparkling waters, is in itself reward for the inevitable costs of controlling domestic and industrial emissions.

13

GROWTH AND AGEING

Patterns of Growth

The General Growth Curve

If the course of child development is assessed in terms of a general criterion of body size such as height or weight, the resulting growth curve shows rapid progress over the first two years, a period of rather steady development for the next six or more years, an acceleration before and during puberty, and a final deceleration as the adult size is reached (Figs. 75, 76).

In early childhood, girls are marginally smaller than boys of a similar age, but because they reach puberty earlier, the girls also show an earlier "growth spurt," becoming heavier and taller than the boys between the ages of twelve and fourteen. If averaged data for an entire population is considered, the "growth spurt" is not a very impressive phenomenon, particularly in

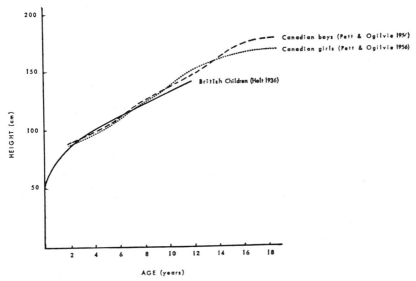

Figure 75. Relationship of standing height to age.

371

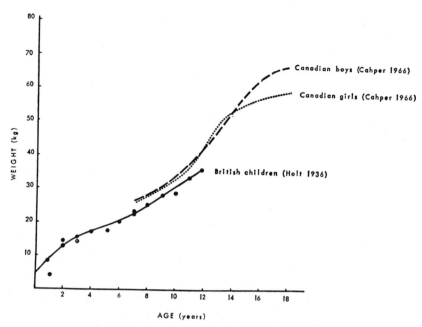

Figure 76. Relationship of body weight to age.

terms of standing height (Fig. 75). The reason for this is that the growth spurt occurs at different ages in different children; when the average is calculated, the deceleration of growth in the early developers masks the spurt in those who mature more slowly. If the growth of an individual child is studied year by year, the height increases by 5 cm/yr between the ages of five and ten, and 7–8 cm/yr immediately prior to puberty; thereafter there is an exponential decline of growth rate to near zero velocity at seventeen to eighteen years of age.

Regional Development

Individual tissues grow at different stages in an individual's development. Some 90 percent of growth in the *brain and head* occurs in the first five years of life, and development of this region is virtually complete at the age of ten. This is related in part to the course of ossification. Up to the age of eighteen months, the individual bony plates of the skull are separated at the fontanelles, and it is relatively easy for an expansion of the brain cavity to occur. Between the ages of two and ten some growth is still possible at the "sutures" between individual bony plates, but thereafter further expansion can only occur if bone is eaten away from the inner surface of the skull and deposited on its exterior.

The *thymus gland* and *lymphoid tissues* also show an atypical growth pattern, reaching almost twice the adult size at puberty; the functions of the thymus gland are still somewhat obscure, but it appears to play an important role in the development of immunity to foreign proteins.

The *reproductive tissues* remain relatively dormant until just before puberty; very rapid growth then occurs, and the mature size is reached in the space of four or five years. In boys, the first sign of puberty is an accelerated growth of the testes and scrotum; this occurs between the tenth and the thirteenth years. About a year later, accelerated growth of the penis begins, and this is accompanied by the height spurt. Pubic hair begins to appear between the tenth and the fifteenth years, and grows more vigorously with enlargement of the penis; axillary and facial hair first develop some two years after pubic hair. Enlargement of the larynx and breaking of the voice occur when growth of the penis is almost complete, and at this stage there is a marked development of strength relative to standing height. In girls, the breasts first begin to develop between eight and thirteen years, and the growth of pubic hair, the development of the uterus and vagina and the height spurt run roughly parallel with breast growth. The first menstrual period (menarche) occurs between the tenth and the sixteenth years, towards the end of the pubertal changes. The girls do not show a strength spurt; on the contrary, the rate of increase in strength slows at the time of puberty. It is uncertain how far this is a true constitutional effect, and how far it reflects social pressures and expectations.

Body fat shows a rather interesting growth curve; there is a substantial (10%–20%) increase of subcutaneous fat between the time of birth and about nine months of age; then, as the child becomes more mobile, the percentage of body fat decreases, and a minimum is reached between six and eight years of age. Girls are on average slightly fatter than boys even in

early childhood, and the difference between the two sexes becomes more marked after the age of eight.

Not only are there differences in the rate of development
between different tissues but there are also differences in the
growth rate of the same tissue in different parts of the body.
Thus in the upper limb, the hands develop earlier than the forearms, and the forearms are in turn consistently closer to their
final adult size than are the upper arms. The same type of growth
pattern (feet > lower legs > upper legs) is shown by the lower
limbs.

Physiological Development

Aerobic power has been studied from the age of four through
to adult life; most investigations have been "cross-sectional," but
there is no reason to suppose that a longitudinal study would
yield a different answer. In boys, there is a steady growth of
absolute readings, so that if data are expressed relative to body
weight, the maximum oxygen intake maintains a constant reading of about 50 ml/kg min STPD. Swedish students tested by
Åstrand showed some improvement in late adolescence, reaching an aerobic power of almost 60 ml/kg min. However, most
other laboratories have not found this; possibly his students
were of above average fitness. Åstrand also found a very high
maximum heart rate in his boys (210–215/min); few North
American authors have found maxima greater than 195–200/min.
All laboratories seem agreed that the terminal blood lactate in
exhausting effort (80 mg/100 ml of blood) is less in children
than in young adults. This may reflect difficulty in reaching a
true plateau of oxygen consumption (p. 412); only about half
of a typical group of schoolchildren show an oxygen plateau.
In young girls, the maximum oxygen intake is almost as high as
in boys, but a deterioration sets in at about ten years of age. This
seems more marked in North America than in Scandinavia, and
teenage girls in the United States and Canada have as low an
aerobic power as adult women (i.e. about 40 ml/kg min).

Submaximum tests. The aerobic power can be predicted from
submaximum exercise tests, as in the adult (p. 415). At the
first visit, anxiety may increase the exercise pulse rate, leading

to a ten percent underestimate of maximum oxygen intake. Interpolated tests such as the PWC_{170} may also be used (p. 421); these again show a regular development with age, normal values averaging about 14 kgm/kg. min in boys, and 11 kgm/kg. min in girls.

Oxygen Conductance. Individual links in the oxygen transport chain (p. 105) develop roughly in proportion to body size. However, there is some evidence that alveolar ventilation accounts for a larger proportion of total ventilation in children than in adults, and that the maximum cardiac output and heart size of a child are smaller than would be expected from body weight. The haemoglobin concentration is also less than in the adult, ranging from about 12 gm/100 ml at one year to 14 gm/100 ml at puberty; in the girls, there is no further increase in either haemoglobin concentration or red cell count, but in the boys a peak haemoglobin of more than 16 gm/100 ml is reached at the age of eighteen, the red cell count increasing from the pubertal value of 4.6×10^6 cells/mm^3 to as much as 5.4×10^6 cells/mm^3.

Strength. People commonly talk of children outgrowing their strength. There is some support for this popular view in the sense that the boys' growth spurt (associated with a lengthening of the long bones) precedes the strength spurt. In the girls, also, height continues to increase beyond the age of twelve to thirteen years, although there is little further development of muscular strength. However, the growth of size prior to strength is a normal feature of adolescence and should not cause alarm or restriction of activity.

Assessment of Maturity

If one wishes to evaluate the result of either a physiological test or a performance measurement in an adolescent child, it is necessary to decide whether the child in question has reached or passed the period of accelerated growth. Scales have been developed for quantitation of sexual development, but the most reliable indices of overall maturity are bone growth as assessed from radiographs, and eruption of the teeth (Tables VIII and IX). In radiographs, attention is directed to the appearance and

TABLE VIII
ASSESSMENT OF SKELETAL AGE FROM RADIOGRAPHS OF THE
WRIST AND LONG BONES

Skeletal Age (Yr)	Carpal Ossification	Other Bones Showing Centres of Ossification
1	Os magnum (capitate)	Head of femur
2	Unciform (hamate)	Lower epiphysis of radius, tibia & fibula
3	Cuneiform (triquetral)	Patella, head of humerus
4	—	Lower epiphysis of ulna, upper epiphysis of fibula and greater trochanter
5	Trapezoid, Semilunar	Upper epiphysis of radius
6	Scaphoid	Centres in head of humerus coalesce
10		Upper epiphysis of ulna Tuberosity of os calcis
12	Pisiform	

TABLE IX
ERUPTION OF TEETH IN RELATION TO DEVELOPMENTAL AGE

Age	Teeth Erupted
	("*Milk*") *Deciduous Teeth*
6– 9 months	Lower central incisors
8–10	Upper incisors
15–21	Lower lateral incisors and first molars
16–20	Canines
20–24	Second molars
	Permanent Teeth
6 years	First molars
7	Two central incisors
8	Two lateral incisors
9	First premolars
10	Second premolars
11–12	Canines
12–13	Second molars
17–25	Third molars

size of centres of ossification, and the extent to which the epiphyses have fused with the shafts of the long bones. The precision of the "development age" thus calculated varies with the calendar age of the child, but at puberty it can be estimated to within about half a year. The dental age has a similar precision; account is taken of both the number of teeth that are visible, and the completeness of their eruption.

In general, girls are more advanced in skeletal and dental development than boys; further, if children of either sex are classified in terms of developmental age, those who are in advance of their calendar years shows greater intellectual and emotional maturity and an earlier puberty. On the other hand, if account is taken of the larger size of those maturing early, then developmental age contributes relatively little to the description of physiological variables such as aerobic power and muscular strength.

Control of Growth

Hormonal Regulation

The prenatal regulation of growth is still somewhat obscure, but it is known that the Y chromosome stimulates the development of the testes from about the seventh week of intrauterine life, and that from the twelfth week the testicular cells produce androgens that lead to differentiation of secondary sexual characteristics. An adequate secretion from the foetal thyroid gland is also necessary to growth, particularly growth of the brain.

After birth, the main regulatory mechanism is a polypeptide "growth hormone" secreted by the pituitary gland, this hormone promotes the incorporation of amino acids into tissue protein, and leads to the formation of muscle and bone rather than fat. The continuing presence of thyroid hormone is also important to growth, and if the thyroid secretion is deficient, development is delayed. The adolescent growth spurt is a response to androgens, secreted by the adrenal cortex in both sexes, and by the testes in the male. Testosterone is probably responsible for the increase of muscle strength and red cell count in boys following puberty. The secretion of these androgens is triggered by "gonadotrophins" liberated from the pituitary gland; the release of the gonadotrophins is in turn held in check by the hypothalamus until an appropriate stage of development has been reached.

Environmental Factors

The relative importance of environmental and constitutional factors in determining the rate of maturation and ultimate body size is still debated. One possible approach is to compare identical and nonidentical twins. The age of menarche differs by an average of two months between identical twins, and by ten months between those that are not identical. This suggests that genetic factors influence the situation, but is perhaps unfair to environment, since twins normally share rather similar living conditions, and a certain variance of environment is a necessary prelude to demonstration of an effect.

A second approach is to compare children of differing social class. It has been recognised for many years that social status is associated with greater growth and earlier maturation; indeed, differences were more obvious in the last century than at the present time, when the traditional social boundaries are breaking down. In the Great Britain of the 1870s, a growing boy with "labouring" class parents was 10 cm shorter than a boy whose parents were not manual workers, and he was also 12 cm shorter than students attending the very privileged "public" school system; the differences were smaller, but still quite obvious (3 and 5 cm respectively) when data for early manhood were considered. In the 1950s, the children of parents falling into British Social classes I and II (professional and semiprofessional groups) were still 2–3 cm taller than the national average. Factors contributing to the greater growth of those at the upper end of the social scale probably include better nutrition, a larger home and thus more adequate sleep, a generally better organized pattern of life, and possibly (at least for students attending British "public" schools) more deliberate exercise.

The specific effect of nutritional deficiencies is seen in data from Germany; the average height of German children increased by about 10 cm between 1920 and 1940, but decreased by 3 cm during the subsequent war period. Animal experiments have also demonstrated the need for first-class protein if growth is to be maintained; the body is unable to synthesize certain amino acids (Table X), and if these are lacking from the diet then an animal fails to gain weight at the speed of its control litter mates. One important criticism of many strenuous animal training experiments is that the exercised group fails to show a normal rate

TABLE X
AMINO ACIDS ESSENTIAL TO GROWTH

*Threonine	Lysine
*Valine	*Methionine
Leucine	*Phenylalanine
*Iso-leucine	*Tryptophan
Arginine	Histidine

* Essential for maintenance of body weight.

of weight gain, presumably because the food intake has been inadequate. Unless malnutrition is prolonged, the main effect of a restricted diet is to delay rather than limit development, and if observations are extended for a long enough period the affected men or animals reach the same size as well-fed controls. Chronic illness leads to a retardation of growth, but it is less certain whether this is a specific effect or a secondary consequence of the accompanying restriction of food intake.

Psychological factors can influence growth. This was well-demonstrated by Widdowson in a study of two German orphanages. In one, growth was much slower than in the second, and this was traced to a stern and rather unpleasant ward sister; when she was transferred to the second orphange, the children at the first establishment gained rapidly in both height and weight, while the development of those at the second orphanage was drastically slowed. (Fig. 77).

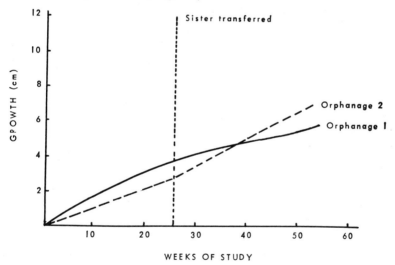

Figure 77. The influence of psychological environment on growth (based on an experiment by Widdowson). A stern and unpleasant sister was transferred from Orphanage 1 to Orphanage 2 at the point indicated by the broken line.

Chronological Trends

One interesting aspect of growth is the progressive increase in body size over the years. A casual visit to an armoury such as that of the White Tower in London is enough to convince the cynic that the present generation is taller than the knights of the middle-ages. In Norway, statistics go back to 1740; there was apparently little change of stature between 1740 and the early 1800s, but over the immediate past century there has been a progressive increase of standing height. In prepubertal boys this amounts to about 1 cm per decade for those with professional parents, and 1.5 cm per decade for those with labouring parents; the adult stature has also increased progressively, the rate of change being about 0.5 and 0.8 cm per decade for the two social groups. The time of puberty has also advanced over the last century; this is best documented for girls, where the age of menarche has changed by about 0.35 years per decade. Maturation remains earlier in those with professional class parents, particularly if they are living in large cities.

What factors have contributed to the faster and greater ultimate growth of the world population? In the poorer classes, improved nutrition and a reduction in the incidence of disease have undoubtedly played a large role. A further factor affecting all classes of society has been a change in marriage patterns. Two hundred years ago it was uncommon for a man to marry outside his immediate village. However, with the development of transport facilities, an ever-increasing range of marriage partners has been available, and the resulting genetic hybridization has almost certainly contributed to greater growth.

Athletic records have developed progressively over the past century, and the rate of improvement is currently showing no sign of slowing; thus the olympic and world record times for the 5000 metre track event have decreased by about 2 percent per decade over the last fifty years, and despite the smaller potential margin for improvement the progression of records has accelerated since 1950. In many athletic events including running and jumping, the increase of average stature has made a large contribution to the improvement of records. Other possible factors include an increase in the total world population, a more complete searching of this population for potential athletes, improvements in training techniques, and in some specific sports improvements in equipment and facilities.

Growth and Performance

Normal Development

In the first four months of life, a baby shows a progressive decrease in reflex and rhythmic movements. Between four and eight months, voluntary activity develops in the upper part of the body, commencing with head raising and progressing to sitting. In the following six months voluntary movement also develops in the lower part of the trunk, and the child learns to walk. Finally, between fourteen and twenty-four months of age, the child acquires movements of a conditional and symbolic type, especially speech. Delay in motor development is often associated with mental deficiency, but this is not necessarily the case; a fair range of sitting and walking ages are compatible with normal mental health.

Coordination develops quite rapidly between the second and the fifth year of life. An average child can jump off the floor at twenty-eight months, stand on one foot at twenty-nine months, jump from a twelve inch step at thirty-seven months, hop at forty-nine months, and throw a ball into a basket at five years. The scatter in the course of development is shown by Gutteridge's data for United States children aged five and seven respectively:

PERCENT OF GROUP WITH PROFICIENT PERFORMANCE

	Age *5 yr*	*Age* *7 yr*
Jumping	58%	84
Hopping	33	84
Skipping	14	91
Galloping	43	92
Throwing	20	74

Balance has commonly been assessed by ability to walk along a narrow board. Unfortunately the dimensions of the board and the method of scoring have varied with the investigator. Bayley used a board 2.5 metres in length, 6 cm wide and 10 cm high. He found that a child of twenty-eight months could walk with one foot on the board; at thirty-one months he could stand on the board, and by fifty-six months could walk the entire length with alternate steps. At five years, the entire length was walked in six to nine seconds, and this decreased progressively to less than three seconds at seven years.

The coordination of older children has been assessed by the Brace test of general motor ability. This consists of a series of twenty graded stunts such as jumping in the air and clapping the feet together; each stunt is either passed or failed. The battery includes items that are intended to sample agility, control, balance, and flexibility. One problem in test administration is that the stunts are not sufficiently difficult for the skilled performer, and some students gain the maximum possible score of twenty. Boys improve rather steadily from an average score of six at the age of six to sixteen at sixteen years; however, there is some slowing in the increase of score at puberty, reflecting the popular impression that boys become clumsy at this age. Young girls score about the same as the boys, but improve little beyond the age of twelve; at this stage they are superior to the boys only in tests that require careful control of body position and static balance.

The CAHPER and AAHPER performance tests (p. 405) show a similar pattern of motor development. Prior to puberty, the girls have marginally poorer scores than the boys, but whereas the boys continue to increase their performance steadily to seventeen years of age, the girls improve little beyond the age of twelve or thirteen years. This presumably reflects a deterioration of motivation as much as a true physiological impairment.

Age and Training

Protein synthesis is promoted by pituitary growth hormone and by androgens. One would thus anticipate that a training regime would be most successful in inducing hypertrophy of cardiac and skeletal muscles if it were carried out during the period of adolescence, when the growth promoting hormones were present in the highest concentrations. Unfortunately, it is difficult to organise suitably controlled experiments to test this hypothesis.

In some animal experiments, quite exhaustive exercise has been applied, for instance, running the equivalent of five miles per day for fifteen years. This has led to difficulties in maintaining adequate nutrition; further, the stresses have plainly been unequal for exercised and restrained animals. Rats have shown a similar pattern of response to physical training at the equivalents of two and six-teen human years. The overall size of regularly exercised animals has not exceeded that of control litter mates, but internal organs such as the heart have accounted for a bigger proportion of total body weight. Unfortunately, experiments have not been carried out on older animals.

Experiments in dogs have suggested that forced inactivity may retard the growth of the long bones by as much as 20 percent to 25 percent. A similar effect can occur in man; thus the dominant arm is longer than its partner, and this difference is more marked in school-age children than in those aged one to four. Studies of tennis players again have shown substantially greater bone development in the dominant arm, and one epidemiological investigation showed that poor negroes who had worked hard for twelve hours per day during their adolescence were taller than nonworking negroes of a slightly higher social class. Such modifications of skeletal growth can only occur prior to closure of the epiphyses.

It is still uncertain how far cardiac and muscular bulk can be increased by training, and the influence of age upon response is also uncertain; many authors have shown that middle-aged men will respond to an appropriate training regime, and it seems likely that the lesser inherent trainability of those who are older is to some extent counteracted by a lower initial level of fitness.

Limitation of Performance for Children

At one time, it was held that excessive effort was dangerous for growing children. In fact, there seems little evidence to support this contention. The large heart of an active child is a healthy manifestation of the training response, as is the development of firm and adequate musculature. Fears of "athlete's heart," of becoming "muscle bound," or (in the female) of masculinization and damage to the reproductive organs are unwarranted. One possible exception to this generalisation is the repetitive lifting of heavy weights, either at work or in the gymnasium; if excessive loads are carried before closure of the epiphyses, this can lead to deformation of the long bones and the pelvic girdle. The International Labour Organisation has recommended boys aged sixteen to eighteen years should not lift more than 20 kg, and that the limiting load for girls of this age should be 15 kg.

These remarks do not imply a wholesale endorsement of competitive athletics for young children. Major competitions subject the young to undesirable psychological and social pressures, and detract from the primary educational purposes of a school or university.

Patterns of Ageing

The Normal Ageing Process

Ageing is associated with a progressive deterioration of all bodily functions. Individual cells deteriorate, and in many organs a part of the active tissue becomes replaced by fibrous and fatty tissue.

In male subjects, many physiological variables reach their peak values between the ages of twenty and twenty-five years; thereafter, there is a progressive decline, leading to some 30 percent loss of function at sixty years, and more rapid subsequent deterioration (Fig. 78). In the female, the peak values are

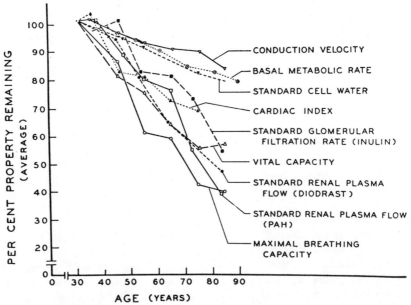

Figure 78. Changes in physiological variables with increasing age. Reproduced from *Proceedings of International Symposium on Physical Activity and Health,* by permission of the author (N.W. Shock) and publishers of the *Canadian Medical Association Journal.*

reached at the time of menarche, and it is by no means clear how far subsequent events are dictated by physiology, and how far by social expectations. We shall thus confine our remarks on ageing to the male. Even with this restriction, there remain a number of obstacles to precise study. What is a normal population? At the age of twenty, relatively few suffer from chronic disease, but at the age of seventy, as many as 50 percent of a population may have some medical abnormality. In general, those who volunteer for testing are the fit and healthy residue. Some of the least fit have been eliminated by death. The true rate of ageing can only be established by painstaking longitudinal investigations; most of the current information is approximate data based on cross-sectional study of age decades. In some instances, the situation has been further complicated by the fitting of linear regressions when the data plainly conform to a curve.

Aerobic power declines from 40–50 ml/kg min at the age of twenty to perhaps 25–30 ml/kg min at the age of sixty; this is due partly to a reduction of absolute aerobic power, and partly to an increase of body weight that commonly occurs between the ages of thirty and forty. There is an associated decrease in the maximum heart rate, from 195 in a young man to about 160 in an older person. The reason for this is obscure. The most logical explanation is a depression of the cardiac pacemaker by a relative oxygen lack within the heart muscle. However, the maximum heart rate of an older person is not increased by the breathing of oxygen during activity. Over the age of forty, an increasing proportion of the population show ECG abnormalities while performing maximum aerobic work; these changes include an increasing horizontal or downward-sloping depression of the ST segment (p. 73) and ventricular extrasystoles. The maximum cardiac output is certainly reduced by the normal, age-related decrease of maximum heart rate. Sometimes both heart rate and cardiac output are limited further by the development of anginal symptoms; however, the stroke volume decreases relatively little with age. The lactate accumulation during a maximum oxygen intake test drops from 100 mg/100 ml of blood in a young person to about 60 mg/100 ml at the age of sixty;

it is uncertain whether this change represents poorer motivation on the part of the older people, or whether there is some physiological basis such as a lesser total store of muscle glycogen.

The mechanical efficiency of submaximal effort is relatively independent of age, and there is thus little change of oxygen consumption, ventilation or pulse rate in response to a given intensity of moderate work. In just submaximum effort, rather more lactate may accumulate in the blood of an older person, and over the range 70 percent to 90 percent of aerobic power, ventilation tends to be greater than in a young person. The rate of adaptation to exercise (the "on-transient") may also be rather slower in an older person.

Oxygen Conductances. Individual links in the oxygen transport chain all show some impairment with age. Stiffening of the joints in the thoracic cage and an increase of airway resistance due to some chronic bronchitis and emphysema reduce the maximum voluntary ventilation from 200 litre/min to 120 litre/min or less. The work of breathing is also increased several fold, and probably for this reason the maximum exercise ventilation is reduced to about 80 litre/min at sixty-five, and to less than 50 litre/min at seventy-five years of age. We have no precise figures for the alveolar ventilation of old people performing maximum work, but it is likely that age is associated with a progressive deterioration of function as has already been documented for rest and light work. The maximum carbon monoxide diffusing capacity decreases progressively with age; this reflects a failure of gas to reach the exchanging surface, the effect of chronic diseases on the lung membrane and alveolar capillary bed, and a smaller maximum cardiac output.

The haemoglobin level theoretically changes little with age. However, in practice, many old people live on rather restricted incomes, or are too lonely and dispirited to prepare nourishing meals; a nutritional anaemia, sometimes exacerbated by atrophy of the gastric mucosa, is thus a not uncommon complaint in the elderly. The tissue "diffusing capacity" also deteriorates. This is partly a reflection of changes in tissue structure, the mucopolysaccharides of the amorphous intercellular substance being replaced by fibrous tissue; there is also a progressive reduction of the maximum capillary bed within the muscles.

Lastly, there is a decrease in the maximum arteriovenous oxygen tension difference. This may reflect in part a diminished ability of the active cells to use oxygen, and in part a decrease of tissue diffusing capacity; however, the major cause is probably that in an older person a smaller percentage of the total cardiac output reaches the active tissues. This in turn may be attributed to the smaller total output, and to the increased blood-flow requirement of tissues other than muscle.

Muscle strength shows a rather extensive age plateau (Fig. 53, p. 189), but the values for a man aged sixty are only some 70 percent of peak readings for a younger person. There is undoubtedly a parallel decrease of muscle bulk. However, the recorded isometric force is limited mainly by a central inhibition of muscular contraction and the apparent loss of strength is undoubtedly influenced by the diminished expectations and the greater fears of over-exertion in the aged.

Blood Pressure. The resting systemic blood pressure rises progressively as a person ages; this is related to a decrease of elasticity in the great vessels, and systolic pressures change to a greater extent than diastolic. Both isometric and prolonged rhythmic work can be limited by an exercise-induced rise of blood pressure. The maximum isometric force and the isotonic endurance of an older person may thus be reduced both by initial hypertension, and also by an unusually rapid rise of systemic pressure as exercise progresses. Reflex adjustments of systemic blood pressure, such as those that occur on standing, are less effective in an older person; this reflects in part a diminution of all reflexes, in part a poorer responsiveness of the capacity vessels, and in part a lower level of cardiorespiratory fitness.

Employment of the Ageing Person

Opinions on the optimum age of an employee vary in almost direct proportion to the age of the person making the judgment. Much depends on the type of work and the criteria of performance that are to be applied. In a desk task, age brings caution, experience, and cumulative skills in the handling of people; on the other hand, creativity and initiative are lost. In neurophysiological terms, one may envisage a progressive decrease in the pool of functioning neurones, but the establishment of an increased number of functional connections; this pattern of change gives both "experience" and "rigidity" of attitudes.

What of tasks calling for physical effort? A worker aged fifty may have much weaker muscles than an employee of thirty, and the aerobic power may also have deteriorated to the point where quite light work represents 50 percent of maximum effort. Nevertheless, unless he is stricken by disease, a fifty-year-old man is well able to continue in his employment. Skill is developed, so that heavy work can be performed more economically. The oxygen cost of the heaviest tasks is further reduced by performing them more slowly. Moreover, the study of overall population statistics may give the misleading impression that all men of fifty are physically weak. In fact, loss of fitness probably occurs more slowly in those who perform heavy work regularly. Unfortunately, the heaviest tasks in a modern factory fall to the "odd-job" man, and the older worker may be relegated to this role when advances in technology have out-dated a traditional and more sedentary craft. The most satisfactory answer to a growing sociological problem seems the development of courses to teach new skills to those displaced by technical advances. In some instances an increase in the physical demands of employment may be unavoidable, and then the 20 percent gain of aerobic power promised by a formal programme of physical training may do much to minimize industrial fatigue.

Ageing and Athletic Performance

In athletic competitions, the average age of successful contestants is markedly influenced by the relative requirements of a given event in terms of agility, physiological power, and experience. Activities such as roller-skating, gymnastics, and speed events are performed best in the late teens. Endurance runners and cyclists, football and tennis players reach their peak in the middle twenties, and a skillful soccer player may remain a useful member of a professional team until his early forties. Sports such as golf and bowling make limited demands on the physiology of the body, and they are performed best in the early thirties.

Ageing and the Training Response

It is now quite well-established that older sedentary men (40–60 years of age) can improve their aerobic power by 10 to 20 percent if they follow a suitable training regime for a period of three months or more. However, this probably represents a regulatory rather than a structural response (p. 446). Body fat may be diminished by as much as 20 percent with a one year programme of regular exercise, but it is less clear how far hypertrophy of heart and skeletal muscle can be induced at this stage of life. A number of longitudinal studies have compared athletes who have persisted with their training and those who have reverted to a sedentary pattern of life. Some of these studies have shown a slower rate of ageing in the continuing athlete, but this has not invariably been the case. Further, the so-called "favourable" rate reported for the continuing athlete has been rather an unfavourable rate for those abandoning an athletic career. Toronto working men apparently lose 23 percent of their aerobic power (—8 ml/kg min) between the ages of forty-five and sixty-five, very similar to the 25 percent loss (—14 ml/kg min) of the continuing athletes studied by Grimby and Saltin. Despite these discouraging figures, the continuing athletes have two practical consolations—(a) their rate of ageing would be worse than that of a sedentary person if they stopped exercising, and (b) while they continue in their athletic endeavors the margin of aerobic power for meeting emergencies remains larger than that of a habitually sedentary individual.

References

Espenschade, A.: Motor development. In Johnson, W.R. (Ed.): *Science and Medicine of Exercise and Sports.* New York, Harper, 1960.

Rarick, G.L.: *Exercise and Growth.* In Johnson, W.R. (Ed.): *Science and Medicine of Exercise and Sports.* New York Harper, 1960.

Buskirk, E.R., and Counsilman, J.E.: Special exercise problems in middle age. In Johnson, W.R. (Ed.): *Science and Medicine of Exercise and Sports.* New York, Harper, 1960.

Åstrand, P-O.: *Experimental Studies of Physical Working Capacity in Relation to Sex and Age.* Copenhagen, Munksgaard, 1952.

Åstrand, I.: Aerobic work capacity in men and women with special reference to age. *Acta Physiol Scand: 49, Supp 169,* 1960.

Shephard, R.J.: The working capacity of schoolchildren. In *Frontiers of Fitness.* Springfield, Thomas, 1971.

Demirjean, A., and Sapoka, A.: Première Réunion Canadienne sur la Croissance et le developpement de l'enfant. Quebec, Ste Marguerite, 1969.

deMath, G.R., Howatt, W.F., and Hill, B.M.: The growth of lung function. *Pediatrics, 35,* Supplement, 1965.

Adams, F.H.; Linde, L.M.: Hall, V.E., and Fowler, W.M.: Exercise fitness tests: Their physiological basis and clinical application to pediatrics. *Pediatrics, 32,* Supplement, 1963.

Harrison, G.A., Weiner, J.S., Tanner, J.M., and Barnicot, N.A.: Human biology. *An Introduction to Human Evolution, Variation and Growth.* London, Oxford University Press, 1964.

Heald, F.P.: *Adolescent Nutrition and Growth.* New York, Appleton-Crofts, 1969.

Sjöstrand, T.: *Physical Fitness in Relation to Age and Sex.* Riksidrotts-förbundets Poliklinikkommitté, Sweden, 1962.

Comfort, A.: *Ageing. The Biology of Senescence.* New York, Holt, Rinehart & Winston, 1963.

Eighth International Congress of Gerontology, Washington, D.C., 1969.

Dacso, M.M.: *Restorative Medicine in Geriatrics.* Springfield, Thomas, 1963.

PART THREE

CHRONIC EFFECTS OF EXERCISE

14

CONCEPTS OF FITNESS

THE DEFINITION OF FITNESS

The average student with a rather limited concept of fitness often conceals his ignorance by asking the question "fitness for what?" In a sense, he is right to do so. The pursuit of "positive health" is the legitimate goal of both physician and physical educator, but it is a very diffuse subject, covering the whole field of human ecology—the physical, social, and psychological interaction between man and his environment.

The type of fitness sought by the individual is markedly influenced by age, sex, occupation, personality, and cultural factors. In childhood, the level of habitual activity is sufficient to maintain the function of the cardiorespiratory system, and fitness is valued mainly in the context of ability to perform complex motor skills requiring speed, coordination, and agility. By the time he has reached the age of twenty, a well-educated western man may already have suffered some deterioration of cardiorespiratory fitness, and he wishes to regain a sufficient level of endurance to gain a place on the varsity team; a working-class youth, on the other hand, may seek the bulging muscles that will enable him to perform feats of prodigious strength, impressing both his peers and his girl friends. At the age of thirty, desires have changed; exercise may now be an outlet for the accumulated frustrations and aggressions of the working routine, or a means of controlling a spreading waistline. By the age of forty, ageing and heart disease is common amongst a man's colleagues; the search is now for a level of fitness that will slow the onset of old-age and reduce the likelihood of a heart attack. At the age of fifty, senescence catches up with the subject himself. Tasks that were previously easy (such as fitting a pair of snow-tyres on a car) become quite exhausting, and the hope is now to recapture a level of fitness that will permit performance of the day's duties, leaving a margin of energy for leisure, recreation, and—if we dare mention a three letter word—sex. The family is now fully grown, and recreation may also provide new sources of interest and companionship.

The average woman is influenced by few of these considerations. Her main objectives are a good figure, posture and carriage. Even students of physical education are frequently disturbed when they find that physical training leads to a disappearance of fat from the breasts, hips, and thighs and an increase in the girth of the calf muscles. Nevertheless, the basic needs of the body are not greatly dissimilar in the two sexes, and many older women have the problems of being exhausted by minor household chores and of succumbing to heart attacks.

A further problem in arriving at a universally accepted definition of fitness has been the existence of quite marked cultural differences between those making the measurements. Observers trained in schools of physical education have concentrated on the development of physical performance tests batteries, including such items as running, jumping, throwing, hanging, back-bending and so on. These test batteries have been designed to sample various facets of "motor fitness"—a concept that embraces elements of strength, endurance, speed, power, agility, coordination, balance, and flexibility. Physicians, on the other hand, have been interested in the physical working capacity, as assessed by tests of cardiac and respiratory performance, in the body weight relative to normal standards, and in the normality of the electrocardiogram; the size and strength of the muscles, if measured, has usually been a secondary consideration. Differences in the training and licensing of the two groups still preclude a common approach to the problem, but fortunately as testing equipment becomes more widely available to both the physical educator and the family physician, differences in the methods of assessment are lessening and there is an increasing emphasis on objective measurement of physiological variables.

In assessing the importance of individual variables to health and fitness, one must take account of the likely duration of activity to which the subject will be exposed. Many athletes engage in bursts of very intense effort lasting ten seconds or less. A soldier on a route march or a marathon runner may sustain continuous exercise for as long as seventy-two hours. But most of the activities undertaken by the average citizen occupy from one to sixty minutes. Exercise of this order is usual in sport, and it also seems the most practical type of activity for countering obesity and cardiovascular disease. Careful observation shows that few industrial activities last longer than one hour. A nominal four hour shift is interrupted by many pauses for conversation, cigarettes, and other nonproductive uses of time. Muscular strength and endurance, mechanical efficiency, and body weight all have some influence on performance during the first sixty minutes of activity; however, the main factor limiting effort of this duration is the oxygen conductance (p. 105) achieved by the cardiorespiratory system.

There is a close relationship between oxygen conductance and working capacity and for this reason the response to effort of the "fit" individual differs from that of the unfit in at least three respects: (a) the maximum rate of working is greater, (b) the various cardiac and respiratory parameters concerned with oxygen transport show a much smaller displacement from their resting values at any given rate of working, and (c) the rate of return of physiological variables to the resting state following a standard exercise is more rapid. Unfortunately, these differences are not uniquely dependent on fitness; thus (a) depends also on motivation, while (b) is influenced by anxiety and clumsiness, reflecting the habituation of the subject to the laboratory and his state of motor learning.

I recently defined *endurance fitness* as "the ability of a man to maintain the various processes involved in metabolic exchange as close to the resting state as is mutually possible during the performance of a strenuous and fully learnt task for moderate time (1–60 minutes), with a capacity to reach a higher steady rate of working than the "unfit," and to restore promptly after exercise all equilibria which are disturbed."

Tests of Fitness

Fitness for Brief Activity (0–1 min)

Objective tests that sample individual determinants of fitness for brief activity have been discussed in previous sections. *Reaction times,* both simple and complex, are readily measured by standard reaction testing equipment (p. 222).

Static strengths are assessed by hand-grip and other dynamometers, and by various types of tensiometer (p. 185). The *dynamic strength* can be tested by simple weights and pulleys or by more complex torque generators and force platforms (p. 187).

Posture (p. 206) is important in many brief activities. *Speed* and *accuracy* are sampled by a wide range of psychomotor tests such as pursuit meters (p. 220). *Coordination* and *steadiness* can be measured by tapping tests (p. 222) and various forms of tilt-board such as the stabilometer (p. 222).

Motivation plays a large role in performance, and is difficult to evaluate. One approach is to incorporate an element of performance into the test itself, leaving the speed or maximum loading to the choice of the subject; the working limit selected can then be related to the appearance of the subject, as rated by an experienced observer, and to associated physiological changes such as the pulse rate at exhaustion. Alternatively, a subject may be presented with a load that is a standard percentage of his maximum power, and be asked to rate this on a suitable scale, ranging from "very very easy" to "very very hard" (Fig. 79). Finally, the outward intensity of an individual's effort may be rated by his peers.

POINTS	SENSATION
6	
7	very very light
8	
9	very light
10	
11	fairly light
12	
13	somewhat hard
14	
15	hard
16	
17	very hard
18	
19	very very hard
20	

Figure 79. A scale of perceived exertion, adapted from Borg.

Methods for the study of *anaerobic "capacity"* and *power* have attracted the interests of Margaria and his colleagues in Milan. Traditionally, the investigation of anaerobic metabolism has involved the measurement of oxygen consumption during the first fifteen to thirty minutes of recovery from vigorous exercise, and a calculation of the excess oxygen consumption relative to initial resting readings (Fig. 1, area BCD). The difficulty with this approach is that the resting oxygen consumption itself is increased after exercise, due to such factors as the rise of deep body temperature, the liberation of catecholamines, and the cost of added cardiac and respiratory work. There is thus a long "tail" to the area BCD where repayment of the oxygen debt has really been completed, but appears to be continuing. If the repayment time is arbitrarily limited to a specific period such as fifteen minutes, to the total debt thus calculated (about 5 litres) is much smaller than if the oxygen consumption curve is followed until the initial resting level is fully restored. If the repayment of the oxygen debt is followed semilogarithmically (Fig. 80), two components may be distinguished. One (the *alactate debt*) has a volume of about 1.9 litres and a twenty-two

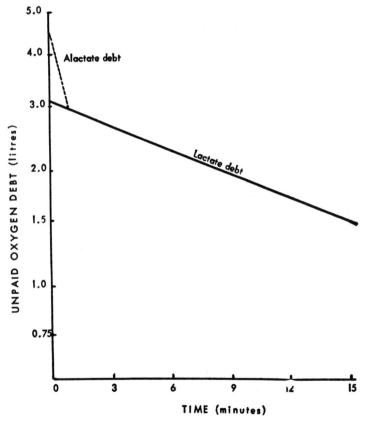

Figure 80. The total oxygen debt remaining unpaid at specific intervals after ceasing exercise. Data plotted on a semilogarithmic scale.

second half time of repayment; this corresponds to (a) regenera-
tion of the high energy phosphate bonds (adenosine triphosphate and creatine phosphate) within the active muscles, and
(b) replenishment of various oxygen stores (p. 152). The other
component, the *lactate debt,* has a volume of about 3.1 litres,
and a repayment time of ten to fifteen minutes; this corresponds
to the oxidation of a portion of the lactate to CO_2 and water,
with the resynthesis of the remainder to glycogen (p. 166).

The recovery curves are difficult to interpret, and unfortunately the rates of repayment do not coincide with the maximum
rates at which the corresponding debts can be incurred. Thus,
Margaria has suggested examining the time course of the forward reactions (Table XI). The alactate debt is largely incurred

TABLE XI

A COMPARISON OF OXYGEN DEBT AND STEADY OXYGEN CONDUC-
TANCE, SHOWING THE MAXIMUM POWER OUTPUT, TOTAL STORED
ENERGY, AND MINIMUM TIME TO EXHAUSTION
(Based on studies of Margaria and his associates)

Energy Source	Maximum Power (in Terms of Oxygen Equivalent)	Total Stored Energy (in Terms of Oxygen Equivalent)	Minimum Time to Exhaustion
Alactate Debt	165 ml/kg min	1.9 litre	8 sec
Lactate Debt	68 ml/kg min	3.1 litre	40 sec
Oxygen Conductance	45 ml/kg min	Infinity	Infinity

before there has been any increase in oxygen consumption or
accumulation of lactic acid. It can be evaluated by having a
subject run swiftly up a flight of stairs; some three seconds are
allowed for acceleration (15 nine inch steps or 30 horizontal
yards), and the rate of ascent over the next two seconds (a
further 10–15 steps) is timed by means of light-beam relays.
The work performed is known from the body weight and the
speed of ascent, and if a mechanical efficiency of 25 percent is
assumed (p. 209), the corresponding oxygen consumption may
be calculated. In a normal young man, alactate power is equivalent to an oxygen consumption of about 165 ml/kg min; in athletes, this rises to 215 ml/kg min, and in an old person it drops
to 100–110 ml/kg min. The total stored energy ("capacity")
can be found by integrating the power developed over the eight
second period prior to exhaustion; it is equivalent to an oxygen
store of some 22 ml/kg body weight, and coincides fairly closely

with predictions based on the known concentrations of ATP (5 mM/kg) and creatine phosphate (15 mM/kg) in human muscle. The enhanced alactate mechanism of athletes reflects largely their greater relative muscle mass; changes in the specific characteristics of unit volume of muscle (p. 444) are of lesser importance.

The maximum rate of lactate production can be approximated by plotting the observed blood lactate level against the intensity and duration of the preceding effort. The metabolism of lactate is sufficiently slow that blood samples can be collected three to five minutes after exercise, thus allowing equilibration throughout the body water. Maximum production occurs with work that is exhausting in forty to fifty seconds. The equivalent power, expressed in units of oxygen consumption, is about 68 ml/kg min. Very similar figures are yielded by athletes and by sedentary men. The "capacity" of the reaction is equivalent to about 45 ml/kg, being somewhat greater in athletic than in nonathletic individuals. The limit seems related to the maximum tolerated blood lactate (100–150 mg/100 ml), and the athlete thus gains some advantage from a larger mass of active muscles and a larger blood volume.

Margaria has argued that the "capacity" of the lactate mechanism is also influenced by the size of muscle glycogen stores, and thus by diet, habitual activity, and the rate of insulin secretion. However, his conclusion is debatable. Let us suppose that during exhausting work 20 kg of muscle are called into action. Their initial glycogen content is 1.5 gm/100 ml so that a total of 300 gm of glycogen may be broken down to pyruvate, with subsequent formation of lactic acid. If the material had been oxidized completely to CO_2 and water vapour, the total energy expenditure would have amounted to about 1200 kcal, since 1g of carbohydrate liberates approximately 4 kcal of energy. With incomplete and anaerobic metabolism, the yield of ATP per mole of hexose is only three molecules instead of 39 (p. 166); the effective energy expenditure is thus $3/39 \times 1200 = 93$ kcal, equivalent to an oxygen consumption of 18.6 litre, or in a man of 75 kg weight 248 ml/kg. This is about six times the observed "capacity" of the glycolytic reaction. Thus, unless we assume the active muscle weighs no more than 3–4 kg, we cannot explain the ceiling of lactate formation in terms of exhaustion of glycogen stores.

The measurement of *muscle strength* has been discussed previously (p. 185). The simplest approach is to test the grip strength, using a hand-grip dynamometer. However, there is some question as to whether this gives an adequate impression of overall body strength, and it is useful to supplement such information by testing the static strength of the limb muscles (for instance, knee extension) and trunk extension or trunk flexion). The cooperation of the subject is usually apparent from his general demeanour and the reproducibility of his efforts. If cooperation is poor (as in some compensation cases), static strength readings can be taken in conjunction with electromyography and soft tissue radiographs (p. 185). For some applications, the dynamic strength may also be of interest; a force platform is commonly used to test this aspect of fitness.

Muscle endurance can be assessed from the tolerance of repeated "isotonic" contractions; note is taken of the period of time over which a given set of weights can be raised and lowered, using a pulley system. Isometric endurance is expressed as the period of time for which a specified fraction of maximum isometric force can be sustained. The end-point of both isotonic and isometric effort is largely psychological and depends to a great extent upon motivation of the subject.

Flexibility can be assessed under passive and dynamic conditions, using various types of goniometer (p. 227).

Fitness for Activity of Moderate Duration (1–60 min)

Some Older Cardiorespiratory Tests. The resting pulse rate. Athletes have a much slower pulse than sedentary individuals. Rates of 28–30 beats/min have been described in some athletes, compared with 75–80 beats/min in a typical unfit University student. The difference is due largely to the much greater resting stroke volume of the athlete. The resting metabolic demands of sedentary and athletic individuals are rather similar, and are met by a cardiac output of about 3.5 litre/min per square metre of body surface area. If the body surface is 1.7 m², this implies a total output of 6 litre/min. The cardiac output is the product of heart rate, f_h, and stroke volume Q_s; thus

$$\dot{Q} = Q_s \times f_h$$

For the athlete, $6.0 = 0.2 \times 30$, while for the sedentary student, $6.0 = 0.08 \times 75$; in other words, the athlete has a resting stroke volume of 200 ml, while that of the sedentary student is only 80 ml.*

The measurement of resting pulse rate might seem to provide a useful test of fitness and an indirect method of assessing cardiac stroke volume. Unfortunately, the pulse readings are rather labile. Results are influenced by emotional factors, effective environmental temperature, posture, recent physical activity, consumption of cigarettes, beverages, and foods and many other variables. There is also a diurnal rhythm of pulse rate that parallels the daily variation in body temperature, the highest readings being obtained in the late afternoon and evening, and the lowest values in the small hours of the morning.

Many of these sources of variation can be minimised or avoided if the pulse rate is measured during sleep. Values may be high for the first two or three hours after retiring, particularly if the subject was physically active during the evening, but the pulse rate in the early hours of the morning is quite consistent, particularly if periods of disturbing dreams are avoided. Physiologists are not always welcome visitors in the bedrooms of the nation, but with the development of devices such as the portable tape-recorder, and the electrochemical integrator (p. 28), objective measurements of nocturnal pulse rate can now be obtained without disturbing the subject. As such devices become more widely available, the measurement of resting pulse rate may find increasing use in the assessment of cardiorespiratory fitness.

The Resting Pulse Pressure. The magnitude of the systemic pulse pressure depends largely on the cardiac stroke volume and the elasticity of the aortic vessels. Thus, if one assumes a value for aortic elasticity, the stroke volume can be derived from a simple measurement of pulse pressure.

Unfortunately, the aortic elasticity is not a constant, and indeed is influenced by many of the same variables that disturb the resting pulse rate, including anxiety, recent exercise, and arteriosclerotic disease. The pulse pressure is thus an unreliable index in many of the situations where we would like to measure stroke volume, and very limited fitness information can be obtained from pulse pressure readings.

The Cameron heartometer is a device for measuring blood pressure and obtaining a mechanical tracing of the pulse wave.

---

* For simplicity, we have here assumed that the arterio-venous oxygen difference is similar in athletes and sedentary students.

In general, subjects who are fit produce large oscillations of the heartometer record, while those who are unfit yield much smaller oscillations. Some authors have carried out very elaborate manipulations of the heartometer "signal," including differentiation (recording the rate of rise of pulse pressure), double differentiation (recording acceleration of the rise in pulse pressure), and estimation of the duration of isometric activity. However, such procedures seem unwarranted. Not only is the signal transmitted a considerable distance from the heart to the brachial artery, but the subsequent method of recording is very indirect. The form of the pulse tracing depends on how firmly the brachial artery is tethered, the distortion imposed by overlying muscle, fat and skin, and the care with which the sphygmomanometer cuff has been fitted. Taking account of these many sources of error, it seems best to regard the tracing merely as a graphic presentation of the pulse pressure, useful for demonstration to a patient, but adding little scientific information to the more usual sphygmomanometer readings.

The heartometer includes a system of lights that signal the appearance and disappearance of the Korotkov sounds (p. 85). Unfortunately, there is a certain mechanical lag in the operation of these signals, and the readings are somewhat inaccurate; certainly, the heartometer offers little advantage over simple auscultation.

Postural tests such as the Crampton Index and the Schneider test are based on the changes of pulse rate and blood pressure that occur when a subject is moved rapidly from the supine to the vertical position. Unfit individuals show a marked increase of heart rate and fall of blood pressure; on the other hand, the blood pressure of a well-trained athlete may rise slightly, with little change of heart rate. The differences of postural response in the well-trained individual reflect partly a larger total blood volume, and partly a more rapid reflex adjustment of the capacity vessels to added gravitational stress. Postural tests are no longer included in the usual fitness assessment. This is partly because pulse rate and blood pressure vary in response to so many extraneous influences, and partly because individuals with a poor postural response also have a poor response to standard tests of physical working capacity. The syndrome of a poor postural response and a limited tolerance for physical work is sometimes dignified by the name neurasthenia.

Breath-holding tests were once popular for the selection of aircrew. It was reasoned that tolerance of a falling oxygen pressure during breath-holding would indicate an equal tolerance of oxygen lack at altitude. The breaking point of a breath-hold is reached when the stimuli of increasing CO_2 pressure and oxygen lack outweigh the individual's capacity for voluntary inhibition of breathing. The rate of change of gas pressures during breath-holding depends partly on the rate of metabolism, and partly on the volume of gas within the lungs. The duration of voluntary inhibition varies greatly with motivation (p. 149), and unless a subject is to be assessed for some event that specifically requires prolonged breath-holding (for instance, swimming underwater), there would seem little virtue in this type of test.

The *Flack test* was also popular in the early days of the British Royal Air Force. In this test, the subject was required to blow a column of mercury to a height of 40 mmHg, and to maintain this pressure for as long as possible. Successful performance depended partly on the power of the chest muscles, partly on the ability to withstand the unpleasant sensation of breath-holding at a positive pressure, and partly on the reactions of the circulation to the increased intrathoracic pressure. Flack's test is now largely abandoned for the general assessment of fitness, but it may have some value in assessing aptitude for specific tasks where the intrathoracic pressure is raised, as in the lifting of heavy weights.

The *vital capacity* was once considered an important measure of fitness. More recent analysis has played down the role of ventilation in oxygen transport (p. 48), and it would be surprising if there were a strong relationship between endurance performance and the various derivatives of vital capacity. On the other hand, the vital capacity may exceed the predicted value if the individual under test has well-developed chest muscles. This is partly because he is able to reduce the initial amount of blood in the chest by a Valsalva type manoeuvre* and partly because he can exert great power in final compression of the thoracic cage.

The Approach of Factor Analysis. With the advent of large computer facilities, there have been numerous attempts to develop improved indices of fitness. The usual approach has been to take a rather heterogenous bunch of data-performance times, heartometer curves and the like, and to partition the overall variance of this data between a number of new and mutually independent variables, using the techniques of factor and principal component analysis. Criticism of such studies has centred on (a) the heterogeneity of the input data, and (b)

* Forced expiration against a closed glottis.

the limited precision of the measures evaluated. Often, the authors concerned have engaged mainly in an unwitting partition of the error of their data, and even where the statistical significance of the isolated "factors" has been demonstrated, the physiological meaning has been obscure on account of the heterogenous nature of the original data.

> One of the first of these analyses (McCurdy and Larson, 1935), antedates the big computers. They started with seven assorted measurements, and by multiple correlation and multiple regression techniques reduced their list to five items which were suitably weighted before combining as a single "fitness index." The five items selected are typical of prewar fitness tests—sitting diastolic pressure, breath-holding time twenty seconds after exercise, the difference of standing pulse rate at rest and two minutes after exercise, the sitting pulse pressure, and the standing pulse pressure.
>
> The present author has himself carried out a number of analyses of this type, but has not been particularly impressed with the usefulness of the resultant information. Three examples may be quoted, as follows: (a) The fitness status, as assessed by activity questionnaires, is more closely related to cardiac measurements than to respiratory data. (b) Statistically independent components or factors describe the initial response to exercise, and modification of this response by physical training. (c) When dealing with a relatively homogenous population, a surprisingly large component of the variance in responses to a standard exercise load can be attributed to individual differences in habitual activity as assessed on a simple four point scale.

Performance Tests. Until recently, many physical educators have assessed fitness by means of a battery of "performance" tests. The batteries usually comprise six or seven procedures, arbitrarily selected to sample characteristics that are thought important to activity of brief and moderate durations.

The *Kraus-Weber test* deserves mention, if only because a large number of United States children have failed it! All items in this test battery (two types of sit-up, two types of leg-lift, a prone trunk-lift, and a forward bend) must be passed. The majority of unsuccessful students were unable to touch the floor on forward bend without flexing their knees. Although commonly regarded as a measure of strength, in reality forward bending is influenced more by flexibility and the ratio of trunk to leg length.

At the present time, the two best-known and most widely used batteries of tests have been devised by the American Association of Health, Physical Education and Recreation (AAHPER) and its Canadian counterpart (CAHPER). The individual tests will now be discussed in a little detail:

One minute speed sit-up. This is commenced from the supine position. In the Canadian version, the elbows are clasped behind the head and brought forward to touch the bent knees. The feet are held on the floor by a partner, and the total number of sit-ups is counted over a sixty second period. As in most performance tests, the score depends substantially on attention to details of positioning. In the United States version of the test, the event is untimed, presumably because most children are exhausted in less than a minute. The knees are kept flat on the floor and the trunk is twisted; a maximum score of fifty is allowed to the girls, with a maximum of one hundred for the boys. There are so many differences between the United States and Canadian versions of the test that a comparison of scores has little real meaning.

Standing broad jump. The landing point of the heel of the foot nearest the take-off line is measured to the nearest inch. The subject is encouraged to bend his knees, hips and ankles, and to take off at 30–45°, swinging his arms as he jumps. The best of two trials is recorded in the Canadian test, the best of three in the United States.

Shuttle-run. The child starts from a lying position (standing in the U.S.!), and runs forward thirty feet to pick up a wooden block and place it behind the starting line. He then returns for a second block and places this alongside the first. The best of two trials is reported to the nearest tenth of a second.

Flexed arm hang. In the Canadian test, the subject grips a bar with his palms facing inwards, and pulls himself to eye level. The time for which this position can be maintained is recorded to the nearest second. The United States girls are required to lift their chin level with the bar, while the United States boys are required to carry out a series of pull-ups.

50-yard dash. This is started from either a crouch or a standing position, and is recorded to the nearest tenth of a second.

300 yard run. The Canadian test is a three hundred yard run. The length of the average gymnasium is much less than three hundred yards and thus the event is timed as a series of six fifty yard runs with turns (outdoor running is undesirable on several counts, since the temperature, wind-speed, weather, and running surface are all beyond the control of the investigator). The present author has examined the time lost per turn, and finds this is almost exactly proportional to the corresponding loss of kinetic energy. The introduction of turns thus penalizes both the fast and the heavy members of a class.

In the United States, the corresponding event is a 600 yard walk-run. Both CAHPER and AAHPER have been hesitant to include a longer run in case this should be dangerous to the child. However, other authors have used endurance running. Balke measured the distance a man could run in fifteen minutes, and more recently Cooper has measured the distance covered in twelve minutes. The latter author suggests an average man should be able to run 1.5 miles in twelve minutes, and he relates the distance covered to the maximum oxygen intake as follows:

Distance covered in 12 Min.	$\dot{V}_{O_2\ max}$
<1.0 miles	<28 ml/kg min
1.0 –1.24	28.1–34.0
1.25–1.49	34.1–42.0
1.50–1.74	42.1–52.0
>1.75	>52.0

Cooper finds a good correlation between the running distance and $\dot{V}_{O_2\ max}$ in well motivated men and boys ($r = 0.9$),[*] but a much poorer correlation in women ($r = 0.7$), presumably because their interest in the test is less.

Softball throw. This is excluded from the Canadian test battery. When a comparison was made between United States and English children, the softball throw was the one item of the AAHPER test where United States children excelled. The explanation seems that the softball is rarely used by boys in Europe.

There are many problems to the interpretation of the AAHPER and CAHPER performance tests. One is that scores depend very much on procedural details. Enough description has been given to show that if the printed instructions are followed carefully, few of the United States and Canadian tests are comparable. Much also depends on the skill of the test administrators. The published normal standards are based on large and randomly selected populations (11,000 children in the Canadian survey), and inevitably data collection has been

[*] A correlation coefficient of unity ($r = 1.0$) would be anticipated if the distance run was perfectly matched with $\dot{V}_{O_2\ max}$.

deputed to children attending the selected schools. Results are also greatly influenced by learning of the required tasks. United States children scored much better in 1965 than in the original survey of 1958, and one would suspect this is due more to frequent use of the test procedures than to any improvement of national fitness between 1958 and 1965. Performance scores are particularly misleading when they are obtained on adults who have been away from gymnasia for a long period.

Some authors in the United States have claimed that a suitably weighted group of four AAHPER type performance tests will predict the aerobic power of adults with an accuracy of about 12 percent. In evaluating this claim, one must first look at the variance of the basic data. This is no more than 20 percent. In other words, the performance tests have described 8 of the 20 percent variance in $\dot{V}_{O_2 \; max}$. This in itself might seem a useful contribution. However, Cumming has pointed out that if account is taken of height and weight, then the measurement of performance contributes nothing to the prediction of a child's maximum oxygen intake. In other words, the performance tests are merely an elaborate way of finding out how tall and heavy a child is. The present author has tested the same hypothesis in adults, where height and weight are relatively constant, but aerobic power ranges more widely. Again, if account is taken of a few fundamental observations such as age, height, weight, and skinfold thickness, performance tests do not contribute to the description of $\dot{V}_{O_2 \; max}$. Certainly, the performance scores include an element of variation not attributable to age, height, weight and obesity, but this reflects such imponderable sources of error as motivation and recent familiarity with a gymnasium and does not yield any useful expression of the fitness of the individual.

Performance tests have many superficial attractions—they are simple, require little apparatus, and can be applied quickly to large samples of a population. But with the possible exception of the distance run in twelve to fifteen minutes, their interpretation is very obscure.

   The Tuttle Pulse-ratio Test. The Tuttle pulse-ratio test is a relative antiquity that has much in common with such procedures as the Astrand nomogram. It is mentioned at this point because it can be applied not only to standarized endurance work such as stepping, but also to performance tests such as a sequence of pull-ups. The ratio indicates the rate of exercise needed to achieve a pulse rate $2\frac{1}{2}$ times the resting value (in other words, a figure close to maximum pulse rate). It is calculated from the formula

$$E_{2.5} = E_a + \frac{(E_b - E_a)(2.5 - r_a)}{r_b - r_a}$$

where $E_{2.5}$ is the required rate of stepping, pull-ups or other activity, E_a is the rate of activity at the first attempt, E_b is the rate at the second attempt, and r_a and r_b are the respective pulse ratios for the first and second attempts. To take a real example, a man has a resting rate of 80, a pulse of 120 at 10 steps/min ($r_a = 1.5$) and a pulse of 160 at 20 steps/min ($r_b = 2.0$). Thus

$$E_{2.5} = 10 + \frac{[20 - 10][2.5 - 1.5]}{2.0 - 1.5} = 30$$

Recovery Tests. The majority of the early tests of fitness were made on either resting or recovering subjects. This presumably reflects the difficulties encountered in making physiological observations on a moving subject.

Dill, working at the Harvard Fatigue Laboratory, suggested that the pulse measured in the first ten seconds of the recovery period corresponded closely with the immediately preceding exercise reading ($r = 0.96$, implying that more than 92 percent of the information content of the exercise pulse rate was contained in the recovery data). Unfortunately, considerable skill and coordination are needed to start a pulse count at the instant a subject ceases to exercise, and if an interval of perhaps thirty seconds elapses before the count is made, the coefficient of correlation between exercise and recovery readings is only 0.8; 36 percent of the information content of the recovery pulse is now unrelated to the exercise response.[*]

The rate of recovery of the pulse is clearly faster in an athlete than in a nonathlete, but the form of the curve is influenced by many factors, including:

1. the relative intensity of exercise stress
2. the age of the subject

[*] The proportion of unwanted information is given by $(1 - r^2)$.

3. the rise of body temperature during exercise, and the rate of cooling permitted during recovery
4. the extent and rate of repayment of any oxygen debt
5. the depletion of blood volume during exercise, and the posture and rate of restoration of blood volume during recovery.
6. the extent to which exercise tachycardia has been mediated by the cerebral cortex
7. elevation of the metabolic rate during recovery, due to such factors as liberation of hormones, a continuing elevation of body temperature, and increased work of breathing.

Some authors have found it useful to evaluate the form of the pulse recovery curve. The well-known *Harvard step test* is one example of this approach. The subject is required to climb a twenty inch bench thirty times per minute until he is exhausted (maximum duration 5 minutes). The pulse rate is then counted 1–1½, 2–2½, and 4–4½ minutes following exercise, and an empirical fitness index is calculated according to the formula

$$\text{Fitness Index} = \frac{\text{Duration of test (sec)} \times 100}{2 \times \text{pulse sum } (1\text{--}1\tfrac{1}{2}) + (2\text{--}2\tfrac{1}{2}) + (4\text{--}4\tfrac{1}{2})}$$

Brouha, the originator of this test, reasoned that the three pulse readings would give a good description of the pulse recovery curve. An index of less than 55 indicates poor fitness; 65 is average, 80–90 good, and >90 is excellent.

The Harvard test is still sometimes used in the evaluation of Olympic athletes; indeed, in some laboratories it has given a better prediction of endurance performance than the measurement of maximum oxygen intake. One reason is that the Harvard test also measures motivation. The gross metabolic cost of climbing the twenty inch step (45–50 ml/kg min) is relatively high even for a young man and many subjects give up before the five minute period is completed. A lower step (17 inches) is commonly used for testing girls and older men, while if the subjects are superbly fit the effort can be increased 20 percent to 25 percent through wearing a 20 kg pack (the *Harvard pack test*).

A second test widely used by clinicians is the Master step test (see also page 75). The patient is exercised by climbing back-

wards and forwards over a double nine-inch step. The rate of
ascent is specified according to age, sex and weight. The extent of
the suggested adjustment can perhaps be made clear by some
examples. A man aged thirty to thirty-four climbs at 18 ascents/
min if he weighs ninety-five pounds, but the rate decreases progressively to fourteen ascents/min if he weighs two hundred fifteen pounds. The approximate gross oxygen costs for the two subjects are thus 29 ml/kg min and 21 ml/kg min, respectively. In
women, the weight corrections are larger; the speed of ascent for a
woman aged thirty to thirty-four ranges from 18 ascents/min at a
weight of ninety-five pounds to 9.3 ascents/min at 215 pounds. The
adjustment for age also varies with weight. In the lightest men, the
required rate of stepping decreases by 21 percent from age twenty-
five to age sixty-five, while in the heaviest men it decreases by 35
percent from age thirty-five to age sixty-five; the corresponding decreases in women are 26 percent and 21 percent respectively. These
few examples are enough to show that the age, sex and weight corrections are rather arbitrary. The required effort is commonly 40 to
50 percent of aerobic power in a young man, but the relative stress
differs widely from one individual to another. Clinicians are interested primarily in the recovery electrocardiogram. This is studied
for ten minutes following the completion of stepping. Perhaps
because the duration of the Master test is short, ($1\frac{1}{2}$ min for a
"single" test, 3 min for a "double" test) some of the more striking
electrocardiographic abnormalities do not appear for at least five
to six minutes after completion of exercise. This is in marked
contrast to a nine to twelve minute progressive step test, where
ECG changes are maximal in the first thirty seconds of the recovery period. Master also examined the rate of restoration of the
normal resting pulse and blood pressure; he stipulated that both
should have returned to within ten points of the initial value two
minutes after ceasing exercise.

Endurance Time and Maximum Performance. A second
method of avoiding the need for physiological measurements
during exercise is to record either the endurance time at a load
which is exhausting in five to fifteen minutes, or the maximum
amount of work which can be completed in a given time (uphill
running distance or work performed on a bicycle ergometer).

The difficulty with this approach is that the point of exhaustion is influenced by many variables, including not only the
maximum oxygen intake, but also the ability of the circulation
to perfuse active muscles, the tolerance of the tissues towards

lactic acid accumulation, possibly the extent of initial glycogen reserves, and the general reactions of the body to a variety of unpleasant sensations.

Very large improvements of endurance time may be brought about by physical training. However, this does not imply a corresponding physiological improvement. A small gain of maximum oxygen intake with some improvement of muscle strength greatly reduce the rate of lactate accumulation at any given rate of working. Training also produces an inevitable habituation to the unpleasant sensations of vigorous exercise. In consequence, the endurance time may change from five to sixty minutes—a 1200 percent "improvement"—although the maximum oxygen intake has only increased by 10 to 20 percent.

Maximum Oxygen Intake. Most authors are now agreed that the best approach to the assessment of cardiorespiratory fitness is to examine the various components of the oxygen transport chain *during* the performance of a well-standardized exercise task, such as uphill treadmill running, pedalling a bicycle ergometer, or stepping.

The continuous monitoring of exercise heart rate has become much easier now that the electrocardiogram is widely available. True, a skilled observer can measure the exercise heart rate by auscultation over the apex beat, or by palpation of the carotid artery in the neck. However, the electrocardiogram greatly expedites the measurement of heart rate, and at the same time it provides a continuous check on the safety of the test procedure.

The least equivocal measure of oxygen conductance is a direct determination of *maximum oxygen intake.* The principle of measurement is to increase the work load progressively every second minute until the oxygen consumption either fails to show an increase or actually declines (Fig. 81). In order to define a "plateau," the oxygen cost of three successive work loads must agree to within 2 ml/kg min STPD. Other subsidiary criteria of a good maximum effort include a pulse rate close to the anticipated value for the individual's age, a respiratory gas exchange ratio of 1.15 or more, and a high arterial lactate level (100–150 mg/100 ml in a young man, 80 mg/100 ml in a child, and 60

Alive Man!

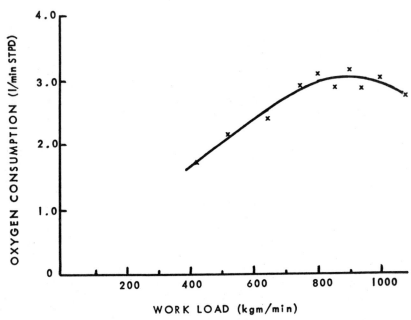

Figure 81. To illustrate the technique of measuring the maximum oxygen intake. The work-load is increased progressively every two minutes until three successive increments change the oxygen consumption by a total of less than 2 ml/kg min.

mg/100 ml in an older man). With young, athletic adults, there is little difficulty in reaching a plateau, and results are reproducible to within 4 to 5 percent. However, the procedure is less satisfactory for children and older adults. As many as 50 percent of children fail to achieve a clear-cut plateau. This may be a problem of motivation; certainly, children give up rather quickly as exhaustion is approached, and the body must be driven into a substantial oxygen debt if a plateau is to be demonstrated.

Details of procedure have recently been reviewed by an international working party. If the maximum oxygen intake were limited simply by cardiorespiratory performance, one might anticipate a common result for any mode of exercise that involved activity of the large body muscles. In fact, the highest values are obtained during uphill treadmill running. The maximum oxygen intake is 3 percent smaller during a step test, 7 percent smaller when exercising on a bicycle ergometer, and as much as 20 percent smaller when using an arm ergometer. The poor results with arm work are due partly to a pooling of blood in the inactive veins of the legs. The second problem with both leg and arm ergometers is a tendency for peripheral rather than a central (cardiorespiratory) limitation of effort. With uphill treadmill running, a subject's face becomes blue and then ashen grey as exhaustion is approached; he may complain of nausea and dizziness, and is seen to be acutely breathless, with impaired coordination and a confused response to questions. On the other hand, a subject working on an ergometer complains specifically of weakness, pain, and exhaustion in the active muscles.

A major part of the ergometer work is performed by a relatively small proportion of the body musculature, and performance is thus limited by local factors such as muscle blood flow, strength, and glycogen stores rather than by the oxygen conductance of the cardiorespiratory system. From the physiological point of view, the *treadmill* is thus the preferred form of maximum exercise. Its main disadvantages are cost, bulk and noise. If a subject trips, he can also be thrown a considerable distance; an emergency hand rail and safety matting should be available, and the observer should give unobtrusive support as the subject nears exhaustion. If a *step test* is to be used for maximum effort, it must be relatively high (at least 18 inches), so that the subject does not have to climb too quickly; a compromise is usually drawn between a comfortable height of stepping and a rate of ascent that may cause the subject to trip. A padded hand support is welcomed by older subjects, particularly during rapid climbing. The main advantages of the step are that it is simple, cheap, and readily portable. If maximum exercise is to be performed on a *bicycle ergometer,* it is important to choose a design with a racing saddle and handlebars and appropriate gear ratios; most ergometers are designed for relatively slow and leisurely operation. The main advantage of the bicycle ergometer is that the subject is relatively immobile; this facilitates the collection of ancillary data such as measurements of blood pressure and cardiac output.

Irrespective of the mode of exercise, careful *preparation* of the subject is important if consistent results are to be obtained. No strenuous physical activity should be permitted in the previous twenty-four hours. A very light meal should be taken at least 1½ hours prior to testing, and stimulants (tea, coffee, alcohol, nicotine and other drugs) should be avoided in the more immediate pre-test period. The room temperature should be comfortable (about 70°F) and all observations should be made in a quiet and unhurried manner; the procedures should be fully explained to the subject, and any unwarranted fears should be allayed.

The technicalities of *oxygen consumption* measurements must be controlled rather precisely. In two recent experiments, volunteers have travelled from one laboratory to another for repeat measurements of aerobic power. Both studies revealed systematic discrepancies in the results reported by the cooperating laboratories, some differences being as great as 25 percent. One problem is the accuracy of gas analysis. The oxygen extracted from inspired gas is no more than 2 to 3 percent, and although it is easy to reproduce oxygen analyses to 0.02 percent, absolute results can differ by 0.3 percent or more from the true value; this in turn can lead to an error of 10 percent in the measured oxygen consumption. Similar problems arise in the determination of carbon dioxide concentrations; some laboratories thus report systematically erroneous respiratory gas exchange ratios, and make a correspondingly inaccurate correction for the difference of volume between inspired and expired gas. There is commonly a failure to check that the equipment used in gas collection offers a low resistance to breathing (p. 129), and the observer may also overlook a leakage of gas at the mouthpiece as the coordination of the subject deteriorates. There are other small but equally important details of procedure, and oxygen consumption readings can only be interpreted in absolute terms if the techniques of measurement are immaculate and have been checked against results obtained in a suitable reference laboratory.

Maximum effort tests are traditionally preceded by a warm-up. There is some evidence that this increases the maximum oxygen intake (p. 190) and minimises the risks of tendon injury during the exercise period. The pulse rate and oxygen consumption can be measured during these preliminaries in order to predict the work load at which the definitive test should be commenced (suitable prediction procedures are discussed in the following section). The simplest maximum effort test commences at 90 to 100 percent of predicted aerobic power, and the work load is increased by 5 to 10 percent every two minutes until the subject is exhausted. The more traditional approach calls for the patient to return to the laboratory on several occasions; at each visit, effort is sustained at a fixed work load for as long as possible, preferably at least three to four min. A curve relating oxygen consumption and work load is drawn and a plateau is progressively defined. This can prove very tedious for both the investigator and the subject, and offers no real advantage over a progressive test. The direct measurement of maximum oxygen intake is still not a common laboratory procedure. Several reasons may be advanced for this. Apart from the immediate risks of muscle trauma and injuries secondary to tripping, there is an appreciable likelihood that the very vigorous effort may induce ventricular fibrillation (p. 76). For this reason, the presence of a physician familiar with techniques of cardiac resuscitation is mandatory, and a defibrillator and other emergency equipment should be at hand. It is then likely that the occasional case of fibrillation will be treated successfully. However, even with good organisation, a proportion of patients developing a ventricular arrhythmia die, and for this reason it seems unjustified to require the more vulnerable older people to undertake such intense exertion. Even in those who are younger, motivation to maximum effort may be a problem. Maximum effort testing would seem logical for athletes, but in practice the results are still disappointing. Contestants sometimes hold a little "in reserve" for an upcoming competition and they also find difficulty in reaching maximum effort during an unfamiliar form of activity.

The directly measured maximum oxygen intake is best reserved (a) for patients where an accurate oxygen conductance value is required for treatment or prognosis, and (b) for research studies on young volunteers, particularly the validation of indirect procedures for the prediction of maximum oxygen intake.

The Predicted Maximum Oxygen Intake. Most investigators use submaximum exercise when evaluating older patients. The results are commonly used to predict the individual's maximum oxygen intake. Most prediction procedures are based on the linear relationship between pulse rate and oxygen consumption over the range 50 percent to 90 percent of aerobic power (Fig. 2); this relationship is extrapolated to the theoretical maximum pulse rate of the individual, and the corresponding oxygen consumption is then read from the abscissae.

The main difficulty with this approach is that the line relating oxygen consumption and pulse rate can be displaced to the left by a number of factors such as anxiety, a high environmental temperature, and a recent meal. The maximum pulse rate of the individual is also modified by altitude, age, disease, and possibly physical fitness. Lastly, the oxygen consumption may show

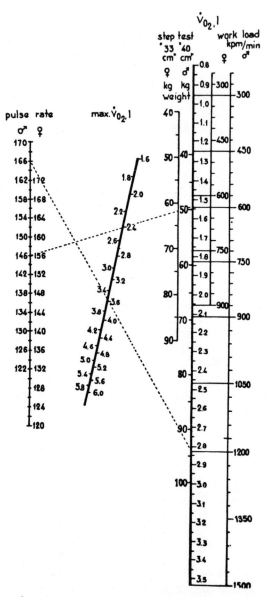

Figure 82. The Åstrand nomogram for prediction of maximum oxygen intake. Submaximum exercise is performed for six minutes. The pulse rate and oxygen consumption are measured in the final minute, and a line is drawn joining the two readings (e.g. 166, 2.82 litre/min STPD); the intercept on the central scale then indicates the maximum oxygen intake (3.56 litre/min STPD). In the case of older subjects, an age correction must be applied (Table XII). If oxygen consumption is not measured, then

an asymptote—a final increase of 0.2–0.5 litre/min $\dot{V}_{O_2}$ with no matching increase of pulse rate. For these various reasons, predictions show a substantial scatter about the true value, and they also have an appreciable systematic error. Some authors have set the latter as high as 25 percent, but if measurements are made with reasonable care, it is more usual for the prediction to underestimate the true $\dot{V}_{O_2}$ max by 0 to 10 percent, with a standard deviation of some ten percent about this systematic error. The precision is not as great as could be achieved by direct measurements on cooperative young subjects, but it is often adequate for survey purposes.

The *Astrand nomogram* (Fig. 82) is perhaps the best known of several prediction methods. It is based on single pulse and oxygen consumption measurements obtained in the sixth minute of bicycle ergometer or stepping exercise; the required intensity of effort is such as to produce a pulse rate in the range 125–170/min. The authors in effect assume that there is a linear relationship between pulse rate and oxygen consumption over the range 50 percent to 100 percent of aerobic power. They further assume that the pulse rates at 50 percent of aerobic power are 128 in men and 135 in women, while the corresponding pulse rates at 100 percent of aerobic power are 195 and 198 respectively. The formulae for calculation of maximum oxygen intake are thus

$$\text{For men, } \dot{V}_{O_2} \text{ max} = \dot{V}_{O_2} \text{ (observed)} \times \frac{195 - 61}{\text{Pulse} - 61}$$

$$\text{and for women, } \dot{V}_{O_2} \text{ max} = \dot{V}_{O_2} \text{ (observed)} \times \frac{198 - 72}{\text{Pulse} - 72}$$

The original populations tested by the Åstrands were young and relatively athletic people, and the question of a decline in maximum pulse rate with age thus did not arise. Subsequently, the procedure was extended to older groups, and it became necessary to introduce an empirical correction factor ranging from 1.00 at age twenty-five to 0.65 at age sixty-five (Table XII). Field workers may still find it convenient to use the Åstrand nomogram as such, but the laboratory worker now finds it more convenient and more accurate to program the formulae for a small "desk-top" computer. If facili-

---

the rate of working on a bicycle ergometer, or the body weight at a standard rate of stepping may be used to predict oxygen consumption (reproduced by permission of Dr. Irma Åstrand).

TABLE XII

EMPIRICAL CORRECTION FACTORS TO BE APPLIED TO MAXIMUM
OXYGEN INTAKE AS PREDICTED BY THE ÅSTRAND NOMOGRAM*

Age (Yr)	Factor
25	1.00
35	0.87
45	0.78
55	0.71
65	0.65

* Figure 82.

ties for the accurate measurement of oxygen consumption are not available, the equivalent rate of working can be substituted, with some loss of accuracy (page 23). A net efficiency of 16 percent is assumed for stepping, and 23 percent for bicycling.

The *Margaria nomogram* (Fig. 83) is based on ascent of a standard 40 cm step at two pre-selected rates (15 and 25 ascents/min); the "steady-state" pulse response to the two loads is noted, and a line drawn to join the appropriate points on the 15/min and the 25/min scales. The intercept is read from the scale with the most appropriate maximum pulse rate (160, 180, or 200/min).

The *Wyndham extrapolation* is based on four pairs of oxygen consumption and pulse readings; Wyndham obtained these measurements during stepping exercise, but the same principle can be applied to bicycle ergometer or treadmill effort. The work loads originally suggested were rather low, and it is better to obtain four evenly spaced readings over the pulse range 120–170/min. A line is fitted to the four points either statistically or visually, and is extrapolated to maximum heart rate. Partly because Wyndham's laboratory is in Johannesburg, at an altitude of six thousand feet, it was initially recommended that extrapolations should be made to a constant heart rate of 180 beats/min, however, most authors who use this procedure now extrapolate to the anticipated maximum of the population they are studying.

At a first glance, one might anticipate that the relative accuracy of the three prediction methods would be directly proportional to the number of observations used (that is, Wyndham > Margaria > Åstrand). In practice, the difference in accuracy is slight. The gain of precision with N observations cannot exceed $\sqrt{N}$. Further, all readings are not of equal merit; much depends on the placement and accuracy of individual observations. If the Åstrand data are obtained at a high work load, little extrapolation is required, and the error is in consequence quite small. On the other hand, the Wyndham procedure may evaluate four readings

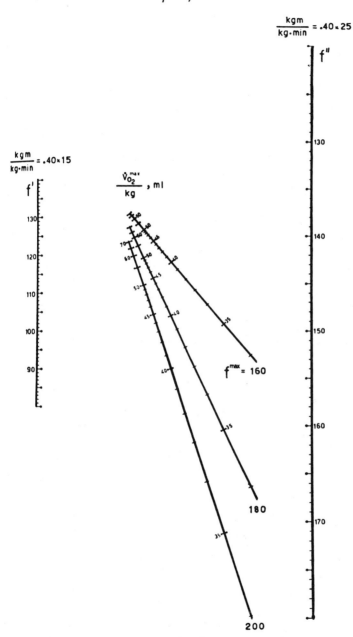

Figure 83. The Margaria nomogram for the prediction of maximum oxygen intake. Reproduced by permission of Prof. R. Margaria.

obtained at relatively low work loads, so that substantial extrapolation is needed; further, in calculating the slope of the oxygen consumption/pulse rate line, undue account is taken of the lowest of these four work loads, where physiological responses are very variable and markedly influenced by environmental factors.

A multistage test may be desired on grounds of safety (p. 509). It can be performed in either a progressive manner (where the work load is increased every three or four minutes), or as a series of discontinuous tests each of five to six min duration. Results are essentially similar with the two approaches, and the progressive procedure is usually preferred since it conserves the time of both subject and investigator.

The preparation of a subject for submaximum exercise should be as thorough as for a maximum test. Anxiety can be reduced by (a) the choice of a familiar type of activity (a shallow step is preferable to a bicycle ergometer or a treadmill) and (b) habituation (p. 444) to the laboratory environment through one or more "dummy" runs. If oxygen consumption cannot be measured, the task should also be fully learnt, so that efficiency is close to the assumed value. A step test has many attractions for a field study, but if detailed ancillary investigations are required, the bicycle ergometer may be preferred because of the relative immobility it confers upon the subject.

Issekutz and his associates have used the *respiratory gas exchange ratio* (R) to predict the $\dot{V}_{o_2}$ max. These investigators noted a progressive increase of R from the resting ratio of 0.83 to a value ~ 1.15 in maximum effort. They found a linear relationship between the work rate and log ΔR (ΔR being the observed ratio $- 0.75$), and on this basis they derived a formula for the prediction of maximum aerobic work rate ($\dot{W}$ max):

$$\dot{W}_{max} = \dot{W}_{observed} \left(\frac{\text{Log } 0.4 - \text{Log } 0.08}{\text{Log } \Delta R - \text{Log } 0.08} \right)$$

In order to convert $\dot{W}_{max}$ to $\dot{V}_{o_2}$ max, it is necessary to assume the efficiency of effort, and to add the resting energy expenditure. The Issekutz prediction works fairly well if one is dealing with experienced volunteers leading well-regulated lives, but the gas exchange ratio is very susceptible to changes of diet, and to anxiety. Further, the maximum value of R sometimes exceeds 1.15. Finally, rather careful gas analysis is needed to determine R with the necessary accuracy. For all of these reasons, most workers prefer pulse prediction methods.

Interpolated Results. The prediction methods discussed so far are based on extrapolation of data. Critics point out that the information content of a set of observations is reduced rather than increased if it is extrapolated. Is it not preferable to report interpolated, or at worst briefly extrapolated results?

The best known interpolation is the PWC_{170}. This measure was originally described by Wahlund and was subsequently popularized by Sjöstrand and his associates. It is the rate of working ("physical working capacity") that can be sustained for six minutes with a final pulse rate of 170/min. It is usually determined by carrying out a series of six minute rides on a bicycle ergometer, although it can be estimated rather more conveniently by a single "progressive" test in which the work load is increased at three minute intervals. The main objection to the PWC_{170} and similar tests is that the imposed stress varies with the age of the patient. At twenty years, the effort required is moderate (about 80% of aerobic power), but at sixty years it is exhausting in one or two minutes. For this reason, some authors also describe a PWC_{150}, to be used on older and hospitalized patients.

Cotes has recently advocated reporting the pulse rate corresponding to an *oxygen consumption of 1.5 litre/min;* again, this represents a mild effort for a young man, but exceeds the aerobic power of some elderly people.

In Germany, the *Leistungs-puls-index* (LPI) and the *oxygen pulse* are popular concepts. These are basically the slopes of the work/ pulse and oxygen consumption/pulse lines, and they are usually measured on a special bicycle ergometer devised by E.A. Müller, during his period of research at the Max-Planck Institut in Dortmund. The LPI ergometer incorporates a permanent magnet which can be progressively driven into the range of a steel flywheel; the rate of displacement of the magnet is so adjusted that the work load increases by 60 kgm/min with each minute that the bicycle is operated. The pulse rate and oxygen consumption are measured while the subject pedals against the rising load. There are several criticisms of Müller's approach. Normal values for the LPI vary with age. Because of the continually changing work load, neither pulse rate nor oxygen consumption reach a steady response to any given load; thus "working capacity" readings obtained from this machine are systematically lower than those derived from the usual progressive or steady-state ergometer test. Finally, the early part of the O_2 consumption/pulse rate line is assumed to be linear; however, this is unlikely to be true between 10 percent and 50 percent of aerobic power, since at this stage the stroke volume is increasing.

The most recent approach to interpolation is the use of age-related *target pulse rates* (Table XIII). The selected targets cor-

TABLE XIII

TARGET PULSE RATES CORRESPONDING TO APPROXIMATELY
75 PER CENT OF AEROBIC POWER

Age (Years)	Pulse Rate (/min)
20–30	160
30–40	150
40–50	140
50–60	130

respond to an arbitrary percentage of the individual's aerobic power; for instance, if 75 percent of maximum aerobic effort is required, the target pulse rate would be 160 at an age of twenty-five years, 150 at thirty-five, 140 at forty-five, and 130 at fifty-five. Figures are now available (Table XIV) showing what loading *should* produce the target pulse rate, given the age and body

TABLE XIV

NUMBER OF ASCENTS OF AN EIGHTEEN-INCH STAIRCASE
PER MINUTE CORRESPONDING TO A WORK LOAD
75 PERCENT OF AEROBIC POWER*†

Age (Years)	(a) Male Patients Body Weight (Pounds)											
	110	120	130	140	150	160	170	180	190	200	210	220
20–30	20	20	20	21	21	21	21	21	21	21	21	21
30–40	18	19	19	19	19	19	19	19	19	20	20	20
40–50	16	16	16	17	17	17	17	17	17	17	17	17
50–60	13	13	13	13	13	13	14	14	14	14	14	14

Age (Years)	(b) Female Patients Body Weight (Pounds)											
	80	90	100	110	120	130	140	150	160	170	180	190
20–30	16	17	17	17	17	18	18	18	18	18	18	18
30–40	16	16	17	17	17	17	17	18	18	18	18	18
40–50	14	14	14	15	15	15	15	15	15	15	16	16
50–60	10	10	10	10	10	10	10	10	10	10	10	10

* Figures apply to patient of average cardiorespiratory fitness for his age.
† Table reproduced from *Frontiers of Fitness*, Springfield,Thomas, 1971.

weight of the individual. The table can be used in two ways. In the simplest type of assessment, the subject exercises for five minutes at the specified loading, and the final pulse rate is compared with the target value; if the target is exceeded by 10–20 beats/min, the man is unfit, while if the final pulse is 10–20 beats/min less than the target, he is of above average fitness. A single stage test of this type is quickly performed, but it has several disadvantages—there is no "warm-up," no warning is obtained of the likelihood of an arrhythmia developing with exercise, and the final pulse rate differs from one individual to another, depending on the fitness of the person concerned. An alternative procedure is to commence exercise at perhaps half the specified loading, and to approach the 75 percent value through one or two further intermediate stages, each of three minutes duration. The test can then be halted if the ECG shows unfavourable changes, and the final loading can be adjusted so that the intended target pulse rate is closely approximated. The ECG appearances and other relevant data are then reported at a stress intensity that is consistent from one individual to another.

Reliability and Validity of Tests. The various measures of cardiorespiratory fitness must be assessed ultimately in terms of their reliability and their validity. The majority of exercise tests such as the direct measurement of maximum oxygen intake, the Åstrand prediction, and the PWC_{170} have a good reliability. When measurements are repeated over the course of several days or weeks, the coefficient of variation is often no more than 4 to 5 percent, so that the test/retest correlation coefficient is 0.97 or better. The main problem arises in terms of validity. We have noted already that submaximum predictions show a systematic discrepancy of (0–10%) ±10% relative to the directly measured oxygen intake. Unfortunately, it is also debatable whether the maximum oxygen intake is the ultimate criterion of fitness—particularly if one is concerned to predict athletic performance. In some trials, the coefficients of correlation between maximum oxygen intake and the results of an athletic contest have been as low as 0.6–0.7; such results compare unfavourably with Harvard step test data, where correlation coefficients of 0.9 and more have been reported. This may reflect partly the zeal and care with which the maximum oxygen intake is measured. Cooper has reported an equally close correlation (0.9) between the twelve minute distance and the maximum oxygen intake per unit of body weight. It is also possible that a recovery test gives added information on such factors as the reflex component of tachycardia, the rise of deep body temperature, and the oxygen cost of breathing. These features of the exercise response could well be important to fitness in an athlete, if not in an ordinary citizen.

Fitness for Sustained Activity (> 60 min)

Glycogen Stores. In maximum anaerobic work the muscle glycogen stores are depleted in a few minutes (p. 399). However, with vigorous rhythmic activity, glycolysis is sustained for an hour or more. The initial concentration of glycogen within the active muscles undoubtedly influences tolerance for sustained effort, and since the development of needle biopsy by Hultman, many biochemical studies have been made.

The main objection to biopsy is that in order to obtain sufficient tissue for analysis, a broad gauge needle (3–5 mm outer diameter) must be used. If the sample is taken from a large muscle such as the vastus lateralis, the procedure is tolerated remarkably well; many subjects have had ten to twenty biopsies performed, both at rest and during exercise, with no complaints other than a mild discomfort that persisted for about twenty-four hours. Nevertheless, repeated muscle trauma of this order seems undesirable, and there have been occasional reports of injury to vital structures such as a major artery or nerve.

Blood Volume. During exercise, fluid is lost both by exudation into the active tissues, and also by sweating. The initial blood volume is therefore an important determinant of tolerance for prolonged effort, particularly if the environment is hot and/or the intake of fluids is restricted (p. 316). The blood volume is usually measured by dilution, following injection of a known volume of "marker". If a dye is used, it should be stable and not metabolized, excreted or lost into the extracellular water; the compound T1824, which attaches itself to the plasma albumin meets most of these criteria. Alternatively, one may inject a suspension of serum albumin tagged with radioactive iodine (I^{131}).

Marker concentrations are determined after allowing ten minutes for mixing; this represents a compromise between completion of mixing and the gradual loss of albumin from the circulation (4%–6% per hour).

Suspensions of red cells marked with radioactive phosphorus (P^{32}) or radioactive chromium (Cr^{51}) may be used to estimate the red cell volume. Whether the plasma or the red cell volume is determined, the data must then be related to a haematocrit reading in order to estimate the total blood volume. Unfortunately, the relative proportions of red cells and plasma vary in different parts of the circulation. The dye techniques thus indicate a larger total blood volume than tagged red cell methods.

A third approach quite commonly used in fitness laboratories is to determine the total haemoglobin. A measured dose of carbon monoxide is inhaled over fifteen to thirty minutes, and the resulting increment of carboxyhaemoglobin is noted. This is proportional to total body haemoglobin. If the haemoglobin content of unit volume of blood is known, the blood volume may then be deduced. Unfortunately, 5 to 15 percent of the inhaled carbon monoxide escapes from the circulation to combine with myoglobin, and this approach thus over-estimates blood volume. Because the total haemoglobin includes information on both blood volume and haemoglobin concentration, many authors consider it one of the best single indices of fitness.

Heat Tolerance. A third factor limiting prolonged effort is a progressive rise of deep body temperature. A well-trained individual has a lower body temperature for a given cumulative stress, and often he also has an ability to reach a higher core temperature before exhaustion.

> Mouth thermometers cannot be used to study the *deep body temperature* during vigorous exercise, because the tongue is cooled by extensive mouth-breathing; if a man is exercising hard in a cool room, the oral temperature can be reduced by as much as 1° to 2°F. At one time, the rectal temperature was a popular index of deep body conditions. The results obtained from the rectum are reasonably representative of core conditions when a man is sitting at rest in a hot climatic chamber, but during exercise the rectal temperature is boosted above the core value by warm venous blood returned from the active muscles of the lower limbs. The recorded tempera-

ture also varies with the depth of rectal penetration (5–20 cm). Some subjects find repeated rectal examinations distasteful. Wolff has devised a radio-transmitting capsule that will report gastro-intestinal temperatures for up to three days. For shorter periods, a thermocouple can be passed into the oesophagus; this gives quite an accurate indication of overall body temperature if carefully positioned, but it can be a little unpleasant to retain during activity. Probably the most practical method of estimating core temperature in an active man is to pass a thermocouple into the auditory meatus until it is resting on the tympanic membrane. Reliable readings are obtained if the external auditory meatus is well insulated, and the recording probe has the advantage of being in close proximity to the regulatory centres of the hypothalamis.

Heat dissipation during exercise depends mainly on sweating (p. 308). Well-trained individuals sweat earlier and in greater quantities than those who are unfit. The *rate of sweating* is determined quite readily if a subject is weighed on a beam balance accurate to 5 to 10 gm. The sweat rate can be as much as 2 litres per hour (p. 311), so that weighings at fifteen minute intervals have an accuracy of 1 percent to 2 percent. In calculating sweat loss, account must be taken of fluid intake, urination, and (particularly if the air is dry) respiratory water losses.

In the industrial setting, the best evidence of poor adaptation to the combined stress of hard physical work and a high environmental temperatures is a progressive *rise of pulse rate* over the course of the working day. If this is observed, the intensity of activity must be reduced and/or the rest pauses lengthened until the individual concerned has achieved a greater level of fitness.

Other Aspects of Fitness

Medical Fitness. A high level of fitness is unlikely to be achieved while a person has overt disease. This is obvious for some of the more acute maladies, but is equally true of many chronic diseases. Recent studies have emphasized that even such a benign condition as varicose veins can lead to a substantial diminution of aerobic power because excessive quantities of blood are pooled in the tortuous varicosities.

A thorough medical examination is thus essential not only on grounds of safety, but also as an integral part of a fitness assessment. If one is dealing with young subjects, the possible distortion of a sample by inclusion of unhealthy individual's is slight. But in older populations as many as 50 percent of those tested may be affected by one or more chronic diseases.

The medical examination may reveal not only past or current diseases, but also the likelihood of future disease. In particular, examination of the exercise electrocardiogram, together with determinations of serum cholesterol and triglycerides, blood and urine sugar levels and glucose tolerance curves may indicate an increased liability to cardiovascular disease.

Where disease is already present, many of the exercise tests proposed above must be performed more cautiously, and their interpretation must also be more guarded. This is particularly true of procedures for predicting aerobic power; these assume both a linear oxygen consumption/pulse relationship and a maximum heart rate that conforms to the population average. Linearity is by no means certain with many diseases, and the theoretical heart rate may not be attained because of incapacitating symptoms. In some instances, physiopathological factors such as a reduced arterial oxygen pressure also lead to lower maximum heart rates than would be anticipated in normal subjects of the same age.

When assessing reasons for lack of fitness in a specific patient, it may be helpful to make a detailed study of those links in the oxygen transport chain that are likely to be affected by the disease process.

Nutrition. The average North American is conditioned to regard overnutrition as the major health problem of our present generation. But there are still many areas of the world where fitness is restricted by lack of food. Children in Nazi-occupied Europe showed a significant retardation of growth as food became scarce, and more recently Wyndham has found gross body weight a useful index of the tolerance of Central African natives for heavy physical work. When the Central Africans first reach Johannesburg, they are substantially below the expected weight for their height, and this deficit is made good as they are provided with adequate foods and participate in a strenuous training programme.

Even in North America there are still many groups who show varying degrees of undernutrition. Examples include (a) ghetto children, (b) old people living on restricted incomes, (c) women who attempt "crash" dieting, (d) alcoholics (particularly those who have a low total calorie intake due to inactivity), and (e) other food faddists (including some athletes).

Perhaps the simplest measure of general nutritional status is the blood haemoglobin level. This is particularly important in the context of fitness, since a low haemoglobin concentration inevitably restricts oxygen transport (p. 48).

Overnutrition is reflected in an excess body weight relative to actuarial data (Table XV) and commonly in high serum cholesterol and serum triglyceride readings. Other aspects of fitness such as maximum oxygen intake and muscle strength are often expressed relative to body weight. This imposes a heavy penalty on those who are obese, but in the context of fitness it is a fair penalty, since the muscles of a heavy person must perform more work, and the oxygen cost of almost all physical activities is also increased by obesity (p. 433).

Drugs and fitness. Note should be taken of the consumption of alcohol and of cigarettes; in making such assessments, the patient's statements should be viewed with caution! The effect of these and other drugs upon physical performance is discussed on pages 327–368.

Present Levels of Fitness

Even if information were available on all the aspects of fitness discussed above, it would not be practical to cover present standards in a book of this length. We shall thus focus our interest on three of the more important areas—aerobic power, obesity, and strength—testing the hypothesis that lack of physical activity has led to a deterioration of fitness in the present generation.

Current Inactivity

It is generally assumed that the people of Western Europe and North America are currently inactive. We think in terms of our immediate friends and acquaintances, and it is perhaps surprising that after World War II only *half* of the families in the "affluent" United States owned *one* car; in 1965, 21 percent of United States families were still without a car, although by this time 24 percent of families owned two or more cars.

The level of community activity is perhaps reflected best in per capita food consumption. Again examining figures for the United States, the estimated usage of food was 3440 kcal/day in 1930, and this dropped progressively to 3130 kcal/day in 1965. There is no easy means of deciding whether the apparent 310 kcal diminution of energy expenditure represents the loss of thirty minutes vigorous activity (12 kcal/min), or a smaller reduction in the cost of many common tasks. However, we may suspect that a reduction of walking and cycling, a greater use of elevators, and mechanization in the home and factory have all played a significant part in bringing about this change.

Personal activity records (p. 28) support the view that the average person makes no great physical demands on his body. Pulse rates greater than 120/min are a rarity, and indeed in many city-dwellers the pulse does not exceed 100 beats/min for more than 10 percent of the day. In sedentary employment, the only activities causing a significant elevation of the resting pulse rate are the climbing of stairs and walking; both are increasingly uncommon phenomena. Even in the so-called heavy industries, it is rare to find tasks that call for energy expenditures of more than three times the resting level, Thus, irrespective of the type of employment, fitness must be sought in deliberate leisure activity. Less than a half of the North American populace make any pretence at deliberate exercise, and in less than 10 percent is there a substantial effort to improve or even maintain personal fitness.

Aerobic Power

There is now abundant data on the aerobic power of selected populations (Figs. 84 and 85). If results are expressed in ml/kg min, young boys in different parts of the world achieve

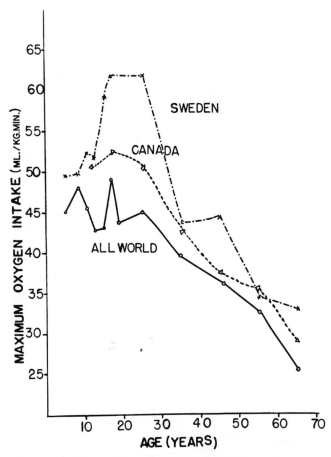

Figure 84. The aerobic power of male populations in different parts of the world (reproduced from Shephard, R.J.: *Endurance Fitness*, University of Toronto Press, by permission of the publishers).

remarkably consistent readings of 48–50 ml/kg min. In most countries, there is a progressive deterioration from the late teen years, and by the age of sixty some 40 to 50 percent of the initial aerobic power has been lost. However, the data from Sweden do not conform to this pattern; indeed, the aerobic power of young Swedish adults is actually greater than that of the children.

It could be argued that this is a problem of subject selection. Few authors have studied random cross-sections of the community.

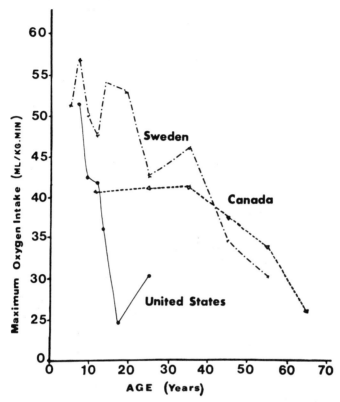

Figure 85. The aerobic power of female populations from different parts of the world (reproduced from Shephard, R.J.: *Endurance Fitness* Toronto, University of Toronto Press, by permission of the publishers).

Sometimes those who have volunteered for testing have been individuals concerned about a personal loss of fitness or a possible risk of coronary disease—these have been the poorer representatives of a community. In Sweden, on the other hand, many of those tested have had direct or indirect connection with gymnastic institutions. However, the differences between Sweden and other parts of the world persist if one compares men of the same age, following the same occupation. Thus Swedish soldiers have the very high aerobic power of 64 ml/kg min, compared with about 46 ml/kg min in the United Kingdom, 44 ml/kg min in Canada, and 38 ml/kg min in the United States. Industrial workers average 53 ml/kg min in Sweden, compared with 44 ml/kg min in Norway, Canada, Australia and Holland. University students average about 50 ml/kg min, compared with 44 ml/kg min in Norway, 40 ml/kg min in Canada, and some even lower figures from the United States. There are many social, cultural, and climatic differences between Scandinavia and the rest of the world, but it is tempting to attribute at least a part of the greater aerobic power of the Swedes to a greater level of habitual activity. I have been impressed that when Swedish colleagues have visited my laboratory, they have not asked "which is a good restaurant," but rather "where can I go for my run." Further, on visiting conservation areas, they have been uniformly horrified by the relentless procession of gross women in bikinis. "In Sweden, they would be ashamed ..." was one comment.

Since the inactivity of the North American is a recent phenomenon, it is interesting to compare present standards with prewar data. Robinson tested Harvard faculty in 1938, and he found younger staff (20–30 years) had an average aerobic power of 49 ml/kg min, compared with the current United States average of 38 ml/kg min. What has happened seems largely an acceleration of the natural ageing process. The older staff (50–60 years) had an aerobic power of 38 ml/kg min in 1938, and the United States average at this age is still almost 36 ml/kg min.

Obesity

Obesity has different meanings for different readers. The dictionary defines it as "extreme fatness." It has a pathological connotation for many physicians—the patient has exceeded the normal, expected weight for his height and age by x or more pounds; the process of fat accumulation has therefore become dangerous and must be reversed by active treatment.

When advising the individual, there is perhaps a need for an arbitrary definition such as fifteen pounds of added fat, but for many purposes it is more convenient to regard the accumulation of adipose tissue as a continuous, rather than a discontinuous process, with the distribution of body weights ranging smoothly from the "ideal" value (where mortality is minimal) to extreme obesity. If the concept of a continuous distribution is accepted, then the behaviour of a population can be described simply by departures from the ideal weight (Table XV). More precise methods of measuring the percentage body fat are described on pages 485 and 487.

TABLE XV

AVERAGE "IDEAL" WEIGHTS IN RELATION TO HEIGHT AND SEX
FOR SUBJECTS OF MEDIUM FRAME.

Based on records of individually insured lives over the period 1935–54, from Build
and Blood Pressure Study of Society of Actuaries, 1959.

| Height (no shoes) | Ideal Weight (indoor clothing) | |
	Men	Women
cm	kg	kg
157.5	57.6	48.5
160.0	58.9	49.9
162.6	60.3	51.2
165.1	61.9	52.6
167.6	63.7	54.2
170.2	65.7	55.8
172.7	67.6	57.8
175.3	69.4	60.0
177.8	71.4	61.7
180.3	73.5	63.5
182.9	75.5	65.3
185.4	77.5	66.8
188.0	79.8	68.5
190.5	82.1	
193.0	84.3	—

The standards proposed by the actuaries are based on a large
population (some 5 million U.S. citizens); however, they are
biassed in the sense that only those persons applying for life
insurance were included. The data were collected in the early
1950s, but young Canadian men still conform quite closely
with the "ideal" values. Unfortunately, some 8 kg of weight
are gained between the ages of twenty-five and forty-five, and
there is a matching 4 mm increase in thickness of the average
skinfold (Table XVI); if the "fifteen pound" criterion is applied,

TABLE XVI

THICKNESS OF EIGHT SKINFOLDS

(Data of author and his associates for men and women approximating "ideal" weights
of Table XV. Mean ± S.D.)

Skinfold	Male (mm)	Female (mm)
Chin	5.8 ± 8.7	7.1 ± 2.8
Triceps	7.8 ± 4.1	15.6 ± 6.2
Chest	12.0 ± 7.9	8.6 ± 3.7
Subscapular	11.9 ± 5.1	11.3 ± 4.2
Suprailiac	12.7 ± 7.0	14.6 ± 8.0
Waist	14.3 ± 8.2	15.3 ± 7.5
Suprapubic	11.0 ± 6.4	20.5 ± 8.2
Knee (Medial)	8.6 ± 4.1	11.8 ± 4.2
Average, All Folds	10.4 ± 4.9	13.9 ± 5.1

the average individual has become clinically obese by the time he is forty-five.

Young women already exceed the ideal value by as much as 8 kg. Much of this "puppy-fat" is lost between the ages of twenty-five and thirty-five, presumably as a result of the increased domestic activity associated with child-rearing. However, the burden of excess weight is regained by the age of forty-five. In subsequent years, the skinfold thickness continues to increase, but there is no further increase of body weight; fat is now being deposited in the body at the expense of muscle.

The present fat content of a child's body is greater than in the prewar period, but part of this change can be attributed to earlier maturation. Boys still reach the "ideal" weight as they become adult, and the percentage of body fat found in one sample of ten to twelve-year-old Toronto school-boys (15.6%) does not seem alarmingly high. Girls of the same age already have 20.7 percent body fat, and they exceed the "ideal" weight when they reach maturity; their nutrition must thus be considered excessive relative to activity.

Muscle Strength

Much of the world data on muscular strength refers specifically to static (isometric) measurements. Such figures bear little relation to dynamic strength (p. 187), and the results obtained are greatly influenced by details of technique such as the limb position and the type of recording equipment. Furthermore, data have generally been expressed in absolute* units of force (kg), taking no account of either leverage or the body bulk to be carried.

The handgrip strength we have found for eleven-year-old boys in Toronto (21 kg) is similar to that in Michigan and slightly better than reported for other parts of Canada; on the other hand, it is about 4 kg less than found in California and Denmark. The outstanding performance of the Californians is somewhat surprising, and it may reflect an earlier maturation of

---

* Absolute is used here in an anthropometric rather than a physical sense; relative units would be expressed per kg of body mass.

the boys rather than a greater ultimate strength; a marked acceleration of strength development occurs with maturation (Fig. 53). The performance of Canadian adult males is again somewhat inferior to that of Scandinavians; in Toronto, figures of 50 to 55 kg are found between the ages of twenty-five and forty-five, whereas in Denmark the corresponding figures are 55–65 kg; on the other hand, United Kingdom factory workers (average 44 kg) have an even poorer grip strength than Canadians.

Our 11-year-old girls (hand-grip strength 19 kg) compare closely with those from other parts of Canada, but are weaker than Danish girls (average 25 kg). Our adult women (31 kg) compare favourably with factory workers in the United Kingdom (25 kg), but are inferior to the young women of Denmark (35–40 kg).

International comparisons of the strength of other muscle groups are less reliable because of difficulties in standardizing the measuring technique. However, they support the general conclusion that at the present time the Scandinavians have a better developed musculature than people living in North America. Asmussen's values for fully-grown young people are summarized in Table XVII.

TABLE XVII

STRENGTH OF SELECTED MUSCLE GROUPS IN DANISH CHILDREN
(Data of Asmussen for boys of 170 cm, girls of 155 cm height. Values vary greatly according to details of measuring technique. Note particularly the difference in results for the key and the handle).

	Isometric Force (kg)	
Movement	*Boys*	*Girls*
Trunk Extension	74	50
Trunk Flexion	53	37
Handgrip	44	28
Pronation (Key)	37	26
Supination (Key)	37	27
Pronation (Handle)	106	70
Supination (Handle)	108	70
Downward Pull	45	29
Horizontal Pull	38	25
Upward Push	23	15
Horizontal Push	26	18
Leg Extension	240	170
Hip Flexion	56	43
Hip Extension	42	32

The absolute grip strength of children has increased in the past seventy years; however, if expressed per unit of body mass, current North American data are rather similar to figures reported from St. Louis over the period 1892–1894. This in itself might suggest that the present generation of children have remained sufficiently active to prevent wasting of the body musculature. On the other hand, Scandinavian children seem stronger than those of North America. The greater muscularity of the Scandinavians may be partly a sampling artefact, but it has recurred in a number of independent studies, and as with aerobic power, it seems likely to reflect a superior genetic endowment and/or greater habitual physical activity on the part of the Scandinavian child.

References

Yoshimora, H. and Weiner, J.S.: *Human Adaptability and its Methodology.* Tokyo, Japan. Society for the Promotion of Science, 1966.

Weiner, J.S., and Lourie, J.A.: *Human biology—a guide to Field Methods.* Oxford, Blackwell, 1969.

Andersen, L.A. *et al.: Fundamentals of Exercise Testing.* Geneva, WHO Monograph, 1971.

Shephard, R.J.: Standard tests of aerobic power. In: *Frontiers of Fitness.* Springfield, Thomas, 1971.

Hayden, F.J., and Yuhasz, M.S.: *The CAHPER Fitness Performance Test Manual.* Toronto, Canadian Association for Health, Physical Education and Recreation, 1966.

A.A.H.P.E.R. Youth Fitness Test Manual. Washington, D.C., American Association for Health, Physical Education, and Recreation, 1965.

Cumming, G.R.: Correlation of physical performance with laboratory measures of fitness. In *Frontiers of Fitness.* Springfield, Thomas, 1971.

Borg, G.: The perception of physical performance. In *Frontiers of Fitness* Springfield, Thomas, 1971.

Shephard, R.J.: *Endurance Fitness.* Toronto, University of Toronto Press, 1969.

Mathews, D.K.: *Measurement in Physical Education.* Philadelphia, Saunders, 1963.

Society of Actuaries: *Build and Blood Pressure Study.* Chicago, Illinois, 1959.

Brozek, J.: Body composition. *Ann NY Acad Sci: 110*:1–1018, 1963.

15

TRAINING REGIMES

On Experimental Design

It is appropriate to initiate our discussion of the physiological responses to training by a discussion of the types of experiment from which conclusions have been drawn.

Cross-sectional Comparisons

Many of the older authors were content to compare athletes with more sedentary members of the population. This approach ignores the important contribution that inheritance undoubtedly makes to athletic prowess. A champion cross-country skier may have an aerobic power of as much as 85 ml/kg min. The usual sedentary university student achieves barely one half of this figure, and although performance can be improved by persistent training, the average student can never approach the physiological status of an athlete competitively selected from a vast population.

The relative importance of training and heredity is still vigorously debated; however, if we continue to take as our basis of argument the aerobic component of human performance, a strong influence of heredity is seen. The standard deviation of aerobic power in a typical group of young and healthy men is from 16 percent to 20 percent. Thus, if we search carefully through a population of one million, we should discover the statistical "freak" with an aerobic power 70 percent to 80 percent larger than that of the average person. Training can add further to the performance of this exceptional individual, but it is unlikely to add anything approaching the initial 80 percent advantage of genetic endowment.

The Longitudinal Survey

As with most physiological problems, it is more satisfactory to conduct a "longitudinal" experiment. A "test" group of sub-

jects follows a training regime week by week, and their physiological status is compared with that of a "control" group who
agree not to alter their level of habitual activity.

Although the longitudinal experiment is open to less objection than the cross-sectional, there are still a number of pitfalls.
The type of person who volunteers for any physiological study
is not typical of the general population—he may be concerned
about his heart or some other facet of health, and psychological
tests often indicate a "neurotic" type of personality. The very
existence of a training group alters the life-style of its members
with respect to diet, cigarette consumption and the like, and
depending upon the experimental design the controls may or
may not show parallel changes in their habits. There is a high
percentage of drop-outs (p. 517) and the residual sample is
inevitably even more atypical of the general population than
the entire group who volunteered for study.

The usual experiment takes "sedentary" members of a community, but unfortunately there is no simple objective procedure
to establish just how sedentary the volunteers are at the commencement of a study. Let us suppose that the usual range of
fitness tests is carried out (p. 395) and a volunteer has a poor
showing; this may mean that he is very sedentary in his habits,
but it is also conceivable that he is moderately active with a
very poor genetic endowment. It is thus necessary to attempt
some quantification of the initial level of activity, using retrospective questioning, a diary, or twenty-four hour pulse counts
(p. 28).

Some workers have simply followed the response to existing
training regimes, observing the progress of hockey, football or
swimming teams as they prepare for the competitive season, or
of older men as they join calisthenic programmes at YMCAs and
other gymnasia. This form of experiment has the advantage that
the natural enthusiasm of the participants is given full rein, but
it is exceedingly difficult to quantitate the intensity, frequency,
and duration of activity that is undertaken. It is possible to
persuade the more intelligent subjects to keep an exercise log
(p. 31), and this can be translated into units of activity, using
Cooper's points scheme, or some modification thereof. However,

the process of translation needs a skilled clerk, and is quite time-consuming; further, since the diary or log involves elements of duration, frequency, and intensity, a decision on the relative merits of these training stimuli is an essential preliminary to the translation process.

In order to control the intensity and duration of training more rigidly, the investigator must insist that exercise be performed in the laboratory, using a device such as a treadmill or a bicycle ergometer. The regime can then be boring for the subject, and in a large city much time is lost in driving to and from the exercise machine. Further, if an adequate sample of subjects is to be tested, an undesirably large part of the laboratory day becomes occupied with the provision of facilities for routine exercise.

Physiological Changes Induced by Training

Overall Changes

Repeated vigorous activity produces substantial adaptive changes in almost all body systems. From the physiological point of view, it is convenient to summarize many of the observed responses in terms of increments in aerobic power, anaerobic "capacity" and anerobic power (p. 396).

Various authors have succeeded in increasing the *aerobic power* of their subjects by 5 percent to 30 percent. The magnitude of the observed response has depended upon the initial status of those tested, the largest effects being seen in the most sedentary members of a group. In general, the period of observation has been quite short, but in the few instances where studies have been extended to two years or more, changes have not greatly exceeded those attained in a few weeks. On the basis of a twelve to fifteen year longitudinal study, Hollmann claimed that regular exercise inhibited ageing. The functional loss in his active subjects was about 1 percent per year, while in the inactive group it was as much as 3 percent per annum. Unfortunately, his conclusion is suspect, because the inactive group had an unusually rapid loss of aerobic power, while the change in those who were still active coincided rather closely with that generally accepted for a sedentary population. In assessing the results of such long term studies, care must be taken in choosing appropriate units of measurement. Often, there is a change in the body weight of participants, and the alteration in aerobic power is then larger if expressed in relative units (ml/kg/min) than if stated in absolute terms (litre/min).

Training—particularly training of the interval type—may build up a tolerance for lactate by increasing the alkaline reserve of the tissues and raising the pain threshold of the body. The terminal lactate concentrations are commonly higher in the trained than in untrained individuals; however, even if this is not the case, the greater total blood volume and an increase in the alactate component of the oxygen debt give the trained person a greater anaerobic "capacity" and power than his sedentary counterpart. The proportion of anaerobic work performed at any given fraction of aerobic power is also reduced by training, because the muscles are strengthened, and perfusion of the active fibres is less readily impeded during contraction (p. 95).

The *endurance* often shows a dramatic improvement with training. If performance is measured at a constant absolute intensity of effort, this is easily understood—what was a maximal or near maximal response of either a muscle group or of the entire body is now perhaps 80 percent of maximum. There is much less reliance upon anaerobic work, and less chance of either exhausting supplies of glycogen or developing an unfavourable intramuscular and intravascular pH. However, even if effort is held to a constant percentage of the individual's current maximum potential, the endurance of strenuous effort is still extended by training. The respective contributions of psychological and physiological factors have yet to be clarified. There is some evidence that training improves "body image" and diminishes anxiety regarding the possible harmful effects of intense effort. The perception of a given effort is also reduced by its repetition, and there must be some habituation to the sensations accompanying vigorous exercise; however, the present author is not convinced that training produces much change in the perceived effort at a fixed percentage of the current maximum performance. If endurance of a given relative load is improved, then the main explanation is likely to be physiological rather than psychological.

Cardiovascular System

Perhaps the most obvious characteristic of the trained person is a very slow *pulse rate,* both at rest and in submaximum effort. The basis of this bradycardia is still debated. Some authors have postulated that stretch receptors in the dilated and hypertrophied atria are more active than in a sedentary person; however, a rapid rather than a slow heart rate is seen when the atria are distended by cardiac failure. Others have claimed that trained atria liberate more acetylcholine in response to a given vagal discharge. Tipton has reported that the integrity of the vagus nerve is essential to a normal training response, and most workers now believe that the bradycardia is centrally mediated, through an alteration in the balance of sympathetic and parasympathetic discharge. The trained state is also characterized by a more rapid recovery of pulse rate after exercise, but there is little if any change of maximum heart rate. The *stroke volume* is increased both at rest and in all levels of activity, particularly if the subject is standing erect; this is in part a consequence of a general increase in *blood volume,* and in part a reflection of an increased tone of the leg veins and thus a greater *central blood volume.* Chest radiographs show an increase of *heart volume* after training; the greater stroke volume is achieved mainly by an increase of myocardial contractility, with greater cardiac emptying, so that the increase of heart volume reflects an increase of cardiac muscle mass. Postmortem examination of an active person confirms hypertrophy of the cardiac musculature, with many of the microscopic changes anticipated in trained skeletal muscle (p. 444). Once hypertrophy has occurred, it regresses rather slowly; former athletes often retain quite large hearts for a number of years, and even pathological hypertrophy (as in congenital pulmonary stenosis) may persist after relief of the valvular obstruction. Hypertrophy is associated with an increase in the cross-sectional area of the major coronary vessels. The capillary density is also increased by training, but there is disagreement as to whether development of the coronary col-

lateral circulation occurs (p. 519). The *haemoglobin* content
of unit volume of blood is unchanged or increased; the blood
may also show a small gain of *alkaline reserve,* particularly if
there has been an emphasis upon interval work. There is a widening of the *arteriovenous oxygen difference* in near maximum
effort; this probably reflects a decrease in skin perfusion with
development of alternative methods of heat dissipation such as
greater sweating. The resting *cardiac output* is usually unchanged by training; in submaximal work, it may be a little
reduced, but in maximum effort it is increased, roughly in proportion to the gain of aerobic power.

There may be some widening of the *pulse pressure* as stroke
volume increases (p. 401). Some authors have also claimed that
regular exercise lowers the mean *systemic blood pressure,* but
it is difficult to dissociate this effect from an inevitable habituation to the laboratory environment as training proceeds.

Respiratory System

Training has a relatively little influence upon the static lung
volumes of an adult; if there is specific development of the chest
musculature, it may be possible to compress the residual thoracic
volume and also to force a little more blood from the pulmonary
vessels, thereby increasing the *vital capacity* by a few hundred
ml. Whether larger changes of thoracic dimensions can be induced by regular exercise in childhood or adolescence remains
an open question. Some authors have described a 10 percent to
20 percent increase of *maximum voluntary ventilation* with training. To the extent that this test depends on the force developed
by the chest muscles, the change may be a genuine response
to some types of training. However, it is difficult to rule out
practice effects, which can in themselves produce a large increase of MVV. Training sometimes leads to adoption of a slow
and deep *pattern of breathing* during moderate exercise; this
feature is seen particularly in swimmers and others who exercise
with periods of breath-holding. There is an associated greater
extraction of oxygen from unit volume of respired gas (that is,
the trained individual has a small *ventilatory equivalent* for oxygen). At any given level of submaximal work, the *respiratory
minute volume* is less in the trained than in the untrained per-

son; this reflects three adaptations—(a) an increase of mechanical efficiency, and thus a lower oxygen cost for a given effort, (b) a centrally mediated decrease of ventilatory equivalent in moderate exercise and (c) a lesser production of lactate in more severe work (the faster adaptation of the cardiorespiratory system to a given load and the improved peripheral circulation during continuing exercise both diminish the need for anaerobic metabolism). The respiratory volume developed during maximal work increases roughly in proportion to the gain of aerobic power brought about by training. Some studies have reported a large *pulmonary diffusing capacity* in athletes, both at rest and during physical activity; this is in part a genuine finding, attributable to their larger central blood volume, but part of the apparent increase is an artifact due to their slower breathing pattern (p. 137). If care is taken to avoid artifacts, then the maximum diffusing capacity increases by no more than would be anticipated from the increase of aerobic power. It presumably reflects an increase of diffusing surface with the increase of maximum cardiac output.

Musculoskeletal System

Training leads to a strengthening of all active bones and ligaments. The calcification of the bones is increased, and where necessary their architecture is strengthened through the development of new trabeculae. The articular cartilages are also thickened and become more resistant to compression, and there is commonly an increase in flexibility of the joint capsule.

Muscle hypertrophy occurs, and there is a marked increase of muscle strength, often out of proportion to the gain in muscle bulk. Most of the increase in muscle dimensions represents an expansion of existing fibres, but some authors believe there is also an increase in the number of muscle cells. There is a corresponding increase in the density of muscle capillaries, with an increase in the proportion of muscle occupied by myofibrils as opposed to fat, connective tissue and supporting proteins. Within the individual fibres there are increases* in mitochon-

---

* It is not yet clearly established that these "increases" do much more than keep pace with the increase in fibre size. Certainly, the anaerobic power per unit of muscle mass is not remarkable in most athletes.

dria, respiratory enzymes, and such biochemical constituents as adenosine triphosphate, creatine phosphate, myoglobin, glycogen, and potassium. Exercise is normally associated with the release of certain intracellular enzymes into the circulation; with training, this release is diminished, but it is not clear whether this merely reflects an improved oxygenation of the active myofibrils, or whether there is some more specific change of membrane permeability.

At the same time that the muscles are developing, there is a depletion of fat depots, both within the subcutaneous tissues and elsewhere. If the training regime is sufficiently severe, there is an associated reduction of serum triglycerides, and possibly some reduction of serum cholesterol (p. 499). The net effect is an increase of body density, often with little change in body weight.

Central Nervous System

In addition to readily visualized gross structural changes, the regular repetition of exercise brings about a number of alterations in the functional responses of the central nervous system. Some may be grouped as *learning*. There is a storage of information relating to γ loop settings in either the premotor cortex or the cerebellum (p. 216) with a brisker reaction time and the possibility of a more efficient mechanical performance of a given task (p. 219). In this context, the ordinary person is undoubtedly pleased to achieve an economy of effort, but the athlete may prefer to extend his range of performance even if efficiency is worsened thereby. Training is also associated with the storage of information that permits a more rapid and complete adjustment of the circulation to such stresses as activity and the vertical posture (p. 402). An impaired orthostatic tolerance is a well-recognised complication of bed rest, weightlessness, and lack of cardiorespiratory fitness. Unfortunately, the space-traveller cannot overcome these problems simply by sustained activity; if his cardiorespiratory condition is to be maintained, there must also be a simulation of gravity by the application of negative counterpressure to the legs.

Other adjustments within the central nervous system fall under the heading of *habituation* or negative conditioning; they express the adjustment of the subject to the various circumstances under which the exercise is performed (p. 413). The integrity of the prefrontal cortex seems important to the normal course of habituation. Any emotional response to the exercise is progressively reduced, and at the same time there is less subconscious inhibition of maximum effort.

Physiological Changes With Bed-rest, Whole-body Immersion, and Weightlessness

The deterioration of physical condition with prolonged bed rest has been known for many years, but the problems of enforced inactivity and the removal of normal gravitational stimuli have assumed new urgency because a very similar deterioration of condition occurs in the cramped and weightless quarters of a space capsule. The physiological manifestations are the reverse of those produced by physical training. The *aerobic power* diminishes by 20 to 30 percent over the course of two to three weeks. The extent of deterioration is rather similar in athletes and in sedentary individuals, but once the functional loss has occurred it is apparently more readily reversed in sedentary than in athletic subjects. The basis of the loss in aerobic power seems entirely a diminution in cardiac *stroke volume;* there is no change of maximum heart rate and although the arteriovenous oxygen difference is increased while performing a given submaximum work, it remains at the prebed rest value during maximum effort. It is interesting that the heart rate at any given percentage of aerobic power is unchanged; the usual methods of predicting maximum oxygen consumption (page 415) should thus operate satisfactorily despite the bed rest. The change of stroke volume reflects partly a reduction of total blood volume, and partly an increase of the peripheral at the expense of the central blood volume.

The usual experimental study of bed rest is rather short, and there are then no significant changes of muscle morphology. Longer periods of bed rest are associated with a negative nitrogen balance, muscle wasting, and an increase of body fat. The urinary elimination of calcium is increased, and there is a tendency to decalcification of the long bones with an increased risk of "stone" formation within the kidneys.

If the sensations of weightlessness are simulated by complete submersion of the body, the deterioration of cardiovascular reflexes is rapid; and impaired tilt-table response is seen in as little as six hours.

The performance of physical work while in bed or travelling in a space capsule minimizes the loss of aerobic power. However, it fails to correct either decalcification or the impaired tolerance to gravity. A bed-ridden patient must stand for at least three hours per day to reverse calcium loss; there seems an association between the support of body weight and the maintenance of calcium balance. The regular application of "negative" counterpressure (suction) to the legs and abdomen prevents the development of orthostatic intolerance in either a bed-ridden or "weightless" subject; however, it does not alleviate the more long-term problem of calcium loss.

Types of Training Regime

Some General Principles

Different types of training regime develop different components of the exercise response; unfortunately, there seems no one pattern of training that will develop all physiological systems by an amount appropriate to optimum performance.

Irrespective of the mode of training, two main types of adaptation may be distinguished. One involves *structural* hypertrophy and even hyperplasia. This response can continue for months and even years, although eventually a limit of development is imposed—possibly because the maximum useful cellular size has been reached. The second type of adaptation has been called by Holmgren a *regulatory* response; this involves the establishment of new functional connections within the central nervous system. The time course is quite rapid, and the new patterns of regulation may be fully developed within a few weeks.

Both structural and regulatory changes are produced rather more easily in the young than in the elderly (p. 382).

Performance in most athletic events (Table XVIII) is helped by a development of the oxygen transport system (cardiorespiratory fitness). Depending upon the type of contest and the initial physique, some strengthening of back, abdominal and leg muscles is often helpful; however, if muscle development is disproportionate to the improvements of aerobic power, the added body weight can set an athlete at a disadvantage, particularly

TABLE XVIII

THE AEROBIC POWER OF ATHLETES IN CANADA (CUMMING) AND
SCANDINAVIA (SALTIN AND ÅSTRAND)

	Canada (ml/kg min)		Scandinavia (ml/kg min)	
	M	F	M	F
Cross-country Skiers	—	—	83	63
Distance Runners	66	—	80,77	59
Cyclists	71	—	74	—
Water-polo Players	58	—	—	—
Walkers	—	—	71	—
Swimmers	57	47	67	57
Weight-lifters	56	—	56	—
Tennis Players	55	—	—	—
Boxers	55	—	—	—
Divers	54	47	—	—
Wrestlers	54	—	56	—
Sprinters	53	45	67	56
Basketball Players	53	44	—	—
Volleyball Players	52	42	—	—
Canoeists	52	—	70	—
Hockey (Field) Players	52	—	—	—
Soccer Players	51	—	—	—
Judoists	49	—	—	—
Gymnasts	42	43	60	—
Throwers	38	38	—	—
Table Tennis Players	—	—	59	43

if his event calls for lifting of the body against gravity. In sports where a substantial fraction of the total effort is sustained by a relatively small group of muscles, performance is helped by specific development of the muscles concerned—presumably improvements of the local circulation (p. 216) then make a substantial contribution to the gain in performance. All forms of activity, but particularly tasks involving rapid and skilled movement are helped by an enhancement of mobility. The strengthening of articular cartilage, ligaments and bone is of particular significance is contact sports, where it helps to minimize the incidence of injury.

Continuous Exercise

Laboratory training is usually of the continuous type. The subject reports to the investigator and performs an exercise that involves a large proportion of the body musculature (such as running on a treadmill or pedalling a bicycle ergometer); activity is sustained for a fixed time such as fifteen or thirty minutes per visit. The load may be kept constant from one visit to the next, or it may be increased progressively, so that each bout of exercise is terminated at the same pulse rate.

Continuous exercise may lead to some development of the active muscles. The efficiency of effort is improved, and there is habituation to the test situation. However, the main physiological response is a substantial increase of aerobic power.

One specific advantage of continuous laboratory training is that the amount of work performed is known from direct observation, and the intensity, duration, and frequency of exercise can be measured quite precisely. In a widely quoted study from Finland, Karvonen found that a certain minimum intensity of effort was needed to induce training. He measured intensity in terms of pulse rate, and suggested this should increase at least 60 percent of the way from the resting value towards the figure anticipated in maximum effort. In his young men, the training threshold was thus about 140 pulse beats per minute. Others have reported some training at much lower pulse frequencies; for instance, Durnin's marching soldiers reached a heart rate of only 120/min. Accordingly, a further laboratory investigation was carried out by the present author; this identified initial fitness and intensity of effort as the main factors influencing the response to a cardiorespiratory training regime. A pulse rate of 120/min is a relatively uncommon finding in the sedentary city dweller of North America, and accordingly it provides an adequate initial training stimulus. On the other hand, if an athlete is already exercising regularly at pulse rates of 170 and 180/min, very intense effort will be needed to bring about a further improvement of cardiorespiratory condition. Within the context of the author's study (1–5 sessions per week, each of 5–20 minutes duration), the frequency and duration of exercise were much less important variables than intensity and initial fitness.

There is still a need for closer definition of the minimum stimulus required to develop and maintain aerobic power. Some authorities suggest as many as five thirty minute sessions per week for those wishing to improve their status, with three sessions per week recommended to maintain the status quo. On the other hand, Cooper, author of the popular paperback *Aerobics* implies that if the intensity of exercise is adequate, five minutes per day may suffice. In the hurried world of the business executive, the difference between five and thirty minutes per day has practical significance, and the question deserves early resolution.

If intense rhythmic effort is sustained for as long as thirty minutes without remission, there may be a substantial rise of systemic blood pressure; this is an important point in the planning of a regime for the middle-aged, coronary prone individual. In the context of athletics, continuous exercise has relevance to early preparation—particularly of endurance competitors such as the distance runner and cyclist. The selected daily training period is commonly three to five times the anticipated duration of a race; exercise is preferably performed away from the laboratory, in pleasant surroundings such as a golf course. The speed is adjusted to produce a steady pulse rate of 150 to 160/min and for the first few weeks of training the objective is a general development of the cardiorespiratory system. Once this has been accomplished, the competitor progresses to faster activity (producing pulse rates of up to 180/min), running over distances of about twice the intended range. At each training session, several repetitions may be alternated with perhaps five minutes of walking and jogging. Finally, as competition approaches, work is concentrated over the intended distance, preferably on the actual running track, so that the correct pace is learnt and the mechanical efficiency and habituation of the contestant reach maximum values.

Interval Training

Interval training is widely used as a method of preparation for competitive running; it also has its advocates in the conditioning of sedentary middle-aged men. Basically, it involves a formal pattern of fast activity (such as running) and slower activity (such as walking or jogging). Depending upon the type of competition and the preference of the individual trainer, there is a substantial variation in the distance and speed of the fast runs, the duration and type of recovery activity, and the total number of repetitions per training session.

Slow interval training is used in the early stages of the season, and is recommended to develop cardiorespiratory fitness; a typical regime might involve three repetitions of a seven unit sequence in which three one quarter mile runs (pulse 180/min) were alternated with three one quarter mile jogs, followed by a one quarter mile walk.

The runner later progresses to *fast interval training*, which is thought to develop his anaerobic endurance. There is possibly an increase of glycogen stores and tissue alkali reserves; in addition there are well recognized increments of ATP, myoglobin, and other cellular components that contribute to "alactate" power. A competitor in a one mile event commonly chooses a seven unit quarter mile sequence similar to that recommended for slow interval work, running each quarter mile interval 1 to 2 percent faster than his average competitive speed for the entire mile. However, the experiments of Irma Åstrand suggest that a lengthening of the active phase and/or a shortening of the recovery phase would do more to develop anaerobic endurance (page 451).

Repetition running is a variant of interval training where the active phases are lengthened, and the intervals are also extended to permit fairly complete recovery. This type of regime is best suited to the contestant in long distance events. Whether aerobic or anaerobic power is developed by this form of training depends largely upon the speed attained during the running phases.

Fartlek training is popular in Sweden. It is an informal type of interval training carried out under "cross-country" conditions, and unless carefully monitored may fail to make the necessary physiological demands upon the body.

Roskamm and his colleagues have compared the effectiveness of two interval regimes and one form of continuous training. A 2½ min exercise/2½ min recovery format yielded the largest increase in maximum watt/pulse (that is, the ability to carry out a combination of aerobic and anaerobic work). On the other hand, the pulse rate at 70 percent of aerobic power was least in the group that devoted the training period to continuous exercise.

Irma Åstrand has provided a useful physiological comparison of several possible regimes (Table XIX). With very brief intermittent activity (< ½ minute), the muscles sustain the full workload, but there is no real approach to a steady state. The oxygen consumption during the active phase is only 63 percent

TABLE XIX
A COMPARISON OF RESPONSES TO ONE HOUR OF INTERMITTENT OR
CONTINUOUS EXERCISE
(Based on data of I. Åstrand.)

Loading	Work (min)	Rest (min)	O₂ Intake (l/min STPD)	Resp Min Volume (litre/min)	Heart Rate (/min)	Blood Lactate (mg/100 ml)
Intermittent	½	½	2.9	63	150	20
(2160 Kgm/min	1	1	2.9	65	167	45
During Active	2	2	4.4	95	178	95
Phase)	3	3	4.6	107	188	120
Continuous						
1080 Kgm/min	60	—	2.4	49	134	12
2160 Kgm/min	9	—	4.6	124	190	150

of the possible steady state value, the blood lactate remains low, and the stimulus to the cardiorespiratory system is relatively mild. We may speculate that much of the oxygen cost is being financed by an alactate oxygen debt, and that this debt is repaid during the one-half min recovery intervals; exercise of this type thus seems likely to develop muscle strength, muscle endurance and alactic power.

With rather longer intervals (~1 min), a fair load is imposed upon the cardiovascular system, but there is still a relatively light build-up of anaerobic metabolites. This might seem a good pattern of training to suggest to the coronary prone individual. The more protracted the work interval, the greater the breakdown of glycogen and the greater the accumulation of lactate; with a three minute work period, the terminal lactate concentrations approach the limit of endurance, and it is doubtful if intermittent work of this intensity could be sustained much beyond the one hour period of Åstrand's study. Nevertheless, the total work performed (30×2160 kg) is in marked contrast with the achievement for continuous work (9×2160 kg). Presumably, the recovery intervals permit a more general dispersal of lactate throughout body fluids. Long interval work of this type seems likely to develop the glycogenolytic power of the muscles. However, an equally large build-up of lactate can be achieved with much shorter bursts of activity, providing that the intensity of effort is sufficient, and the recovery period is somewhat foreshortened (as in the case in fast interval work).

There is evidence that any development of anaerobic power is specific to the active muscles, and the wise athlete thus concentrates on the type of activity to be followed in actual competition.

Sprint Training

The sprinter requires a brisk reaction time, explosive strength, experience in moving at the maximum attainable speed ($\sim$25 mph) and a large anaerobic power; however, there is little taxing of anaerobic "capacity." The duration of training sprints should thus be sufficient to permit acceleration to maximum speed ($\sim$6 seconds), but little advantage is gained if the effort is sustained for more than ten seconds.

Very high heart rates are developed by the sprinter—often, these exceed the anticipated steady-state "maximum" heart rates; however, the duration of activity is too short for a full adaptation of the peripheral circulation, and the stroke volume may actually be less than the resting value—particularly if the breath is held during the sprint. For these reasons, sprinting itself has little influence upon aerobic power.

If an athlete wishes to improve his cardiorespiratory fitness, and at the same time to practice the technique of sprinting, he may alternate fifty yard sprints with jogging or walking an equal distance (*"interval sprinting"*); the physiological situation is then analogous to brief but intense intermittent work (Table XIX). A second variant is *"acceleration sprinting"*; here, a typical sequence involves jogging, striding, sprinting, and walking over equal distances. The objectives are twofold—to warm up gradually to maximum effort, thus avoiding the muscle and tendon injuries that might otherwise occur with outdoor work in cold weather (page 191) and to develop maximum speed at each sprint without cumulative fatigue; an extended recovery period is thus essential. Acceleration sprinting is particularly suited to the improvement of explosive strength.

"Hollow sprints" include two maximum efforts, separated by a period of jogging, and followed by a period of walking. The effect of this type of regime is to extend the period of intense activity, while preserving its sprint characteristics; more time is permitted for glycolysis, and greater development of anaerobic "capacity" may be anticipated.

Sports Participation

The popular press commonly equates "getting in shape" with the taking up of some sport such as golf. How much value may be attached to sports participation as a training method?

For the professional athlete, it has little value unless the sport concerned is one in which competition is envisaged. Time is occupied that could be devoted to more effective preparation, and the skills that are learnt may interfere with techniques needed in competition; thus the performance of the tennis player deteriorates if he engages in recreational badminton. Lastly, if the recreation is pursued strenuously, there may be anatomical changes in the body that are undesirable for success in a specific contest. One example from the author's practice concerned a marathon cyclist; he had a fairly satisfactory absolute aerobic power, but was unable to resist a temptation to indulge in occasional sprint cycling. This produced a disproportionate development of the leg musculature, and reduced his relative aerobic power to a modest 48 ml/kg min. Although free of excess fat, he was a very heavy man, and during the marathon races he became tired when cycling up long hills.

At a first glance, recreational sports seem a good basis for improving the fitness of the general population. However, there are again several problems. If an interest is developed in team sports at school or in young manhood, then there is a high probability that the activity will not extend into the all important period of middle and older age. If the sports are played against an individual opponent, the amount of exercise that is taken depends very much upon the skill of the opposing player, and as such it is hard to quantify. Many of the sports popular among the middle-classes—golf, sailing, bowling and the like fail to induce the intensity of cardiorespiratory stress that will develop or even maintain the condition of the heart. Some indication of the relative effectiveness of different sports may be obtained (a) from estimates of their caloric cost (Table XXII), and (b) from the aerobic power of successful contestants in various forms of activity (Table XVIII). Although golf does little for the heart, the extended periods of moderately increased caloric expenditure may be quite effective in reducing obesity. In this context, walking can be preferable to jogging (p. 523).

Cooper's *Aerobics* system is a practical attempt to use a variety of recreational activities as a means of improving cardio-respiratory condition. The objective is commendable, and his book is eminently readable for the general population. However, our experience has been that patients using this system are less persistent in exercise than those enrolled in a formal programme such as calisthenics at the YMCA. A further shortcoming of *Aerobics* is its limited emphasis upon diet; many of the potential users of the system are overweight, and the reduction of obesity achieved by the average student of "Aerobics" is less than that of those following a supervised programme. Details of the points awarded for individual sports may also need some revision. There should be a consistent relationship between the points earnt and the rate of caloric expenditure, and the relative earnings for intensity and duration of activity need further study. Nevertheless, Cooper has made an important contribution by suggesting that a person can elect any one of a wide range of sports, and yet achieve a measurable and effective training stimulus.

Unfortunately, most vigorous recreations are expensive in terms of land usage. In large conurbations, such activities are currently feasible, but this is only possible because a small minority of the population are active. If we accept the thesis that all citizens should participate in regular exercise, then it is difficult to advocate the majority of sporting activities as a means of maintaining fitness. Physicians and physical educators must take a lesson from dance-hall entrepreneurs, and devise modes of recreation that permit maximum utilization of the available floor or field space.

Circuit Training

The concept of circuit training was developed by two English physical educators (Morgan and Adamson). Eight to twelve "stations" are arranged around a gymnasium, and different forms of calisthenics are performed at each. Morgan and Adamson suggested a good circuit should include exercises for the arms and shoulders, back, abdomen, legs, and combinations of these several areas.

The *arm work* may include gripping (hanging, swinging or climbing on a rope), heaving (climbing on beams or ladders, heaving weights on pulleys), pressing (press-ups, parallel bar work, dumb-bell pressing or the use of a chest-expander) and arm raising against resistance (lifting and swinging a dumb-bell). *Back-exercises* should be so devised that the subject cannot use the leg muscles in the stead of the spinal musculature. It is also important to avoid injury to intervertebral discs and ligaments; the load should be borne by a straight back with active extensor muscles, and twisting movements should be avoided (page 210). Perhaps the most effective procedure is to take a load upon the back via the arms—as is commonly the case in real life. *Abdominal exercises*—in leg raising and sit-ups the abdominal muscles have a secondary, fixating role, and there is a danger that the stronger leg muscles may strain the lumbar spine. For this reason, trunk curling is the preferred approach to abdominal exercise. *Leg exercise* is easily arranged as bench stepping, and as jumping and squatting with or without weights. Because of the tendency to move the trunk with the legs, most leg exercises also activate a large fraction of the total body musculature. The *combined exercises* are rather characteristic of circuit work, and involve such items as jump and heave (pull-ups on a parallel bar) and jump and press (push-up to high support position on a parallel bar).

The individual to be trained determines for himself how many repetitions he can make at each station. He then moves three complete times around the circuit, performing half the maximum number of repetitions with each visit to each station. On subsequent days, he attempts to move faster around the circuit, and gradually increases the number of repetitions.

The type of physiological change induced by circuit training depends very much upon the content of individual circuits. A substantial development of aerobic power is possible, particularly if items such as stepping, skipping and running are included. However, from the description given above, it is clear that the usual emphasis is upon muscle building. Roskamm has compared circuit training with continuous exercise and interval training; in his experience, the latter procedures were more effective in developing aerobic power, while the circuit work yielded a larger gain of muscular strength.

Circuit training is quite popular in preparation for contact sports, where muscle bulk is an advantage. It has the merit that an individual is competing with himself, rather than some less suitable external competitor. However, from the viewpoint of the average citizen, the muscle-building emphasis seems undesirable, particularly when this is concentrated upon the arm and shoulder regions, and the implied (but not fundamental) need for gymnastic equipment also limits the general application of circuit work.

Calisthenics

Calisthenics has a long history in physical education—indeed, the discipline may trace its roots to the rhythmic exercises of Swedish teachers such as Salzmann and Ling, and the German Turnverein or outdoor gymnasium. More recently, the popularity of gymnastic work has declined—particularly in North America, perhaps because it has continued to favour the militaristic emphasis originally imparted by German immigrants.

From the physiological point of view, there are a number of objections to calisthenics. As commonly performed, the energy cost is too low to stimulate an improvement in cardiorespiratory condition. Karpovich and his associates found the oxygen consumption in trunk-bending was no more than 20 percent above resting, and the most active of more than forty common exercises yielded an oxygen consumption of only 0.8 litre/min. Karpovich studied convalescent patients. In the British Army, where a more rapid cadence was required, the oxygen consumption reached 1.6 litre/min, but in Swedish gymnastics (where the emphasis is still upon beauty rather than speed of movement), the average oxygen cost is again in the range 0.8–0.9 litre/min. This is not to deny that physical condition can be improved by regular calisthenics; significant changes in strength, body composition, and cardiorespiratory performance can be induced if sufficiently vigorous activity is undertaken. Further, the very existence of a group with an enthusiastic leader is a useful motivating tool, and because of the group support a gymnasium centred programme may achieve results in patients who would soon defect from more solitary modes of activity.

Common criticisms of calisthenics are that the frequent repetition of meaningless movements is boring, and that the demands made on the individual are not related to his capacity. The boredom can be counteracted by a good leader who promotes a spirit of camaradie within the group, and a grading of demand can be achieved by careful initial allocation of the patient to one of a series of progressive calisthenic classes.

The Canadian *5BX and 10BX* plans are personal schemes of progressive gymnastics that require no formal apparatus. Each day is divided between five minutes of the more usual calisthenics and six minutes of stationary running, or longer periods of outdoor running and walking. The starting point in the scheme is individually graded in terms of age and initial attainment. Stanley Brown has assessed the oxygen cost of various 5BX charts by carrying out the specified exercises within a closed-circuit metabolism room; he was sufficiently fit to operate at the top end of the charts, and found that the caloric cost (averaged over 11 minutes) increased from 8 to 16 or 17 kcal/min as he moved from Chart 1 to Chart 6. Certainly, if a person has the athletic prowess to reach Chart 6A, he is doing much to improve his cardiorespiratory fitness. The main item responsible for cardiovascular conditioning is obviously the running period, and the man of thirty who reaches chart 4C, running a mile in 7½ minutes (8 mph) is developing a final oxygen consumption of about 46 ml/kg min; the intensity of effort is good, but its duration is rather short.

The 5BX plan was originally developed for the Royal Canadian Air Force, but it has since become available to the general public as a small paperback volume. A substantial number of copies of this publication have been sold; indeed it has probably reached about 5 percent of Canadian homes; however, it is less certain how many of the pamphlets have been read or acted upon. The twisting exercises proposed in charts 4 to 6 seem liable to precipitate spinal injuries, and although there are no formal statistics, I am told by military surgeons that their practices suggest there may be some truth in this assertion.

Weight Training

Weight training has gained great popularity in recent years, particularly among orthopaedic surgeons, who find it a useful means of stabilizing major joints in players of contact sports. The regular use of weights increases the "static" strength over a wide range of joint angles; it also improves muscular endurance, and if the exercise is extended over many months there is a development of muscle bulk. However, there is commonly a discrepancy between gains in muscle strength and the increase of muscle bulk, whether this is assessed clinically (muscle girth) or radiographically (p. 185). It is probable that part of the increase in both strength and endurance reflects a lesser inhibition of the motor neurone pool.

The largest and most rapid gains of strength occur when the muscle is exercised during "overload." A muscle is said to be in the overloaded condition when the initial fibre length is greater than the optimum for subsequent development of tension (Fig. 48). The daily training routine consists of several "sets," each involving two to ten "repetitions" of the lifting effort. Many regimes have been proposed, usually with inadequate experimental justification; there is no strong evidence against the assertion that three "sets" of ten "repetitions" per day is a suitable regime for optimum results.

Although some physical educators have described weight-lifting as "isotonic" exercise, this is technically incorrect; the subject develops an isometric tension equal to the weight to be supported before any movement is commenced, and this tension is further modified to accomodate changes in leverage as the exercise progresses (Fig. 50). The isometric contraction is of sufficient intensity to occlude or partially occlude the local circulation, and the systemic blood pressure thus tends to rise, with adverse effects upon the work of the heart (p. 66). Many weight-lifters also hold their breath with the glottis closed—a form of Valsalva manoeuvre; this produces a large initial increase of systemic blood pressure, a subsequent dramatic fall due to obstruction of venous return, and a second increase of pressure as the expiration is released, and blood again enters the thorax. The Valsalva effect is unpleasant even for a healthy person, and can be dangerous to anyone with cardiac problems. Although fixation of the chest may be essential at certain points in a weight-lifting manoeuvre, in general, the weight lifter should breathe as naturally as possible.

Despite the potential risks of weight-lifting, practical experience is not particularly alarming. Karpovich found only 494 accidents (1.5%) in a group of 31,702 individuals performing various types of weight training; the majority of problems were due to injuries of the back, shoulders, and fingers, and there were only five instances of hernia and one of sudden death. It is of course unlikely that weight training was popular with the coronary prone in 1950 (when the Karpovich study was conducted).

Weight training does relatively little to improve cardiorespiratory fitness; treadmill endurance may increase due to better perfusion of the strengthened muscles, but there is little gain of aerobic power. The explanation lies in the low oxygen cost of weight lifting. A total of perhaps 3000 kg-m of work may be performed in a training session (30 lifts of a 50 kg weight through 2 metres), but if this is spread over an hour in the gymnasium, the average intensity of activity is no more than 50 kg-m/min (compared with 1200 kg-m/min during a hard bicycle ergometer ride). The athlete no doubt appreciates this point, and also undertakes exercise that will improve his cardiorespiratory endurance, but there is a real danger that the layman will feel he has met the requirements of health using the weights. He builds an impressive shoulder musculature (which has little merit apart from its sexual attraction), and he attempts to carry the increased body mass with an inadequate heart and circulation. As noted on page 383, the development of muscles not needed in a specific contest can be a disadvantage even to an athlete. In addition to the increase of muscle weight, there may be a loss of joint flexibility. These factors undoubtedly contribute to the traditional fear of becoming "muscle bound."

Isometric Training

In isometric training, no appreciable external shortening of the muscle occurs; contractions may be made against a rigid external device such as a dynamometer, or the muscles may be tensed against their natural antagonists; this last possibility is of interest to the surgeon, since it offers a possibility of maintaining muscle strength while the limb is immobilized within a plaster cast; if the patient is unwilling to contract the muscles voluntarily, activity may be induced electrically ("faradic stimulation").

> Much of the interest in isometric training was engendered by Müller, a German work physiologist who until recently was director of the Max-Planck Institut in Dortmund. He maintained that large increases of maximum strength could be brought about by as little as one isometric contraction per day. If the contraction was of maximum strength, it needed to be held for only one to two seconds, and if of two thirds maximum strength four to six seconds of activity were needed. The maximum potential training effect could also be attained with more sustained contractions at 40 to 50 percent of maximum strength, but if the intensity was reduced to 20 percent of maximum effort a gradual waning of strength occurred.
>
> Some authors have duplicated Müller's findings, but others have been less successful. Müller has criticized the unsuccessful investigators for using subjects with a low "training potential"; by analogy with cardiorespiratory training, it is reasonable to suppose that the response is greatly influenced by the initial condition of the musculature. On the other hand, there seems a dangerous fallacy in Müller's approach of using a similar device to both produce and measure training. Part of the apparent increase in strength that he has reported could be no more than a learning of technique. In support of this criticism, it has been pointed out that any gains of strength are very specific to a particular movement, executed at a particular angulation of the joint.

Some authors claim that isometric activity is as effective as "isotonic" in the development of muscular endurance, while others claim that "isotonic" activity leads to appreciably greater gains in both endurance and muscle bulk. Part of the difficulty is semantic—it is necessary to distinguish static from dynamic strength, and static from dynamic endurance. If this distinction is drawn, there seems good evidence that "isotonic" activities such as weight-lifting have little effect on static strength or endurance, but give appreciable gains of dynamic strength, and very large increases of dynamic endurance. On the other hand, regular isometric contractions develop isometric strength and isometric endurance, but have little influence upon dynamic strength and dynamic endurance.

If the performance of athletes is compared, distance runners have no greater isometric strength than the average citizen, but they have many times the normal endurance for repetitive "isotonic" work. The athletes with the greatest isometric strength are the sprinters and the throwers; however, the sprinters have a normal "isotonic" endurance, and if the loading is expressed as a percentage of maximum isometric strength, the "isotonic" endurance of the throwers is less than average.

There is little question that the small amount of time apparently needed for isometric training makes this a very attractive regime for the sedentary middle-aged person; it also seems safer than the repeated lifting of heavy weights. However, the physiologist cannot be influenced unduly by convenience. If there is a need to develop the musculature of an older person, much turns upon the type of development that is desired—static strength, or dynamic endurance. This differs from one industry to another, and the exercise prescription must be adjusted accordingly.

The physiological mechanisms involved in any gain of strength or dynamic endurance certainly include a decrease of central inhibition. The intense anaerobic work involved in maximum or near-maximum static contractions may also stimulate the development of alactic power (as in repetitive sprints); however, it would be surprising if a maximum improvement of alactic power could be achieved by one intense contraction per day, as a literal acceptance of Müller's work might suggest.

Eccentric Contraction. Several authors have recently drawn attention to the possibility of training a group of muscles by requiring work to be performed against gravity (eccentric contraction—for instance, lowering weights or running downhill). There is some evidence that this may be a particularly effective training method, and further studies will be awaited with interest.

The Strategy of Training

Type of Training Required by an Athlete

This point has already been discussed somewhat in previous sections. The relative importance of speed, anaerobic "capacity" and aerobic power vary with the duration of the event in which the athlete will compete. A suitable emphasis for runners is illustrated in Fig. 86, and similar graphs can be created for con-

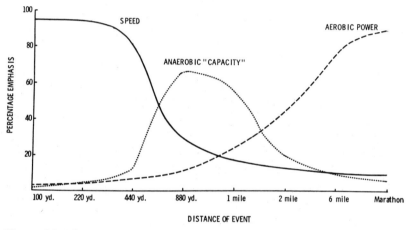

Figure 86. The strategy of training for track events. The relative importance of aerobic power, anaerobic capacity and speed is suggested in relation to distance run.

testants in other types of competition. Repetitive and acceleration sprints develop speed, suitable forms of fast interval work develop anaerobic "capacity," and continuous running or moderate length interval work build up aerobic power.

Plan for a Typical Athletic Season

Let us suppose that the athlete is competing four months in a year. He is allowed a one month holiday in which he enjoys active relaxation, participating in regular endurance-type pastimes such as vigorous swimming; during this time he must prevent a gross deterioration of physical condition and avoid sports that may interfere with his specific acquired skills. When training is resumed, the first three months are spent in the development of aerobic power and strength. Depending on the type of event in which the athlete will compete, there is subsequently an increasing emphasis on the development of speed and anaerobic "capacity." During the competitive season, the quantity of training is adjusted to maintain—and if possible to develop—the physiological status of the athlete, while allowing sufficient rest for optimum performance in competition. Rest is important to the psychological preparation of the athlete. It also allows time for recovery from minor (subclinical) injuries, with the restoration of fluid balance and the replenishment of glycogen stores.

The daily duration of training depends upon the persistence of the individual, but in general is increased as physical condition improves. Except at times of competition, a distance competitor may cover several times his competitive distance, and a speed athlete may make ten to twenty repetitions of his chosen event.

It is uncertain whether there is any physiological basis for the alleged deterioration of performance with *overtraining*. There may be a lack of minerals and glycogen, with a disturbance of fluid balance and a build-up of subclinical injuries. Furthermore, if excessive activity is undertaken to the detriment of necessary rest and recreation, this can become burdensome to the athlete; the diminishing physiological returns upon his investment of time and effort have a negative psychological impact upon competitive performance. The increase of muscle mass at the expense of cardiorespiratory development can be a further hazard for the distance athlete.

Training for the Nonathlete

The typical sedentary person requesting an exercise programme has reached middle-age (40–50 years), is somewhat obese (excess weight 5–10 kg), and may already have had a coronary attack. Specific regimes for the coronary patient are discussed elsewhere (p. 522). The main needs of the sedentary person with no immediate pathology seem a substantial increase of daily caloric expenditure (to help in controlling body weight) with progression to exercise of sufficient intensity to improve cardiorespiratory condition. A preliminary visit to a physician is desirable at this age and a gradual increase in the maximum permitted intensity of activity will avoid minor tendon injuries and the occasional coronary episode that can otherwise have a marked negative influence upon the motivation of an exercise "class."

The development of cardiorespiratory fitness calls for activity that can increase the oxygen consumption to at least 60 percent of aerobic power. Swimming, cycling, stepping, skipping, and running are suitable exercises for this purpose. Formal classes provide a motivational drive and allow closer supervision, but there is then risk of a dangerous competitive spirit between participants. If activities are performed at home, thought should be given to provision of emergency care (for instance, jogging in pairs), and if outdoor activity is contemplated the need for a warm-up should be stressed. A mask that will warm and humidify inspired gas is also quite useful under winter conditions. Brief interval running has the advantage that it stimulates the cardiorespiratory system without accumulation of anaerobic metabolites that could initiate an undesirable rise of systemic blood pressure. Unfortunately, interval training is rather unfamiliar to the usual middle-aged man, and there is a need to test whether such individuals can use this approach successfully.

Some development of muscles in the leg, abdomen, and back may be helpful, although the necessary changes are often brought about by rhythmic activity, without recourse to specific isometric or weight-lifting work. There is no need to induce development of the shoulder and arm muscles unless the nature of the patient's work calls for frequent lifting of heavy objects. An emphasis upon "isometrics" or weight-lifting convinces the patient he is keeping himself fit when he may merely be producing a top-heavy body with a poorly developed heart. Prolapse of intervertebral discs is a common hazard of middle age, and it is prudent to advise against calisthenics that involve vigorous and swift turning movements. Reflexes are also poorer than in a young person, and the bones more brittle; the middle-aged should thus avoid complicated work on gymnastic apparatus, particularly if there is a penalty of bone injury when the necessary skills are lacking. Sports such as golf may be helpful in increasing caloric usage, but it is important that the patient should appreciate their intensity is insufficient to improve cardiac condition. Finally periodic repetition of medical and physiological examination is of value; excessive enthusiasm can be regulated, and if interest is waning, it may be rekindled by a "good" test result. In this context, the dice is loaded in favour of the examining physician. A "good" result is likely even if the patient has not worked too hard, since the response to physiological testing is "improved" by both learning and habituation (p. 219, 444).

The Training Process

The fundamental processes involved in training are poorly understood. The general pattern of adaptation to chronic exercise has many parallels in responses to external stresses. If a man is faced by heat or a low oxygen pressure, then the rate and extent of bodily adjustments depend largely upon his initial condition (including recent and past experience of the stress), and the intensity of environmental change. In the case of heat stress, there even seems some interaction with physical training; the man acclimatized to heat is better able to cope with exercise than one who is not so acclimatized. Presumably, the common factor is a rise of blood temperature, reported by the hypothalamic thermoregulatory centres. Despite such interactions, there are unique features of the bodily response to repeated exercise, and a man cannot be brought to a peak of physical condition by such measures as repeated heat exposure. Many of the training responses are "regulatory"—they involve the establishment of new neuronal circuits within the central nervous system. Examples include habituation and other psychological adjustments to exercise, improvements in the efficiency of movement (conscious and subconscious), the development of new mechanisms of respiratory and circulatory regulation, and the lessening of inhibition at the motor neurone pool. General theories of sensory and motor learning apply, and the processes can be accelerated or slowed by the various techniques familiar to the educator.

The slowly developing structural adaptations—the increase of heart and muscle mass and the expansion of intracellular elements—have perhaps greater interest for the physiologist. Despite much research, the prime stimulus to such development remains uncertain. One of the first possibilities to be investigated was that an intracellular oxygen lack provided a common stimulus to various types of structural adaptation. However, this hypothesis is readily disproved—neither the acute oxygen lack of high altitude exposure nor the life-long oxygen shortage of some forms of congenital heart disease will produce the muscularity of an athlete; again, tissue oxygen lack is more likely in the elderly than in the young, yet it is difficult to improve the structural status of an older person. The influence of age upon training suggests a role for either growth or sex hormones. Testosterone and its derivatives can promote the build up of muscle protein under certain conditions (p. 361), the normal pubertal secretion of these hormones is often adduced to explain the strength spurt of adolescent body (p. 375), and an excessive secretion can lead to Herculean gigantism. On the other hand, there is no evidence that physical activity itself leads to an increased output of sex hormones. There have been suggestions that exercise stimulates the release of anterior pituitary growth hormone; however, it is difficult to accept a fundamental role for this hormone, since training is quite effective in the early forties, at a time when secretion of growth hormone must be less than in the adolescent child. Further, although tumours of the anterior pituitary can lead to an abnormal development of the body musculature, the increase does not necessarily involve the active components of the tissue and there have been reports that work-induced hypertrophy is possible in animals following extirpation of the pituitary gland. Whereas physical activity specifically increases mitochondrial and myofibrillar protein, growth hormone leads to a more uniform increase in all the constituents of a muscle. In other words, growth hormone acts as a "linear amplifier"—it increases anabolic activity throughout the tissue, and there remains some undiscovered trigger, initiated by physical activity, that brings about a selective synthesis of myofibrillar protein.

References

Howell, M.L., and Morford, W.R.: *Fitness Training Methods.* Canadian Association for Health, Physical Education, and Recreation, Toronto, Ont., 1967.

Orban, W.R.: *The Royal Canadian Air Force 5BX Plan,* 2nd ed. Ottawa, Queen's Printer, 1962.

Kasch, F.W., and Boyer, J.L.: *Adult Fitness. Principles and Practices.* Greely, Col., All American Productions and Publications, 1968.

Peebler, J.R.: *Controlled Exercise for Physical Fitness.* Springfield, Thomas, 1962.

Morgan, R.E., and Adamson, G.T.: *Circuit Training.* London, Bell, 1965.

Hettinger, T.: *Physiology of Strength.* Springfield, Thomas, 1961.

Rohmert, W.: *Muskelarbeit und Muskeltraining.* Stuttgart, Gentner Verlag, 1968.

Roskamm, H.: Optimum patterns of exercise for healthy adults. *Canad Med Ass J., 96,* 895–899 (1967).

Massie, J.: Some studies of motivation and attitude in a voluntary training programme. M.Sc Thesis, University of Toronto, 1970.

Klein, K.K.: *The Knee in Sports.* Austin, Pemberton Press, 1969.

Wilt, F.: Training for competitive running. In Falls, H. (Ed.): *Exercise Physiology.* New York, Academic Press, 1968.

16

ACTIVITY AND METABOLISM

The Need for Fuel

Throughout this volume, we have considered the body as an active machine. Like machinery invented by the human brain, the body requires a continuous supply of fuel in order to function properly. This fuel provides energy to meet the needs not only of overt activity, but also of resting metabolism and growth.

Resting Metabolism

The concept of a "basal" state has already been discussed (p. 9). Whether observations are made at rest or under truly basal conditions, the body consumes energy to meet the minimum metabolic requirements of the various tissues (p. 49), and to maintain their integrity. Work is performed in such tasks as pumping air into the chest, pumping blood around the circulation, and transporting materials across cell membranes in opposition to established concentration gradients. Apparently permanent molecules such as tissue proteins are continually being broken down and resynthesized, and since the cycle of breakdown and resynthesis is not 100 percent efficient, energy is needed to maintain a protein pool of constant size. Lastly, heat is lost from the body in most environments, and this loss must be made good if the desired homiothermic condition is to be preserved.

Body Size. The resting energy requirement inevitably varies with body size. The needs of the tissues are almost directly proportional to body weight, but heat loss is more closely related to the individual's surface area. DuBois showed many years ago that a man's surface area could be approximated by the formula

$$B S A = W^{0.425} \times H^{0.725} \times 71.84 \times 10^{-4}$$

where BSA is the surface area (in m^2), W is the unclothed weight in kg, and H is the standing height in cm. Nomograms are available for making this calculation (Fig. 87.), or alternatively it can be programmed for a small computer. The DuBois formula works well for people of average build, and the results are adequate for many purposes; however, the specialist now prefers improved nomograms, particularly when dealing with individuals of extreme body types.

Because of the preponderant effect of heat loss upon resting metabolism, the energy requirement of a resting man is a power function of his body weight ($W^{0.75}$).

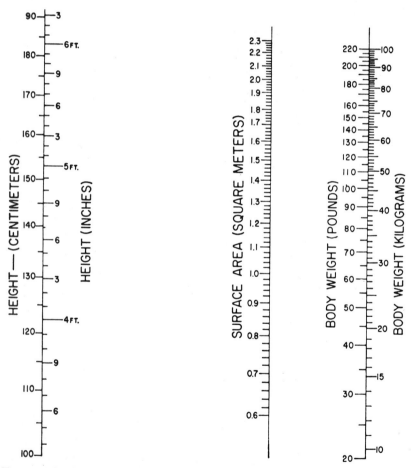

Figure 87. The relationship of body surface area to height and weight. Nomogram devised by DuBois, and based upon the formula

$$BSA = W^{0.425} \times H^{0.725} \times 10^{-4}$$

(By permission of Lea & Febiger, Philadelphia.)

Age. It is well recognized that the activity of the body as a whole is slowed with ageing. The same seems true of individual cells. Thus, the life of the human red cell is approximately one hundred days, but the metabolism of freshly drawn blood is much greater than that which has been stored for perhaps half of its life span. In addition to cellular ageing, active tissue such as muscle is replaced by metabolically less active fat* and connective tissue fibres. The basal metabolic activity thus falls from about 0.83 kcal/min/m² at the age of ten to 0.67 kcal/min/m² in a young adult man, and 0.61 kcal/min/m² in a man aged sixty-five.

Sex. The basal energy expenditure is lower in women than in men, probably because of the greater proportion of insulating and metabolically inactive fat within the female body. Corresponding figures are 0.63 kcal/min/m² for a young woman, and 0.57 kcal/min/m² in a woman aged sixty-five.

Temperature. The metabolic activity of individual cells tends to increase with a rise of temperature, according to the "Law" of Arrhenius (p. 49). On the other hand, the energy requirements of the body as a whole are stimulated by a decrease of environmental temperature.

Early effects of cold include an increase of incidental activity and frank shivering, while with more prolonged exposure there is the possibility that endocrine adjustments may stimulate tissue metabolism.

Endocrine Glands. Pathological conditions of the thyroid gland —involving excessive secretion (thyrotoxicosis) or a deficiency of thyroid hormone (myxoedema) lead to corresponding alterations in basal energy expenditure. The hormone thyroxine stimulates both protein synthesis and the peripheral utilization of glucose, at the same time enhancing the breakdown of glycogen stores in liver and muscle.

Individual Variation. As with any physiological variable, there is a considerable range of normality. A true basal state is hard to attain, and no great significance can be attached to a 20 percent departure of basal metabolism from the anticipated value for age, sex, and body size.

The resting energy requirement is even more variable, since individuals differ markedly in the relaxation that they achieve while nominally sitting at rest.

---

* The metabolic activity of adipose tissue depends upon the method of calculation. If inert fat is excluded, and data is expressed relative to the protein content of the tissue, then fat is seen to have quite a high rate of metabolism.

Growth

Energy is required for the growth of new body tissue in infants, children, and pregnant women; the precise caloric need can be calculated from the energy equivalent of the tissues that are synthesized (see below). Lactating women also require additional feeding; their added caloric needs are equivalent to the energy content of the milk that is produced.

Physical Activity

Techniques for the measurement of physical activity have been considered in a previous chapter (pp. 20, 28). The most reliable method of assessing the energy needed for performance of any given task is to determine the corresponding oxygen cost. Complications introduced by anaerobic work are usually neglected, and a fixed relationship between oxygen consumption and energy expenditure is assumed (1 litre/min STPD = 5 kcal/min); in fact, the energy equivalent of oxygen varies from 4.7 to 5.1 kcal per litre according to the type of fuel that is burnt, but it is difficult to estimate the relative usage of fat and carbohydrate during exercise. Many authors have classified the intensity of activity in terms of the gross energy expenditure required. Understandably, rather different ratings of intensity have been made by nutritionists (who think of a 24-hour-day), industrial physicians (who anticipate 6–8 hours of activity) and sports physicians (who are often interested in very brief periods of intense effort). Table XX is indeed a commentary upon the difficulty of interdisciplinary communication. Fortunately, it is not necessary to reconcile

TABLE XX
RATING OF ACTIVITY IN TERMS OF ENERGY EXPENDITURE

Rating of Activity	Level of Energy Expenditure (kcal/min)		
	Nutritionists (Orr & Leitch)	Industrial Physicians (Brown)	Sports Physicians
Sedentary	1.25	2.0	2
Light	—	2.0–3.3	2–5
Moderate	1.25–2.50	3.3–5.4	5–10
Heavy	2.5 –5.0	5.4–9.0	10–15
Very Heavy	5.0	9.0	>15.0

these divergent viewpoints, since the whole concept of fixed caloric ranges is questionable, particularly with respect to industry and sport. A young and athletic man with an aerobic power of 6 litre/min STPD will find a task of 5 kcal/min quite light work, but the same activity will present an intolerable load to an elderly lady with a maximum oxygen consumption of 1 litre/min. It is preferable to express the intensity of effort as a percentage of the individual's aerobic power; the tolerated percentage then depends largely upon the duration of the intended effort, decreasing in a semilogarithmic fashion as the working period is extended. Bonjer's subjects withstood 62 percent for one hour, 51 percent for two hours, and 33 percent for eight hours. Other factors that further limit effort tolerance include superimposed bursts of high intensity activity, a hot and humid environment, and an awkward working posture.

Typical energy requirements for various industrial, domestic and sporting activities are summarized in Tables XXI and XXII. If the performance of individual adults is compared, we find

TABLE XXI
THE GROSS ENERGY COST OF VARIOUS INDUSTRIAL
AND DOMESTIC ACTIVITIES

	1.25 kcal/min	1.25–2.5 kcal/min	2.5–5 kcal/min	>5 kcal/min
General*	Sleeping Sitting	Standing Walking	Fast walking Playing with children	Running Stair-climbing
		Washing	Dressing	Playing with children
M le ccupations	Office worker Tailor Printer	Shop assistant Painter Carpenter	Rivetter Painter Carpenter	Miner Lumberjack Construction labourer
		Light metal worker Shoemaker	Sheet metal worker Blacksmith	Steel worker Machine fitter Mason Small farmer Postman
Female Occupations	Writer Typist Sewing Knitting Ironing Dishwashing	Sweeping Dusting Washing	Polishing Scrubbing Laundering	

* Values are slightly higher for men than for women.

TABLE XXII
THE GROSS ENERGY COST OF VARIOUS SPORTING ACTIVITIES
(kcal/min)*

Archery	3–6	Dancing	4–8	Table tennis	4–5
Athletics	Up to 20	English football (soccer) 5–12		Tennis	6–9
Badminton	6	Field hockey 9		Volleyball	3–4
Basketball	9	Gardening 3–5			
Billiards	3	Golf (no cart) 5			
Bowls (lawn)	4	Gymnastics 3–12			
Boxing	9–14	Horse-riding 3–10			
Canoeing	3–7	Rowing 4–11			
Climbing (mountain)	7–10	Skiing (cross country) 10–19			
Cricket	5–8	(downhill) up to 10			
Cross-country running	10–11	Squash racquets 10–18			
Cycling	4–20	Swimming 5–15			

* The figures are based on data collected by Durnin and Passmore, and presented in *Energy, Work and Leisure*, Heinemann, 1967. They refer mainly to small numbers of male subjects. No account has been taken of rest pauses.

that the energy cost of a given task E varies as a power function of body weight W, according to an equation of the type

$$E = a + b (W)^n$$

where a is the resting energy expenditure, b is a constant, and n has a value between 0.75 and 1.0. A large part of the interindividual variation is related to the work performed in raising and lowering the centre of gravity of the body; the influence of weight upon energy cost is thus greatest for tasks that involve substantial movement of the centre of gravity of the body.

Children and young adults perform many tasks with unnecessary exuberance, and the metabolic cost of a given activity thus diminishes with age. It is also lower in a female than in a male of the same weight. Cold weather tends to promote exuberant movements; in these circumstances, energy expenditure is further increased by the weight of clothing and (in outside work) by snow-covered surfaces. However, environmental temperature has little influence upon the efficiency of the muscles *per se*, and in laboratory studies, the oxygen cost of effort in cold and hot rooms is remarkably similar.

Industrial and Domestic Activity. Many of the data for industrial and domestic activity (Table XXI) are now hallowed by a certain antiquity. It is hard to find either a blacksmith or a woman who habitually scrubs floors by hand. Even figures for occupations that are still popular must be viewed with caution, since energy requirements have fallen progressively with the introduction of improved tools and packaging and the tuition of more economical working techniques. Simple changes like an alteration in the tyre size or handle-length of a wheelbarrow, improved maintenance of saws, the use of smooth rather than jerky limb movements, the optimization of bench heights and the carriage of loads close to the body have all reduced the effort required of most labourers. Successes of the work-study teams (ergonomists) have been supplemented by automation of many important industrial processes. Some of the figures quoted in the world literature thus have little relevance to our present generation; even traditional "heavy" industries such as mining, farming and lumber work often require an average energy expenditure of less than 5 kcal/min, and there are few remaining occupations that call for more than three times the resting energy expenditure. Self-pacing has become much less frequent. If a labourer chooses his own rate of work, he tends to operate at about 40 percent of his aerobic power; a man of outstanding physique thus adopts an above average rate of working, with shorter rest pauses. However, society is increasingly regulating the rate of production by both conveyor-belts and trade unions; inevitably, the standard output required then falls within the compass of a man having less than average fitness.

Sports Activity. The metabolic intensity of sports activity has varied less dramatically than the cost of industrial work. Nevertheless, the passage of time has been accompanied by alterations in rules, the development of better but heavier protective equipment, and the introduction of new techniques of play. All of these changes challenge the current accuracy of previously reported caloric costs. Perhaps the most extreme example is the use of an air-conditioned motor-driven cart when crossing a golf course. Cycling is a second area of change; most published information refers to the use of narrow 26-inch wheel racing machines, whereas current users are purchasing much smaller wheeled cycles with broad tyres. New sports are also gaining popularity with the increased affluence of the community; water skiing and human kite flying are two pertinent examples in North America.

Even if equipment and rules are held constant, the energy expenditure may differ markedly from one individual to another of similar body weight. Skill is an important variable, and with training the energy expenditure for a given rate of play can fall substantially. A further controlling factor is the intensity of competition offered by an opponent; the energy cost of many games can vary from 5 to 15 kcal/min according to the vigour and enthusiasm of the contestants.

The total caloric requirements of a competitive athlete can be surprisingly large. An active skier or football player may have a regular daily usage of 6000 kcal, and expenditures of up to 12,000 kcal per day have been reported in some marathon cycling contests.

The Sources of Fuel

Energy Equivalent of Foodstuffs

The energy liberated by combustion of pure food products may be recapitulated as follows:

Fat	9.3 kcal/g
Alcohol	7.0 kcal/g
Protein	4.1 kcal/g
Carbohydrate	3.8 kcal/g

Thus, if the composition of a given food is determined in terms of these constituents, the calorie yield may be specified (Table XXIII). Foods such as butter have a high fat content and a relatively low water content; they thus have a high caloric density. On the other hand, carbohydrate rich foods— such as vegetables—have a high water content and a low caloric density. Protein foods in this respect occupy an intermediate position between fats and carbohydrates.

In the past, attempts have been made to assess food intake by inventories and retrospective questionnaires. However, the information thus obtained has been so inaccurate as to be of

TABLE XXIII

THE CALORIC EQUIVALENT OF CERTAIN COMMON FOODSTUFFS,
COOKED WHERE APPROPRIATE (kcal)

1 apple	75	1 egg	75	3 oz pork	285
serving apple pie	330	¼ cup flour	100	10 potato chips	110
2 slices bacon	95	1 tbs. French dressing	60	1 med potato	120
1 banana	90	½ grapefruit	40	serving pumpkin pie	265
1 cup lima beans	150	1 fillet haddock	160	1 cup rhubarb + sugar	385
1 cup pork beans	295	½ cup ice cream	165	1 cup rice (converted)	205
3 oz beef	278	1 tbs jam	55	3 oz salmon	120
1 cup beets	70	3 oz lamb	230	3 oz sardines	180
1 tea biscuit	130	1 tbs lard	125	4 oz sausage (pork)	340
		2 large lettuce leaves	5		
1 slice bread	65	serving lem. meringue	300	3 oz. shrimp	110
1 cup broccoli	45	2 oz liver	120	1 cup spaghetti	220
1 tbs. butter	100	1 cup macaroni/cheese	450	1 cup spinach	45
1 cup cabbage	40	1 tbs margarine	100	1 cup summer squash	35
1 slice angel food	110	1 cup whole milk	165	1 cup strawberries	55
1 slice choc cake	370	skimmed milk	85	1 tbs sugar	50
1 cup carrots	45	1 cup mushrooms	30	1 cup tomato juice	50
1 cup cauliflower	30	1 cup noodles	105	1 tomato	45
1 cup celery	20	1 cup oatmeal	150	3 oz tuna	170
1 oz cheddar cheese	115	1 tbs salad oil	125	1 cup turnips	45
1 oz cottage cheese	25	1 orange	70	3 oz veal	185
1 cup chicken soup	75	1 cup orange juice	110	½ slice watermelon	45
1 cup chocolate	140	1 pancake	60	1 cup white sauce	430
1 cup cocoa	235	1 cup parsnips	95	1 cup wheat flour	400
1 oz codfish	105	1 peach	45		
clear coffee	0	1 tinned peach	79		
1 cup cornflakes	95	1 pear	95		
1 ear corn	85	1 cup tinned peas	140		
1 tbs. whipped cream	50	1 cup tinned pineapple	95		
1 doughnut	135	1 plum	30		

little value. The current approach of a dietetic research team is to live with a family for a period, and to observe the actual food consumption of the individual householders. The food cooked may be assessed by weighing, or (a little less accurately) in terms of portions, and after due allowance for wastage, the results may be converted to kilocalories, using a schema such as that in Table XXIII; the data thus obtained is accurate to about 15 percent.

Calorie tables are eagerly studied by a large number of women who wish to reduce their weight. Weight loss is inevitable, irrespective of diet, if energy expenditure exceeds caloric intake. Lettuce and fruit diets seem attractive in that bulk is achieved with a low total caloric intake; their main disadvantage is that the bulky cellulose component gives a temporary feeling of gastric fullness, but also speeds the emptying of the stomach, leading to a need for further fortification within two or three hours. It is obviously prudent to avoid sugary items such as iced cake and fruit syrups; these not only have a large caloric yield, but are also highly palatable, encouraging overeating. Several artificial sweeting agents such as saccharin and the cyclamates have fallen under medical suspicion, and should at present be avoided. The current tendency of obesity clinics is to recommend to those who can afford it a high meat intake; it is much more difficult to eat an excess of fat and protein than an excess of sugar. Slower emptying of a protein-filled stomach also enables the patient to extend the interval between meals, cutting out the carbohydrate "snacks" which probably led to his or her initial downfall.

Interrelation of Fuels

Diet varies widely with ethnic, geographic and economic factors. In general, protein is expensive, and carbohydrate is cheap. Some groups, such as hunting Eskimoes, have an unusually high intake of fat. In the affluent metropolitan centres of North America, a typical middle-class citizen derives 12 percent to 15 percent of his food* calories from protein, 35 to 40 percent from fat, and 45 to 55 percent from carbohydrate. However, the body is very adaptable, and can readily substitute one source of fuel for another (Figs. 88 and 89). Carbohydrate, fat and protein can all serve as energy sources, and if taken in excess all can contribute to fat storage. If a suitable source of nitrogen is available, the majority of the

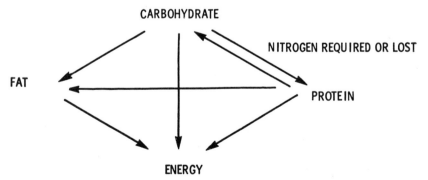

Figure 88. Interrelationships of food supply and energy production. The more detailed biochemical basis of this diagram is given in Fig. 89. Note particularly that fat cannot be converted to carbohydrate or protein.

* In many instances, alcohol provides 15 to 30 percent of calorie requirements.

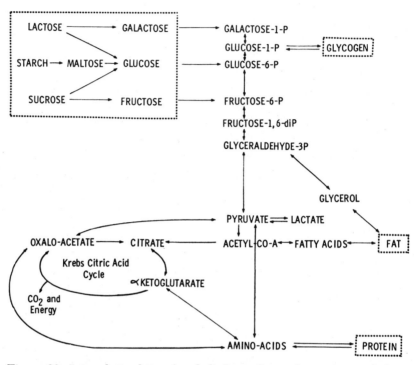

Figure 89. Interrelationships of carbohydrate, fat, and protein metabolism. Note that carbohydrate and nonessential amino-acids are interconvertible, but that because of the point of entry of fat into the Krebs cycle (Acetyl-Co-A/Citrate stage), fat cannot be converted to carbohydrate or protein.

amino-acid constituents of protein can be synthesized from carbohydrate. However, certain amino acids cannot be formed in this way, and they must be included in any diet in sufficient amounts to meet the requirements of tissue formation and maintenance; these "essential" amino acids include valine, leucine, isoleucine, threonine, methionine, phenylalanine, tryptophan, lysine, and (in growing children) histidine and arginine. Fat cannot give rise to carbohydrate, and since the tissues of the central nervous system are unable to metabolize fat, there is an inevitable minimum breakdown of protein if the body is starved of carbohydrate. A certain minimum intake of carbohydrate is also desirable to prevent "ketosis"; when the necessary carbohydrate is lacking, fat tends to be converted to ketone bodies (aceto-acetic acid, β hydroxybutyric acid, and acetone) instead of burning completely to CO_2 and water. Some authors have also postulated a need for small quantities of "essential" fatty acids. These are of the polyunsaturated variety (p. 491), and are thought to play a role in the synthesis of physiologically active prostaglandins.

The Normal Fuel for Activity

Hultman and other Scandinavian workers have used the technique of muscle biopsy (p. 424) to clarify the metabolic needs of active muscle.

Energy is derived from both carbohydrate and fat, but in the well-nourished individual there is no significant contribution from protein. Even in prolonged exercise such as the cross-country skiing marathons of Scandinavia, there is no increase of nitrogen excretion, as would be anticipated with enhanced protein breakdown.

The relative usage of carbohydrate and fat varies with the intensity and duration of effort, and the nature of the immediately preceding diet. If the workload is more than 75 percent of the individual's aerobic power, at least three quarters of the energy usage is derived from carbohydrates. The sugar content of the blood is no more than 6gm (24 kcal), and this is insufficient to sustain vigorous exercise for longer than one to two min. The transfer of glucose from the liver to the skeletal muscles is enhanced by effort, reaching a maximum rate of about 1 gm/min (4 kcal/min). The main nutritional determinant of intense and sustained rhythmic work and the sole nutritional determinant of anaerobic isometric work is the size of the muscle glycogen store; if completely exhausted by aerobic mechanisms, muscle glycogen would provide 1600 kcal of energy (equivalent to 60–90 minutes of intense activity). The glycogen stores can be increased by suitable diet (see below). While this manoeuvre makes little difference to the initial performance of an athlete, the contestant with a large glycogen store is able to sustain his rate of energy output after an hour or more, at the time when his competitors are flagging in their efforts.

At exhaustion, the glycogen content of the active muscles may be reduced from the normal value of 1.5 gm/100 gm to as little as 0.1 gm/100 gm, and if a final sprint is made at this stage, the terminal lactate concentration may be only 50 mg/100 ml of blood, compared with the figure of 120–150 mg/100 ml common in maximum effort of brief duration. The active muscles persist in their attempts to metabolize sugar when other sources of carbohydrate have gone. Initially, the breakdown products of glycolysis inhibit the enzyme hexokinase and thus temper the greed of the cells for glucose; however, this regulating device fails as glycogen stores are depleted. There is also some diminution of insulin secretion during sustained exercise, but at exhaustion, the blood sugar is low. The central nervous system depends on blood sugar for its metabolism, and it is thus possible that central exhaustion rather than peripheral depletion of glycogen may be responsible for the final weakness of a contestant. Certainly, performance can be dramatically restored if an athlete is given a small dose of sugar or glucose at this stage; some workers advocate 200 gm at hourly intervals, but in view of the normal physiological usage of glucose ($\sim$1gm/min), there is probably little advantage in exceeding 100 gm/hour.

Training and a high fat diet both increase the relative usage of fat at a given intensity of effort. This is generally helpful to the athlete, since glycogen stores can then be used over a longer period of activity. Some of the fat is derived from active cells, but there is also an increased uptake from the blood. Thus at the commencement of exercise, the plasma free fatty acid concentration falls. If the effort is sustained, there is a later rise of plasma FFA concentration due to enhanced mobilization of fat from adipose tissue. Immediate responses to exercise must therefore be distinguished carefully from any more permanent changes of serum lipids induced by increased activity (p. 499). The stimuli to release of depot fat include the secretion of hormones (adrenaline, noradrenaline, and growth hormone) and a fall of blood sugar. Release is inhibited by high plasma concentrations of insulin, glucose, or lactate. Recent experiments suggest that carnitine, a well-recognized betaine found in muscle extracts, is an essential cofactor for the intracellular metabolism of fat; however, there is no reason to suppose a deficiency of this factor in anyone receiving a normal protein diet, and there is no evidence that carnitine plays any specific role in the greater fat usage of the trained athlete.

The Optimum Fuel

The interconvertibility of the various foodstuffs is such that whether the patient is an athlete or a sedentary worker, little other than psychological advantage is gained by departure from an ordinary well-balanced diet. Such a diet is adequate to provide essential amino-acids, to avoid ketosis, and to supply any essential fatty acids that may be needed.

Supplies of mineral elements (particularly iron and calcium) and vitamins such as A and thiamine rise in almost direct proportion to the total caloric intake. Thus, although it can be argued that athletes need above average quantities of both minerals and vitamins, most workers accept the fact that their requirements are met automatically as the food intake is increased. Nevertheless, there are occasional reports such as a recent Australian study which noted a low intake of thiamine in Olympic athletes who performed poorly. Some athletes have a low serum iron concentration, but this is hardly justification for iron therapy unless the haemoglobin level is also reduced. Indeed, problems of anaemia, dental caries, osteoporosis, and vitamin deficiencies are more likely in sedentary members of the population, because their total caloric intake is low; such deficiencies are a particular hazard to the sedentary alcoholic, and some nutritionists have advocated the fortification of alcoholic beverages with minerals and vitamins.

The glycogen content of the muscles can be increased if a high carbohydrate diet is taken for a few days prior to an important athletic contest; however, a nice judgment must be used, since if the tissues become accustomed to using carbohydrate rather than fat, the tolerance for prolonged work may be diminished rather than enhanced. The optimum regime seems a bout of vigorous exercise several days before a contest, a short period on a protein/fat diet, and then when the muscle cells have developed a maximum hunger for glycogen one or two days of a high carbohydrate diet.

A heavy meal should be avoided for several hours prior to competition, since digestive activity diverts blood from the muscles to the gut. The optimum arrangement seems a light and not too sugary meal between two and three hours before

an event. If the exercise is prolonged, the ability to maintain
a high power output is enhanced by regular (hourly) doses of
a dilute sucrose or glucose solution; although subjectively, some
athletes prefer quite high concentrations (up to 40% glucose),
these are unphysiological and delay gastric emptying. Water,
sodium and potassium losses should also be made good, particularly in a hot climate (p. 316).

An Excess of Fuel

Causes of Obesity

If foods are eaten in excess of energy requirements, then
storage occurs. Liver and muscle can accumulate small quantities of glycogen (to a maximum of about 100 and 400 gm
respectively) but the main site of energy storage is the adipose
tissue. This consists of 86 percent fat, 12 percent water and
2 percent protein. In obesity, there is a marked increase not
only in fat, but also in the protein component; hyperplasia of
the adipose cells has occurred, and this contributes to difficulty
in subsequent dieting.

> Fat has several virtues as a storehouse of energy. It is stable, and
> fits readily into body spaces, protecting and insulating the tissues.
> It is also easily mobilized, with a large energy yield (7 kcal/gm).
> Carbohydrates, in contrast, store a substantial weight of oxygen
> (which the body could have derived from the atmosphere), and
> because of associated water molecules some carbohydrates such
> as glycogen have an effective energy yield of no more than 1 kcal/
> gm.

The excess food consumption of an obese person is often
small; indeed he may complain that he eats less than his slimmer colleagues. Typically, the accumulation of 10 kg of fat
occurs at a rate of no more than 1 kg per year. Since the energy
equivalent of fatty tissue is 7 kcal per gm, the excess food consumption is no more than 7000 kcal per year—an overeating of
less than 1 percent. Obesity often runs in families, but it is not
clear how far this reflects the influence of constitution, and how
far it is due to the poor eating and activity patterns current in
certain households. Once an individual has become fat, he

certainly tends to restrict physical activity, and the insulating layer of fat also reduces heat loss from the body; thus at this stage, food needs may be genuinely less than those of a slimmer person. Recent film studies show that obese subjects have a low level of activity, both at work and during recreation.

Hypothalamic centres regulate the balance between food intake and activity; suggested mechanisms for the feedback of information to the hypothalmus include food sensors in the gastrointestinal tract, receptors that report on the availability of glucose to the cells (i.e. combined information on blood glucose and insulin levels), sensors of body temperature, and possibly some as yet unexplained long-term control from body fat depots. Mayer suggests that the various regulating mechanisms are very successful in maintaining a constant body weight over a wide range of activity, but that a failure of regulation occurs during either extreme inactivity or exercise to exhaustion (Fig. 90). Unfortunately, many obese patients appear to operate in the zone of extreme inactivity, outside the competence of the regulator. Psychological factors may play a role in the failure of regulation. Obese people tend to be "habit" eaters, consuming all that is readily available; leaner individuals on the other hand,

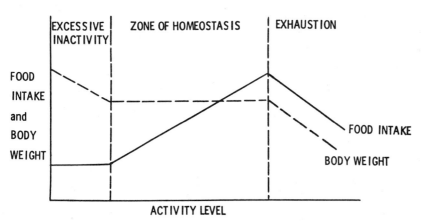

Figure 90. Illustration of the relationship between physical activity and food intake. Over a wide range of activity, body weight is held remarkably constant, but in extreme inactivity, the weight rises, while if exercise is pursued to exhaustion it is no longer possible to maintain body weight. Based on studies of Mayer.

are more readily influenced by their level of satiety, and by past and anticipated activity. The replacement of a cigarette habit by a food habit is a common finding among patients attending smoking withdrawal centres. A weight gain of 5 to 10 kg may occur in the first year that smoking is stopped—a specific illustration of the importance of the psyche in regulating food intake. A further factor influencing the completeness of the body's control over its food supply is excretion. Not all of the ingested calories are retained within the body; a variable loss of complex organic molecules occurs in the faeces, and (as urea and ketone bodies) in the urine. On a high fat diet, 18 percent of ingested calories are lost to the body, but on the high carbohydrate diet enjoyed by many obese persons this loss drops to 6 percent. Gastrointestinal hurry and secretion of hormones favouring fat metabolism may thus be factors that keep down the weight of a slim person.

Excess Weight

Obesity is essentially an excess of fat or adipose tissue. However, it is commonly assessed in terms of overall excess weight (p. 433). This is relatively satisfactory for population studies., but provides limited information on the status of the individual. Keys has documented three very different types of weight gain as follows:

Cause of Weight Gain	Composition of Weight Gain		
	Fat	Cells	Extracellular Fluid
Gluttony	66%	20%	14%
Gluttony + indolence	109%	−20%	11%
Physical activity	−38%	120%	18%

If a patient has an excessive weight relative to the ideal figures (Table XV), this may reflect development of cells (muscle) or fat. Nevertheless, in a statistical sense excess weight is associated with an increased risk of death from a number of diseases, particularly cardiac and cerebral vascular conditions, diabetes, and abnormalities of the digestive system (Table XXIV). If a man of forty-five is of average weight for his age, he will live 1½ years less than if he is of the ideal

TABLE XXIV

THE INFLUENCE OF OBESITY UPON MORTALITY. DEATH RATES OF
GROSSLY OBESE* MEN AND WOMEN AGED 15–69, EXPRESSED AS A
PERCENTAGE OF STANDARD VALUES.
Based on data of Build and Blood Pressure Study (Society of Actuaries, 1959).

Condition	Men	Women
Diabetes	629	250
Vascular Diseases of Brain	215	210
Heart and Circulation	185	217
Pneumonia and Influenza	242	—
Digestive Diseases	298	225
Kidney Diseases	298	—
Accidents and Homicides	120	—
Suicides	142	—
All Conditions	168	178

* Grossly obese subjects drawn from category F of Society, with exception of diabetes in women, where in the absence of this information the average of values for categories D and E has been taken.

weight, and if he is 20 percent above average weight, he will shorten his life expectancy by a further 2½ years. Furthermore, if an obese patient is persuaded to reduce his weight, then his risk of death returns towards the ideal value. Unfortunately, the average Western man tends to exceed the ideal weight as he ages. However, the adverse trend is not inevitable; in fact, it is rare among active primitive peoples.

Other Methods of Assessing Obesity

The fact that a given individual has an excessive weight is of limited significance unless it can be shown how much of the increased weight is due to fat. The appearance of the patient provides a simple subjective guide, but inevitably decisions made on this basis differ markedly from one examiner to another. Anthropometric measures used in somatotyping may also provide some guidance; for instance, muscle leads to an increase in breadth of the chest and the proximal parts of the limbs, while fat tends to increase abdominal dimensions. Authors such as Sheldon have devoted much time to the description of body types, and refer to *ectomorphs* (long-boned, with little fat and poor muscular development), *mesomorphs* (powerful, thick-set and muscular), and *endomorphs* (round and obese). We are all able to recognise extreme members of these three categories, but unfortunately as many as 70 percent of most populations fall into the "grey" area where characteristics of two if not three body types are present.

The measurement of skinfold thickness is simple and can be quite informative; the objective is to determine the thickness of a double layer of skin and fat, excluding underlying muscle. The fold is formed parallel to the natural skin creases and it is supported between the forefinger and the thumb while it is measured by a standard caliper; this should exert a pressure of 10 gm/mm^2 over an area of 35 mm^2. Unfortunately, the readings obtained by this technique can differ by 25 percent from one observer to another, and a calibration of staff is essential to meaningful results. Some authors measure as many as eight folds, but most of the necessary information can be derived from three sites (triceps, subscapular and suprailiac). Typical normal values are given in Table XVI. A number of formulae are now available to convert such readings to estimates of percentage body fat; however, such mathematical manipulations give an unwarranted sophistication to the data.

A more complex but more satisfactory approach is to determine body density by underwater weighing. If the subject's weight in air is W_A and his weight underwater is W_W, then his external volume V_E can be determined from the weight of displaced water ($W_A - W_W$) and its density at the temperature of submersion. Weighings are carried out following a forced expiration, and the residual volume of gas within the lungs V_R is determined by helium dilution (p. 119). If care has been taken to expel trapped air from the bathing suit and hair, the body density D is given by:

$$D = \frac{W_A}{V_E - V_R}$$

A typical density reading for a young adult falls in the range 1.05–1.06. The body fat content is estimated from this overall density on the assumption that there are two main body compartments—lean tissue (density 1.1) and fat (density 0.9). Active young men and women have respectively some 10 percent and 20 percent body fat. However, in middle-aged North American society fat percentages of 25 percent for men and 45 percent for women are by no means uncommon.

Adults do not normally object to the ritual of a hydrostatic weighing, but infants and young children are less willing to submit to complete submersion while strapped to a chair. In pediatric studies, the external volume V_E can be estimated from the displacement of air within a closed chamber. The fat content of the body can also be determined from its capacity to absorb a tracer substance that is selectively soluble in adipose tissue. Interest is currently focussed on inert gases such as krypton, but details of methodology have yet to be perfected.

Alternatively, it is possible to estimate the lean body mass, and to calculate the mass of fat by difference (Fat = total mass minus lean body mass). Some authors use a whole body counter to determine the body content of the natural isotope K^{40}. Since potassium is located primarily in muscle, the lean body mass can be estimated from this figure. Others study the fluid compartments of the body. By the use of suitable markers such as deuterium or tritium, the intra- and extracellular components of the total body water can be calculated, and after making certain assumptions about the relationship of water to body compartments, the lean body mass can be predicted.

Lastly, some workers examine the urinary excretion of creatinine. The excretion rate (Cr) is primarily related to muscle mass, although it can also be influenced by creatine intake and hormonal changes. The ratio of Cr to height (H) and weight (W) is sometimes used to describe population characteristics: Cr/H reflects the muscle mass per unit height, or muscularity, while Cr/W reflects the proportion of the total body weight that is muscle, and hence is an index of obesity.

A Shortage of Fuel

Minimum Caloric Need

If the food consumption is inadequate, activity must be reduced or the body tissues will be used to meet energy requirements. The output of manual workers with a limited diet (for example, men living in prison camps or underdeveloped countries) bears a close relationship to the available food supplies. However, even if the work is entirely sedentary, the caloric expenditure cannot be reduced below about 2500 kcal in the case of men, and 2100 kcal in the case of women. When world food requirements were calculated, the Food and Agriculture Organization of the United Nations set a caloric intake of 3200 kcal for their "reference man," and 2300 kcal for their "reference woman" (Table XXV). United States nutritionists work on somewhat lower figures (2900 kcal for men and 2100 kcal for women); however, it is debatable whether the average level of activity in the United States has fallen below the minimum needed for complete health; if this proves to be the case, the nutritionists should press for a combination of more calories and more activity. The requirement of any given population naturally depends upon its age, since both activity and energy needed for tissue maintenance decrease with ageing.

TABLE XXV
THE ENERGY EXPENDITURE OF A REFERENCE MAN (AGED 25
YEARS, WEIGHT 65 KG) AND OF A REFERENCE WOMAN
(AGED 25 YEARS, WEIGHT 55 KG) AT A MEAN
ENVIRONMENTAL TEMPERATURE OF 10°C*

Activity	Reference Man			Reference Woman		
	Duration (Hours)	Cost (kcal/min)	Total per Day (kcal)	Duration (Hours)	Cost (kcal/min)	Total per Day (kcal)
Work	8	2.5	1200	8	1.83	880
Washing & Dressing	1	3.0	180	1	2.5	150
Walking	1½	5.3	480	1	3.6	220
Sitting	4	1.54	370	5	1.41	420
Recreation & Domestic Work	1½	5.2	470	1	3.5	210
Bed Rest	8	1.04	500	8	0.875	420

* Data of Food and Agricultural Organization of the United Nations, F.A.O. Nutritional Studies No. 15.

Composition of Weight Loss

The changes in body composition during a period of weight loss depend upon the initial status of the individual and the level of activity that is maintained while dieting. Keys* has summarized the problem as follows:

Method of Weight Loss	Composition of Weight Change		
	Fat	Cells	Extracellular Fluid
Obese—Dieting Alone	75%	10%	15%
Obese—Dieting Plus Exercise	98	−10	12
Thin—Starvation	50	50	0
Late Starvation	30	90	−20
Terminal Starvation ("Wet")	10	40	−150
Terminal Starvation ("Dry")	2	18	80

Deliberate Dieting

In the early stages of dieting there may be a substantial water loss. The body stores of glycogen (some 500 gm) are mobilized, and since some 3 gm of water is stored with each gram of glycogen, the body weight inevitably drops by 1.5 kg; This fact is exploited vigorously by manufacturers of proprietary foods. The early water loss is made good as the body stabilizes at a new weight and the stores of glycogen are replenished.

* Data from *Human Starvation*. University of Minnesota Press, 1950.

Loss of protein is difficult to avoid with even a small reduction in the caloric intake of an inactive person. However, the problem of tissue wasting is readily overcome if a firm diet is combined with increased exercise. Additional calories are used, the physical appearance is often improved, and activity helps to quell the pangs of hunger through such mechanisms as an altered setting of the hypothalamic glucose receptors and an increase of body temperature. The most effective regime for a typical obese patient is to reduce the food intake by 100 kcal/day (using data such as Table XXIII), and to increase activity by an equal amount. The desired objective is more likely to be realized through a programme of moderate exercise than by short bursts of more intense effort; thus a brisk two mile walk uses about 100 kcal of additional energy, whereas the jogging of a mile in eight minutes adds only 55 kcal to the daily energy expenditure.

The proposed regime of 100 kcal dietary restriction and 100 kcal of new activity per day will produce a weight loss of 0.2 kg per week, or 10 kg over the course of a year. Weight gain is normally a slow process, and except in unusual circumstances (such as a need for early surgical intervention), a slow but steady loss is the optimum mode of treatment, offering time for the modification of attitudes towards both food and activity. A deficit of 500–1000 kcal per day (a loss of up to 1 kg per week, to a total of 5 kg) may be permitted without detailed medical supervision; this requires more rigorous dieting, including the use of skimmed milk, lean meat, less butter, and reduced servings of most carbohydrates, together with increased exercise. "Slimming drugs" such as the amphetamines (p. 353) are potentially dangerous, and should only be used under the immediate guidance of a physician; they probably act by altering the setting of appetite regulating centres in the hypothalamus. Methyl cellulose acts like a green vegetable, giving a sensation of fullness by virtue of its large and unabsorbed bulk; it is open to the same objection as a natural cellulose diet— there is an increased rate of gastric emptying and early satiety is followed by renewed hunger.

Drastic Weight Loss

Very drastic diets are sometimes followed by boxers and wrestlers who wish to achieve a specific weight categorization. Such deliberate starvation and/or dehydration has been roundly condemned by associations of sports physicians; it is hazardous both to the individual who lowers his weight and to the opponent who is faced by an unfair and unequal contest.

Starvation

Anxious young women sometimes find themselves grossly underweight. It is always important to exclude a serious medical basis for a sudden loss of body weight, but often there is no ready explanation other than temperament (anorexia nervosa). The treatment is then to advise a very palatable diet with a high caloric density. Often, the appetite of such a patient is poor, and prolonged medical treatment may be needed to ensure recovery.

Accidental starvation may follow a catastrophe in a remote place (climbing, flying, or sailing). It may also complicate acute medical and surgical emergencies. Reserves of carbohydrate (mainly as glycogen) are exhausted within a day and thereafter energy requirements are met purely from fat and protein. Protein breakdown is essential to supply the blood sugar requirements of the central nervous system. At first, the percentage usage is not great (about 15% of calories, 60 gm per day). There is a reserve of labile protein in all tissues, but particularly the liver. This totals some 300 gm. Once this reserve has gone, tissue wasting is inevitable. It is most obvious in the skeletal muscles. As starvation progresses, the percentage of energy derived from protein increases, and the loss of plasma protein leads to tissue oedema and water retention. Two weeks of starvation is relatively harmless, but after about forty days both fat and protein stores have been reduced to the minimum compatible with survival; tolerance of starvation depends on the initial size of the fat depots, and on the energy that may be expended in trying to reach a place of safety.

The intestine participates in the tissue atrophy, and great care must therefore be taken in rehabilitating starved patients. The first meals provided should always be small and readily digested.

Diet and Heart Disease

Strength of the Association

Many facets of modern society have been blamed for an increase in the incidence of ischaemic heart disease (p. 505).

Inevitably, suspicion has fallen upon a change in dietary patterns. Since fatty plaques are found in ischaemic blood vessels, it has been tempting to postulate that the problem is related to a high intake of animal (saturated*) fat (Fig. 91). The saturation of various common fats and oils is summarized in Table XXVI. Most animal products have a high percentage of saturated fatty acids, while the vegetable oils contain mainly unsaturated fats. The manufacturers of vegetable oils have thus been quite active in promoting the replacement of animal fat

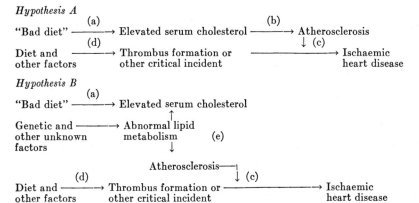

Proof of steps (a) and (c) is well-established. Proof of step (a) rests largely upon the feeding of high cholesterol diets to caged animals; it is a difficult hypothesis to examine in man. Step (d) probably encompasses a number of factors such as increase of cardiac workload by exercise or anxiety. Exercise may also dislodge a clot from elsewhere in the circulation, for instance the lung. The role of diet at stage (d) is suggested by the association between hyperlipidaemia and an increased clotting tendency of the blood.

Hypothesis A is in keeping with epidemiological data, but so is hypothesis B if it is assumed that a number of the unknown factors contributing to abnormal metabolism are by-products of our technically oriented Western Society. If hypothesis A is correct, then a change of diet would have a direct effect on serum cholesterol and thus the extent of atherosclerosis. However, if hypothesis B is correct, little advantage would be gained from a change of dietary patterns.

Figure 91. Some hypotheses concerning the relationship between diet and ischaemic heart disease (after G. Beaton).

* In a biochemical context, fats may be classified as saturated or unsaturated. Unsaturated fats include in their molecule fatty acids with one or more polyvalent carbon linkages. The extent of unsaturation of dietary fat is commonly reported as the "iodine value." The polyvalent linkages have an affinity for iodine, and transition from an animal to a vegetable fat diet may raise the iodine value from perhaps 50 to 100 or more. Polyunsaturated fats (with several polyvalent carbon linkages) apparently slow the rate of atherogenesis more than do monounsaturated fats.

TABLE XXVI

THE TYPE OF FATTY ACID IN SELECTED FATS AND OILS*

Food	Fatty Acids (% of Total)		
	Saturated	Monounsaturated	Polyunsaturated
Bacon	39	51	10
Butter	70	27	3
Chicken	30	48	22
Coconut	97	1	2
Corn	12	33	55*
Cottonseed	26	22	52
Herring	21	0	79*
Lard	40	48	12
Linseed	11	64	25
Olive	9	86	5
Palm Fruit	49	42	9
Palm Kernel	88	11	1
Peanut	19	50	31
Safflower	14	35	58*
Sesame	14	43	43
Soyabean	18	18	64*
Sunflower	12	35	53*
Whale	81	0	19

* Based mainly on the data of Joliffe. The foods marked with an asterisk have a particularly high ratio of polyunsaturated to saturated fatty acids.

by vegetable products. But when stripped of advertising pressures and emotional overtones, how strong is the association between ischaemic heart disease and the use of animal fats?

If the diet of a typical North American is compared with that of a primitive and unacculturated tribesman, several obvious differences are seen. The North American consumes some 50 percent more food than the tribesman; much of this represents wastage in the kitchen and on the table, but the obesity of the typical middle-aged man also reflects an excessive food intake. The average North American eats twice as much protein, and four or five times as much fat as many primitive peoples, together with large quantities of sugar. Civilized communities have shown a particularly dramatic increase of sugar consumption over the last two hundred years; in the United Kingdom of 1770, per capita consumption was about five pounds per annum; by 1870 this had risen to twenty-five pounds per annum, and in 1970 it was one hundred twenty pounds per annum.

Despite the large fat intake of western man, the case against this particular component of diet is not very strong. Some primitive peoples—the Eskimoes, Mongols, and East African tribes such as the Samburu and Masai—have a high fat diet, yet remain relatively free of ischaemic heart disease. Furthermore, the consumption of animal fat by the western world was already high in the early 1900s, and it is difficult to blame the subsequent "epidemic" of ischaemic heart disease upon the relatively small increment of fat consumption since the turn of the present century. Again, if individual patients from the western world are matched in other respects, it is difficult to show a statistically significant association between fat intake and the occurrence of overt ischaemic heart disease.

The main argument advanced by those favouring a low fat diet is that individuals with a high serum cholesterol level (> 250 mg/100 ml) have a greater than average risk of ischaemic heart disease. Certainly, the immediate effect of a low cholesterol diet (Table XXVII) is a dramatic reduction of serrum cholesterol. In one study from the author's laboratory, a small group of healthy young men adhered to a rigid low cholesterol diet for eight weeks. Initially, the serum cholesterol dropped from 170–230 mg/100 ml to around 90 mg/100 ml. However, when the subjects undertook vigorous effort, they were unable to maintain body weight without increasing their intake of sugars, and there was then an associated return of serum cholesterol towards base-line values; it seemed that hepatic synthesis of this material had increased. A much longer pilot trial was recently concluded under the auspices of the United States National Heart Institute. This study covered a span of eight years, and involved eight hundred institutionalized

TABLE XXVII

THE CHOLESTEROL CONTENT OF SOME COMMON FOODSTUFFS, EXPRESSED AS MG PER AVERAGE SERVING*

Beef, raw	84	Lamb, raw	80
Butter (1 pat)	38	Lard (1 tblsp.)	13
Cheese (cheddar)	30	Liver, raw	330
Cheese (skim milk)	0	Margarine (vegetable)	0
Chicken, raw	60	Milk (one cup)	26
Crab	190	(skim)	7
Egg (one)	250	Oysters (6)	1200
Fish	70	Pork	84
Heart, raw	150	Shrimp (12)	150
Ice cream	35	Veal	118
Kidney, raw	375		

* Based mainly on data of Joliffe.

Note: vegetables contain no cholesterol, unless butter, cheese or other animal products are added during cooking.

veterans; half of the group were fed a vegetable oil diet, lowering their cholesterol intake from 653 to 365 mg per day. At
the end of the study, the average serum cholesterol reading
was 18 percent below the initial value. The test group also had
a marginal advantage over the controls in terms of the incidence of ischaemic heart disease. Unfortunately, the study was
beset by a number of the problems that plague long term
prospective investigations—the subjects were relatively elderly
(average age 65)—adherence to the modified dietary regime
was less than 60 percent, and the faithful members of both
test and control groups became more health conscious as the
experiment progressed. Thus, the control group also experienced a substantial (13%) decrease of serum cholesterol, and
it may well be that nonspecific factors rather than the diet of
unsaturated fats were responsible for the improvement in prognosis of the test group.

> In some experimental animals such as rabbits and pigs, it is
> possible to produce plaques resembling (but not identical with)
> human atherosclerosis by feeding massive doses of cholesterol or
> animal fat. However, it is necessary to precondition the animals by
> prolonged cageing and/or alterations of hormonal secretion before
> lesions develop, and the combination of unusual circumstances and
> a highly abnormal food pattern prejudice the relevance of such
> investigations to normal life. At best, it can be concluded that
> animal studies are not inconsistent with a role of cholesterol in
> plaque formation.

A review of the cholesterol balance sheet of the body suggests that there is no fundamental biochemical reason why a
high fat diet should be the only or even the most common
basis of plaque formation. Some 1000 mg of cholesterol are
synthesisized daily by the liver and the intestines. This is
substantially more than the usual dietary intake of 600 mg, and
furthermore the rate of synthesis is boosted by an excessive intake of calories, whether given in the form of fat or carbohydrate. The daily excretion is also large (1000 mg), and blood
cholesterol levels soon reflect any changes in the rate of such
excretion.

Interest has recently focussed on a possible alternative evil
of our western diet—the high sugar intake. This is a rather

attractive hypothesis, since it would link up with the known association between diabetes and ischaemic heart disease, and would explain why exercise reduces the insulin requirements of diabetics. The immediate response of animals to the feeding of large quantities of sugar is an increased output of insulin, but if the sugar diet is maintained, the Islet cells secreting this hormone eventually become exhausted and show irreversible damage. The cholesterol levels of animals may be somewhat increased by a high sugar diet, although typically the change is not very great. The possible role of an excessive sugar intake in human ischaemic heart disease is supported by the retrospective questioning of coronary patients immediately following their first attack and before diet has been modified. Some coronary victims report a sugar intake of three hundred to four hundred pounds per annum, and there is commonly a history of addiction to tea or coffee. The adverse feature of these drinks seems their sugar rather than their caffeine content. Repeated administration of large doses of caffeine has no long-term effect upon the serum cholesterol levels of experimental animals. One immediate effect of caffeine is to precipitate a lipolysis, with an increase of serum free fatty acids; this response is not seen when caffeine is taken with sugar in such forms as sweetened Cola.

Other important variables to be considered in any dietetic experiment are the total caloric balance and the level of habitual activity. The change in status of many control groups and the the ability of primitive peoples to withstand a wide range of diets suggests that an overall excess of food may be necessary before the harmful effects of either animal fat or sugar are revealed. Sugar may be injurious partly because it encourages overeating. Exercise helps to avoid the large rise of blood sugar following a carbohydrate meal, thereby diminishing the insulin required of the pancreatic islets; a larger intake of sugar can thus be tolerated before the Islet cells become exhausted.

Irrespective of mechanisms, the success of any short-term programme of dietary modification is unlikely to be very great. An interest in dieting is rare before early middle age, and Hartroft has pointed out that in North America the deposition of fat in the lining of the blood vessels commences in infancy. It is more pronounced in children, and can be quite advanced in young adults. Postmortem examination of United States soldiers killed in Korea revealed advanced plaque formation in some 15 percent of those studied. A preventive dietary programme should thus commence not in adult life, but immediately upon cessation of breast feeding. Once the atherosclerotic process has progressed to a fibrinoid or calcified state, no dietary regime can be of avail. Again, diet may help but cannot correct any genetically-induced problem in the transport or metabolism of fat. Control of obesity may reduce the load placed upon the heart by a sudden burst of physical activity, but it is unlikely to influence other trigger factors that can initiate an overt episode of myocardial ischaemia once atherosclerosis is present.

Some populations are able to tolerate quite extensive atherosclerosis without a high incidence of ischaemic heart disease. Possibly, they lack the trigger factors that convert a silent lesion to an overt coronary attack. Certainly, it would be profitable to explore why they have this unusual tolerance.

Specific Studies of Serum Lipids

Classification of Hyperlipidaemias. Whether a faulty diet is responsible or not, there is general agreement that the risk of ischaemic heart disease is increased in those individuals who have a high serum lipid level (hyperlipidaemia); as many as a third of all coronary victims are grossly hyperlipaemic, and five out of six have a serum cholesterol greater than 210 mg/100ml.

Early classification of hyperlipidaemia was based upon the apparent cause, and writers distinguished dietetic (fat-induced or carbohydrate-induced hyperlipaemia) from what was thought a genetic condition (essential familial hyperlipaemia).

Current classification is based on the response of the serum to electrophoresis and ultracentrifugation. Typical electrophoresis patterns are illustrated in Fig. 92. The four main types of lipoprotein are as follows:

α (high density) fraction—20% cholesterol, and larger amounts of protein

β (low density) fraction—50% cholesterol

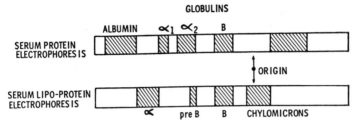

Figure 92. Electrophoretic study of serum lipoproteins. After completion of electrophoresis, the serum protein film is stained with brom-phenol blue, and a fat stain such as Oil-Red O is used to identify the different lipoprotein fractions.

> pre β (very low density) fraction—50% triglyceride, mainly of
> endogenous origin
> Chylomicrons—90% triglyceride, derived from body fat.

The α lipoproteins are unrelated to atherogenesis, and hyperlipidaemias are described mainly in terms of the β and pre β fractions. Using such techniques, Fredrickson and Strisower have each described five patient groups. Group I has an increase of low density lipoproteins, normal or reduced levels of very low density lipoproteins, and yellow xanthomatous deposits of carotene and lipochrome pigments around the tendons and in the eyelids. It has been suggested that the problem in this class of patient is a deficiency in the enzyme responsible for the breakdown of chylomicrons. Certainly, the fat levels in such patients remain uninfluenced by diets low in animal fat and sugar, and there is little response to drugs such as clofibrate (an inhibitor of cholesterol synthesis) and cholestyramine (a bile-sequestering resin which increases the faecal excretion of cholesterol). However, the low density lipoprotein concentrations can be reduced to more normal values by the use of large doses of thyroid hormone. Patients of *Group 2* have a similar lipoprotein pattern, but xanthomata are absent and normal concentrations of lipoprotein can be restored by administration of clofibrate. *Group 3* have an increase of very low density lipoproteins, normal concentrations of low density lipoproteins, and xanthomata; they respond well to clofibrate treatment. *Group 4* have an increase of very low density lipoproteins with a reduced level of low density lipoproteins. They respond well to dietary restriction, but while clofibrate reduces the level of very low density lipoproteins in such patients, at the same time it sometimes increases the level of low density lipoproteins. *Group 5* have elevated concentrations of both types of lipoprotein; pateints of this type respond best to combined thyroxine and clofibrate treatment.

In general, it is easier to modify the concentration of the very low density lipoproteins than it is to change the concentration of the low density fraction. Concentrations of β lipoprotein may even be increased by the administration of drugs. Unfortunately, there is some evidence to suggest that β lipoproteins are the main culprits in atherogenesis.

Some laboratories do not possess equipment for electrophoresis or ultracentrifugation. Fortunately, information on the type of hyperlipidaemia can also be obtained from a consideration of increase in cholesterol and triglyceride levels, as follows:

	Cholesterol	*Triglyceride*
Type I	+	++
Type II	+	±
Type III	++	+
Type IV	±	++
Type V	+	++

Serum triglyceride readings of less than 150 mg/100 ml are usual in slim subjects, and readings greater than 200 mg/100 ml may be regarded as substantially elevated.

Independence of Hyperlipidaemia as a "Risk Factor." Many factors associated with a high risk of ischaemic heart disease have been identified (p. 506). It is less clear how far these factors make independent contributions to the delineation of the coronary-prone individual. A person who has a high serum cholesterol is likely to be a middle-aged male who overeats, is somewhat obese, and has an abnormal exercise electrocardiogram. Again, comparisons of sedentary workers with more active groups such as share-croppers and foundry employees suggest a possible association between lack of physical activity and high blood lipid levels. Thus in many respects the biochemical tests duplicate information that could be obtained by simple questioning. However, they probably contribute some additional knowledge; for instance, not all obese patients have high lipid readings, and the risk characteristic of an aggressive "A-type" personality does not appear to be associated with high lipid values.

Exercise and Serum Lipids. There have been many claims that exercise decreases the serum cholesterol level. Occupational comparisons certainly support such a view, but in those laboratory investigations where a significant drop of cholesterol has been observed, the caloric intake has been inadequate, and a decrese of body weight has occurred. In one study initiated by this laboratory, men were first stabilized on a low cholesterol diet, and were then required to run vigorously on a treadmill for twenty-five minutes per day; the food intake was carefully adjusted to maintain body weight, and under these circumstances there was no change of serum cholesterol. Other laboratories have subsequently reached identical conclusions.

In contrast, exercise will produce a small decrease in fasting serum triglycerides, and since high triglyceride readings are associated with an increased risk of ischaemic heart disease, this change should be beneficial to the patients.

Body weight and Serum Lipids. Even if there is no change of habitual activity, weight loss is usually associated with a fall of serum cholesterol. Conversely, the serum cholesterol rises during periods of weight gain. Once the body weight has stabilized, differences between thin and obese persons are much less obvious.

Should Diets Be Modified? Several national and regional Heart Associations find themselves under frequent pressure from enthusiastic proponents of vegetable fat diets. On the available information, there would seem little justification for attempting to modify the food patterns of an entire nation in this way. At best, the populace would succeed in the rather unpalatable task of eating 40 percent vegetable fat, and there might then be a marginal reduction in both serum cholesterol and the incidence of ischaemic heart disease. However, it is likely that many of the population would replace fat by sugar, and current evidence suggests this could be more harmful to the patient than the original diet of animal fat. It is well recognized that while a low fat/high carbohydrate diet can depress serum cholesterol, it also leads to an increase of serum triglycerides. Again, we have already noted the possible harmful effects of added sugar upon the pancreatic Islets. Finally, it is by no means certain that vegetable fat in itself is devoid of risk, particularly if the majority of the fat is polyunsaturated. Polyunsaturated fats have a tendency to polymerize to a compound called ceroid, and this may provide a rather permanent basis of clot formation; animal fat clots can be broken down by body enzymes, but such enzymes are completely unable to attack the waxy ceroid.

Despite the several objections to the use of a low cholesterol diet by the general population, there may be some advantage in modifying the diet of patients with a high risk of coronary disease; if a man is threatened by premature death, even a small improvement in his prognosis may be worthwhile, and a case can be made for tolerating the inevitable disruption of life in the kitchen and the supermarket. However, it seems unlikely that all "high-risk" patients will be helped by dietary modification, and much further investigation is required to identify the type of person who will benefit most from a change in food habits.

References

Renhold, A.E., and Cahill, G.F.: Adipose Tissue. *Handbook of Physiology,* Section 5. Baltimore, Williams & Wilkins, 1965.

Brozek, J.: Body composition. *Ann NY Acad Sci,* 110:1–1018, 193.

Brozek, J.: *Human Body Composition.* Oxford, Pergamon Press, 1965.

Bogert, L.J., Briggs, G.M., and Calloway, D.H.: *Nutrition and Physical Fitness. Philadelphia,* Saunders. 1966.

Blix, G.: *Nutrition and Physical Activity.* Uppsala, Sweden, Almqvist & Wiksell, 1967.

Sheldon, W.H.: *The Varieties of Human Physique.* New York, Hafner, 1963.

Tanner, J.M.: *The Physique of the Olympic Athlete.* London, George Allen & Unwin, 1964.

Poortmans, J.R.: *Biochemistry of Exercise.* Basel, Karger, 1969.

Hultman, E.: Muscle glycogen stores and prolonged exercise. In *Frontiers of Fitness.* Springfield, Thomas, 1971.

Revell, D.T.: *Dietary Control of Hypercholesterolemia.* Springfield, Thomas, 1962.

Kummerow, F.A.: Metabolism of lipids as related to atherosclerosis. Springfield, Thomas, 1965.

17

ACTIVITY AND HEALTH

Terminology

It may be helpful to the nonmedical reader to commence our review of activity and health by defining some of the terms commonly used in the context of ischaemic heart disease.

Coronary Infarction

This is the "coronary attack" of popular parlance. An area of the heart wall becomes starved of blood (ischaemic), and dies. The cause is often a sudden occlusion of a major branch of a coronary artery, either by a blood clot, or by haemorrhage into a fatty plaque within the vessel wall (p. 66). However, in some patients an infarct develops in the absence of any demonstrable blockage; it is then assumed that at the moment of infarction the oxygen demands of the heart muscle exceeded the supply available from somewhat narrowed vessels. This type of situation is particularly likely when the blood pressure is raised by either sustained isometric activity (page 68) or anger.

If the area of cellular damage is large, the immediate or early demise of the patient is likely. Death results from an abnormality of ventricular rhythm (fibrillation, p. 76), or the onset of cardiac failure (p. 54). A proportion of patients (increased somewhat by intensive care) survive the immediate insult. The infarcted area (infarction means, literally, "stuffed with blood") is gradually replaced by scar tissue, and normal function is partially or completely restored. The likelihood of recovery is influenced by the extent of the *collateral circulation* connecting the two main coronary arteries.

The recognition of a typical coronary attack is not too difficult. The patient has some or all of the predisposing factors to be discussed below, and—often without warning—is afflicted by a sudden very intense vice-like pain in the midline of the chest. This persists without remission for as long as twenty minutes, and the patient is pale, cold, and showing signs of collapse. Immediate admission to a hospital offering intensive care is required, and since many patients die within the first few minutes of attack, an ambulance offering intensive care is also desirable. Ventricular fibrillation and cardiac arrest are likely complications. The carotid pulse rhythm should be monitored prior to arrival of the ambulance, and if the observer has the necessary training, cardiac massage (p. 78) should be given as necessary.

Angina Pectoris

Angina of effort is also due to a relative myocardial oxygen lack; however, oxygen deprivation is less serious than during infarction, and there is no irreversible tissue damage.

As with infarction, there is a midline chest pain or sense of oppression, but this does not last for longer than two minutes, and is not severe enough to cause collapse. Often, the pain may radiate upwards into the root of the neck, or along the inner aspect of the left arm. There is usually a clear precipitating cause—anxiety or a walk uphill (particularly in cold weather, when cutaneous vasoconstriction is maximal, and nerve endings within the airway are stimulated by cold dry air). The symptoms are relieved rapidly by rest and nitroglycerine tablets.

Atherosclerosis

Atherosclerosis is a general condition of the arteries in which the lumina are partially occluded by fat. The earliest changes are probably endothelial; there is an increased content of mucopolysaccharides, and extracellular deposition of lipid, particularly cholesterol. Fatty plaques develop and are enlarged by inflammation, haemorrhage and thrombus formation. If these changes occur within the coronary arteries, they predispose to either angina or infarction.

Atherosclerosis may be coexistent with but should be distinguished from arteriosclerosis; the latter involves a loss of elasticity and a hardening of the vessel walls, often with radiographically visible calcification. *Arteriosclerosis* occurs to some extent in many older people, and if severe it can cause an increase of systemic blood pressure, a narrowing or incompetence of the cardiac valves, and ultimately weakness of the vessel walls.

Ischaemic Heart Disease

Ischaemic heart disease is a composite term referring to the several possible manifestations of relative oxygen lack in the myocardium. It is to be preferred to the term *atherosclerotic heart disease*. Although the latter is sometimes used as a synonym, atherosclerosis may be present for many years without ischaemic manifestations—a second, triggering factor such as an unusual oxygen demand or the lodgement of a thrombus is needed to produce overt ischaemia. Further, as we have noted above, the postmortem evidence of atherosclerosis may be rather slight—the prime emphasis in some episodes of sudden death is ventricular fibrillation or infarction associated with an increased oxygen demand rather than a specific blockage of the coronary vessels.

The "Epidemic" of Ischemic Heart Disease

Much alarm has arisen among middle-aged people over the apparent "epidemic" of ischaemic heart disease that is afflicting Western society. Each year, it seems that "coronary attacks" claim a larger number of the populace, and the age of the victims also seems to fall.

How far is the popular fear borne out by objective statistics? A recent Canadian study by Anderson and LeRiche is fairly typical of figures for other western nations. They collected data for men aged forty-five to sixty-four (Fig. 93). Official mortality statistics showed a 2½ fold increase of ischaemic heart disease between 1931 and 1951; however, part of this apparent increase could reflect changing fashions of diagnosis and certification of death. Accordingly, Anderson and LeRiche reexamined the

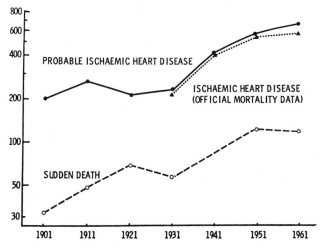

Figure 93. The incidence of sudden death, probable ischaemic heart disease, and deaths classified as ischaemic heart disease in the Province of Ontario. Data for men aged forty-five to sixty-four years, collected by Anderson and LeRiche.

original certificates for the period 1901–1961, and distinguished "probable" cases of ischaemic heart disease; these amounted to about two hundred per 100,000 in 1901, with little increase to 1931, but a sharp subsequent rise to five hundred per 100,000 in 1951. The fact of "sudden death" is hardly susceptible to misinterpretation, and at the age under consideration, it is reasonable to assume that the majority of sudden deaths are caused by ischaemic heart disease. Ontario mortality statistics show thirty sudden deaths per 100,000 in 1901, rising to sixty per 100,000 in 1931, and 130 per 100,000 in 1951. Thus we may conclude that there has been a real increase in deaths from ischaemic heart disease during the present century. However, there are also some indications that the "epidemic" has now reached its peak, particularly in the United States. In 1955, United States authorities reported a death rate from arteriosclerotic and degenerative heart disease of 342 per 100,000 men aged forty-five to fifty-four. Between 1955 and 1967, this age and disease specific death rate increased by no more than 3 percent, compared with increases of 50 percent to 60 percent in some European countries. Finland, with 469 deaths per 100,000 men of this age group now has a worse record than the United States.

The magnitude of the problem is vast. If all ages are considered jointly, then heart attacks take an annual toll of some 700,000 United States citizens, and the resultant economic loss to that country has been set at $31 billion dollars per year. Over a seventy year life span, a man has a 40 percent chance of developing a coronary attack. Many of those affected are of course quite elderly, and it can be argued that with the conquest of major bacterial and viral diseases, it is inevitable that "cardiac" deaths will become more frequent. However, even if we restrict our attention to the middle-aged working population (ages 45–64 years), figures for the province of Ontario (1961) still show an annual "cardiac" death rate of 590 per 100,000 men and 160 per 100,000 women. At this age, it is by far the commonest mode of death for both men and women, and in the men it accounts for almost 50 percent of all fatalities.

It is less certain how far the average age of attack has decreased during the current century. Although much publicity is drawn to occasional "coronary" deaths in relatively young men, clinical manifestations of the disease are still uncommon in patients under the age of forty. Recent statistics show an annual "cardiac" death rate of thirty per 100,000 at the age of thirty-five, and only seven per 100,000 at the age of thirty.

At all ages, the situation is complicated by the existence of much subclinical disease (Table XXVIII). This hampers the

TABLE XXVIII

DEATHS, INCIDENCE AND PREVALENCE OF CORONARY ARTERY DISEASE IN BRITISH MEN AGED FIFTY-FIVE TO SIXTY-FOUR YEARS*

	Annual *Rates Per 100,000 Men*
Deaths from Coronary Heart Disease	500
Incidence of Coronary Heart Disease	1,000
Prevalence of Clinical Disease	5,000
Prevalence of Ischaemic Myocardial Lesions	10,000
Prevalence of Severe Occlusive Coronary Artery Disease	15,000`
Prevalence of Much Coronary Atheroma	20,000
Prevalence of Moderate Coronary Atheroma	30,000
Prevalence of Little Coronary Atheroma	50,000

* Data for the period 1953–1955, as obtained by Morris.

design of experiments that call for known "cases" and "control" subjects. If all stages of the disease process are considered, more than 90 percent of men aged fifty-five to sixty-four years show postmortem evidence of atheroma. On the other hand, only 10 percent show ischaemic scarring of the myocardium, only 5 percent develop sufficient symptomatology for the disease to be clinically recognised, and the annual incidence of new episodes of coronary heart disease in previously healthy people is no more than 1 percent.

The majority of coronary attacks are fatal. In a recent study from Belfast, 25 percent of hospitalized victims died within the first fifteen minutes of attack, almost 40 percent died in the first hour, and 65 percent died in the first twenty-four hours. At the end of four weeks, only 5 percent of patients were still alive. Despite intensive care units, the prognosis remains gloomy unless the attack is a mild one. Thus the development of effective preventive measures would represent a significant medical advance.

Predisposing Factors

The epidemiology of ischaemic heart disease has received extensive study, and a number of predisposing ("risk") factors are well-documented. Their value as screening tools may be assessed in terms of *sensitivity* and *specificity*. Consider, for instance, the serum cholesterol readings. In a community study at Framingham, Mass., 156 of every 1000 men aged forty to fifty-nine had a high serum cholesterol (>260 mg/100 ml); if the reported data is extrapolated to cover a ten year period, thirty-two of these men would develop clinically recognized ischaemic heart disease. The total number of new episodes of ischaemic heart disease over the same period would be 120 per 1000 men. The sensitivity of the test is thus 32/1000 (27%), and the predictive value of a high serum cholesterol reading is 32/156 (21%). A total of 844 men had normal serum cholesterol readings, but 880 would remain free of clinical ischaemic heart disease over the ten year period; the specificity of the test is thus [844−(120−32)]/880 (86%), and the predictive value of a negative result is (120−32)/844(10%).

Assuming that patients were advised as to prognosis on the results of this single test, there would be (156−32) falsely positive diagnoses, and (120−32) falsely negative diagnoses. A number of the falsely positive results would convert to true positive results if the study continued for more than ten years, since further patients with subclinical atheroma would then develop obvious signs and symptoms. However, at the same time there would be some increase in the number of patients with falsely negative results.

The overall value of any given test is conveniently summarized by the *risk ratio*. This compares the predictive value of positive and negative results; for serum cholesterol it amounts to 2.1 (21%/10%).

A second factor predisposing to ischaemic heart disease is a high systemic blood pressure; in the Framingham study, a "casual" systolic pressure of 160 mmHg or more and/or a "casual" diastolic pressure of 95 mmHg were regarded as abnormal. A total of 120 patients exceeded these limits. Again extrapolating results to cover a ten year period, the blood pressure readings have a sensitivity of 18 percent and a specificity of 86 percent, with a predictive value of 15 percent for positive tests and of 12 percent for negative tests. The risk ratio is thus 1.3. If we consider the combined results of blood pressure and serum cholesterol determinations, the risk ratio rises to 2.5, and if either a high serum cholesterol or a high blood pressure are accepted as positive findings, a risk ratio of 2.9 is attained. Other authors have achieved an even better discrimination. Thus, if the data of Morris and his colleagues for London busmen is extrapolated to cover a similar ten year period, the presence of a high serum cholesterol and/or a high systemic blood pressure yields a risk ratio of 5.1.

Many other factors, when considered singly, discriminate significantly between the coronary prone and the coronary resistant individual. However, few of these factors contribute much additional information after patients have been classified in terms of serum cholesterol and systemic blood pressure.

Ischaemic heart disease is more common in men than in women, particularly at ages before the female menopause. This may reflect hormonal influences, or it may be due simply to differences of life style (pressures of work, frequency and intensity of physical activity, cigarette consumption, and so on). The dominant role of life style is suggested by the fact that the difference in incidence between men and women is progressively diminishing in western society.

Death rates from ischaemic heart disease are still very low in "primitive" communities. However, it is difficult to decide how far this reflects a constitutional difference, how far it is due to a more appropriate balance of nutrition and activity on the part of "native" peoples, and how far it reflects an absence of the pressures of modern civilization.

The victims of ischaemic heart disease often give a strong family history of "coronary" attacks and sudden death. Heredity undoubtedly plays some role in predisposing to ischaemic heart disease, but there is also inevitably a more careful searching of family records following an attack. Furthermore, the household environment is shared, and the family concerned may have poor attitudes to such factors as diet and physical activity.

It is difficult to quantitate the stress of living in a large city and working within a giant business corporation. Certainly, ischaemic heart disease does have some predilection for corporate executives, but it is difficult to disentangle executive responsibility from the associated hazards of overeating at business luncheons and lack of physical activity. One study within the Bell Telephone organization suggested that those particularly prone to attack were men with upward social mobility. Their very success in the company was presumably a reflection of an achievement-oriented personality (itself an adverse factor), and because of their working-class parentage, greater stress may well have been encountered in the personal relationships of an advancing business and social career.

Ischaemic heart disease is much more common in heavy smokers (p. 333). The unfavourable influences of obesity and excessive food consumption are discussed elsewhere (p. 485); the specific role of physical inactivity is considered below.

Laboratory tests used to identify the coronary prone individual include a depression of the ST segment of the exercise electrocardiogram (p. 73), elevation of serum cholesterol, triglyceride and phospholipid levels, and a poor tolerance to ingestion of a standard dose of glucose (i.e. diabetes or a prediabetic state).

If information from all possible sources is combined, as many as 50 percent of potential coronary patients can be identified. This is an interesting statistical exercise, and has some value in providing high-risk groups for prospective experiments. On the other hand, it is debatable whether such knowledge is useful to the individual patient. Many of those tested are wrongly classified, and since there is no specific cure, solemn warnings of an impending heart attack may well create a cardiac neurosis. In general, the management of the individual is unchanged. Gross diabetes or hypertension may require appropriate therapy, but with these specific exceptions the same advice is tendered to high and low risk patients—avoid overeating, reduce body weight, take more exercise, smoke less cigarettes, and learn to relax at home and at work. Multiphasic screening brings to light patients with subclinical atheroma; although the individual is aware of his disease for a longer period, and in consequence has an apparently longer period of survival, his age of death remains unchanged.

Physical Activity and Ischaemic Heart Disease

Possible Harmful Effect of Exercise

The majority of studies of physical activity and ischaemic heart disease have been conducted by enthusiasts who have started their investigation with the assumption that exercise is good for a person. It may thus be a useful corrective to consider first evidence regarding the possible harmful effects of vigorous exercise. A casual survey of the daily paper suggests there may be a problem—"man dies shovelling snow"—"student of twenty-three dies in the University gymnasium"—"another death at the Y." Such headlines are naturally misleading, since they take no account of the snow-shovellers and gymnasts who survive in large numbers.

It is possible to approach the question of exercise and sudden death epidemiologically. The day is divided into three periods—work (which in most cases involves relatively light physical activity), leisure (when any significant added energy expenditure is incurred), and sleep; we then collect data on the time of day when coronary attacks occur. Such studies have shown no obvious concentration of attacks in the leisure period, and no unusually low incidence at night. However, it would be rash to conclude from this evidence that physical activity has no immediate effect upon the likelihood of a coronary attack. In the first place, some people do not go to bed to sleep! The physician who is summoned from his home to attend a coronary victim in the wee hours of the morning may well have a shrewd suspicion that sexual exercise has precipitated the attack he is called to treat. A second problem arises from dilution of data. In a typical North American city, less than 10 percent of the adult population are taking significant leisure activity. Any effect that exercise may have upon the time-related incidence of coronary disease is thus obscured by events occurring in the other 90 percent of the population who never exercise. A third difficulty is that a "coronary attack" is a clinical rather than a pathological diagnosis. One patient may die of ventricular fibrillation immediately following an episode of relative myocardial hypoxia; this could well be related to exercise. Another patient lodges a clot in a coronary vessel; again, exercise could play some role by driving the clot into the circulation. A third patient dies of cardiac failure some hours following a large infarction; the initial cause was a complete thrombosis of a major coronary artery, and this occurred while the patient was asleep. These are very different pathological conditions, yet all are classified as acute coronary deaths. When account is taken of these sources of uncertainty, it is hardly surprising that the incidence of "coronary attacks" bears no relationship to time of day.

No one has as yet attempted to correlate heavy snowfalls with coronary attacks. This might be a very profitable line of investigation, although again there would be many variables to control, particularly the wetness of the snow and the ambient temperature while shovelling.

A third approach is to review the experience of gymnasia and fitness-testing laboratories. Bruce has perhaps the most extensive data on this point. He tests a somewhat biassed sample—mainly middle-aged hospital patients. A proportion are undoubtedly "coronary prone." He finds one coronary episode per three thousand maximum effort tests, and one attack for every 15,000 submaximum tests. In general, the patient goes into ventricular fibrillation. Partly because Bruce has a well-trained emergency team at the ready, and partly because the coronary vasculature of his patients is adequate for rest if not for maximum effort, such attacks are not usually fatal in his hands. However, they could well be if the same tests were carried out by less well-prepared staff.

A typical exercise test lasts no more than ten minutes. Are the risks of such exercise really as high as two attacks per one thousand man-hours? Perhaps the case is somewhat overstated. It is more than ten minutes before blame ceases to be attached to exercise. Some of Bruce's episodes of fibrillation developed during subsequent showering. Nevertheless, the risks are in stark contrast with armchair life. A middle-aged bus driver sitting in the padded comfort of his vehicle has a risk of 2.7 attacks per one thousand man-*years*. Maximum exercise increases his chance of a coronary attack by four orders! Even if we were to assume that all of Bruce's patients had suffered previous coronary attacks (and this is by no means the case), the risks of maximum and submaximum exercise would still be respectively at least three and two orders greater than the hazards incurred by sitting at rest.

These alarming statistics should be tempered by several considerations. Firstly, we are not dealing with a normal, random sample of the population. Almost by definition, any North American who decides to undertake deliberate exercise is abnormal. A short visit to the YMCA is sufficient to show that the average fitness class is drawn from the coronary-prone segment of the population—the participants are middle-aged executives, originally of "mesomorphic" build, and now becoming obese. Secondly, we are not looking at the entire life span of our chosen population—we have deliberately focussed attention on the few brief moments they spend in the gymnasium. It may well be that for the remaining 23½ hours of their day, the exercising group have a much lower risk of coronary disease than those who are inactive. If so, exercise has not really increased the risk of ischaemic heart disease—it has merely localized it to the gymnasium; providing that resuscitative equipment is at hand, the patient may be more likely to survive than if he sustains a coronary attack while on his own. This in turn raises important public health problems regarding governmental certification of gymnasia (p. 552); what are the minimum acceptable facilities, in terms of emergency equipment and medical or paramedical staff? Who should be permitted to undertake cardiac massage and/or defibrillation? Internationally acceptable answers to such questions are urgently awaited.

Possible Hazards of Inactivity

Objective Evidence of Laziness. Most people sense intuitively that the present generation is less active that its forbears. How strong is the objective evidence on this point?

If pulse-counting techniques (p. 28) are used to study the habits of the average city-dweller of 1971, it soon becomes obvious that no significant activity is undertaken. Pulse rates of more than 110 beats per minute are rare except during emotional excitement, sexual activity, and the occasional lifting of a heavy item of furniture. The usual day contains nothing more vigorous than a few minutes of leisurely walking, and the ascent of a few flights of stairs. Many of the present generation avoid even these sources of exercise, driving to the door of any building they may visit, and waiting for the elevator rather than climbing any stairs.

Does this attitude to activity represent a significant change of life style relative to the city-dweller who lived thirty or forty years ago? Certainly, the views of the industrial physiologist are changing. When physiologists first moved onto the factory floor, it was appropriate to think of very heavy work as a sustained energy expenditure of more than 9 kcal/min. Now, it is rare to find industrial tasks that call for more than two to three times the resting energy expenditure (3–5 kcal/min), and there is no demonstrable gradient of "fitness"—whether assessed in terms of aerobic power or of muscular strength—between the so-called "heavy" and "light" workers; fitness depends on leisure rather than on working activity. When prescribing maximum permissible levels of effort, the early industrial physiologist thought it prudent to consider the energy cost of travelling to and from work. The present author can remember that before the second world war, th main hazard on industrial stretches of the North Circular Road in London was not an excess of cars but rather a plethora of bicycles. Cycling involved the factory employees in quite vigorous effort, often as much as 10 kcal/min. Now, many of the bicycle factories have closed, and it is commonplace to own two or more cars, particularly in North America (Table XXIX). Even at home, there is much power equipment, and tasks carried out by the handyman thirty years ago are now deputed to the employees of "service" industries. This trend is well reflected by estimates of daily food con-

TABLE XXIX

FAMILIES IN THE UNITED STATES OWNING ONE OR TWO CARS

Year	One or Two Cars	Two Cars
1950	59%	7%
1955	70%	10%
1960	77%	15%
1965	79%	24%

TABLE XXX

DAILY PER CAPITA FOOD CONSUMPTION IN THE UNITED STATES

Year	Total Caloric Value	Carbohydrate	Fat	Protein
1930	3440 KCal	474 gm	134 gm	93 gm
1940	3350 KCal	429 gm	143 gm	93 gm
1950	3260 KCal	402 gm	145 gm	94 gm
1960	3140 KCal	375 gm	143 gm	95 gm
1965	3130 KCal	372 gm	144 gm	96 gm

sumption (Table XXX). The average United States citizen is eating 10 percent less than thirty-five years ago; the main change has been a reduced intake of staple foods such as wheat and milk. If anything, more of the present generation are overweight, and it is also probable that a higher percentage of the apparent food consumption is now wastage. Thus the habitual activity of the present generation is certainly reduced.

Retrospective Evidence. Has this general decrease of physical activity been harmful to cardiovascular health? One very tempting approach has been to draw a parallel between the increasing incidence of ischaemic heart disease and various objective signs of diminishing activity such as vehicle registrations, usage of electrical power, and diminution of food consumption. In some instances, statistically significant associations have been demonstrated, but unfortunately this does not prove a cause and effect relationship. Many features of life have changed in the Twentieth Century; activity has decreased, but there has also been a dramatic increase in the consumption of refined sugars (p. 492) and of cigarettes (p. 328).

A second retrospective approach is to compare the extent of ischaemic heart disease among groups that are presumed to differ in habitual activity. The men compared have included mailmen and postoffice clerks, railway switchmen and booking clerks, white and blue-collar gas company employees, and sedentary and active members of Jewish communal settlements. Epstein has accumulated much data of this type (Table XXXI). Whether comparisons are based upon the extent of postmortem scarring or atherogenesis, upon mortality, or upon the prevalence of clinical and ECG evidence of ischaemic heart disease, the active workers have a more favourable experience than seden-

Alive Man!

TABLE XXXI
THE INFLUENCE OF PHYSICAL ACTIVITY UPON ISCHAEMIC HEART
DISEASE—EVIDENCE FROM AUTOPSY, MORTALITY, AND MORBIDITY
STATISTICS*
(By permission of the author and the publisher of the *Bull NY Acad Med.*)

Criterion	Age	Comparison	Frequency Ratio
(a) *Autopsy Data*			
Large scars	45–70	Light/heavy work	2.9
Large scars	45–70	Light/"active" work	1.7
Small multiple scars	45–70	Light/heavy work	1.7
Small multiple scars	45–70	Light/"active" work	1.5
Severe coronary atherosclerosis	45–70	Light/heavy work	1.1
Severe coronary atherosclerosis	45–70	Light/"active" work	1.3
Coronary atherosclerosis index	30–60	Sedentary/"active" work	1.0–1.2
(b) *Mortality Studies*			
Standardized mortality ratios of	45–64	Sedentary/light work	1.0†/1.1
Californian nonfarm workers	45–64	Sedentary/medium work	1.3/1.3
	45–64	Sedentary/heavy work	1.4/2.2
Death rates for arteriosclerotic	40–64	Clerks/railway switchmen	1.5
heart disease in railway	40–64	Clerks/railway sectionmen	2.0
employees			
Death rates for arteriosclerotic	All ages	Clerks/carriers‡	0.8
heart disease in Washington	to 65	Clerks/carriers	1.2–1.4
post office employees		Clerks/carriers	2.8
(c) *Morbidity Studies*			
Q & QRS pattern on ECG	40–59	Other work/lumberjacks	4.9
T wave changes on ECG	40–59		1.6
Postexercise changes on ECG	40–59		1.3
Prevalence of coronary heart disease	40–59	Clerks/railway switchmen	1.8
Prevalence of angina	40–59		5.0
Prevalence of myocardial infarction	40–59		1.4
Myocardial infarction	40–59	Clerks/factory workers	4.0
Angina	40–59		1.3
Total coronary heart disease	40–59		1.5
Prevalence of coronary heart disease	40–74	Professionals/workers	5.0
Prevalence of coronary heart disease	40–74	Farm owners/workers	2.8
Prevalence of coronary heart disease	40–74	Farm owners/owner-workers	3.5

* Based on data collected by Epstein, Bull. N.Y. Acad. Med, 44; 924-925, 1968.
† First column refers to medium risk patients, second column to low risk patients.
‡ The three comparisons refer respectively to mail carriers with less than 20 years of service, more than 20 years of service, and according to current service.

tary employees. However, the interpretation of such statistics is subject to many pitfalls. Clearly, strong and healthy men are likely to choose such occupations as lumberjack, and in the event that they sustain a "coronary attack" it is probable that they will seek alternative sedentary employment. If angina is used as a criterion of ischaemic heart disease, the very fact of vigorous activity may make obvious what would otherwise remain a clinically silent area of atheroma. Finally, physical activity may give an individual the capacity to live with a certain amount of atheroma or fibrous scarring of the myocardium, even if it is not competent to reverse the disease process. These problems are well brought out in the extensive studies of Morris and his colleagues. They hypothesized that the London bus-driver had a rather sedentary task, while the bus conductor was much more active. The average London bus conductor climbs roughly the height of the Empire State building per day, and use of the electrochemical pulse integrator (p. 32) has confirmed that he is active relative to the driver. The incidence of first attacks of coronary disease is 2.7 cases per thousand man-years for the drivers, and 1.9 cases per thousand man years for the conductors. The mortality rate is also higher in the drivers than in the conductors. On the other hand, the conductors are more liable to angina than the drivers, and at post-mortem both groups have rather similar atheromatous deposits. The main pathological difference between the drivers and the conductors is that the former more frequently show fibrous scarring of the myocardium. Apparently, the exercise of stair-climbing gives the conductors an ability to live with their atheroma. One weakness of the London Transport study, well recognised by Morris and his colleagues, is a lack of initial equivalence of drivers and conductors. Data is available on the sizes of the first uniforms issued to the bus crews, and even at the time of recruitment the drivers were fatter than the conductors. Presumably, the sedentary job appealed to a lazier type of individual. Initial differences between the two groups limit the interpretation of what is otherwise an excellent retrospective survey; unfortunately, the drivers had a greater risk of a manifest "coronary attack" than the conductors on the day that they commenced working for the London Transport System.

A third type of retrospective investigation has compared the longevity of former sportsmen such as Cambridge "blues" with that of the general population. In early studies of this sort, the claim was made that sportsmen lived rather longer than average; however, when account was taken of the economic privileges enjoyed by University graduates, the life expectancy of the athletes was seen to be comparable with that of sedentary scholars graduating from the same institutions. Other fallacies were then exposed. Life expectancy did not necessarily reflect the coronary death rate—in fact, athletes showed an excess of noncoronary fatalities, particularly violent deaths in motor accidents and the like. It was further shown that on leaving University, the "athletes" rarely maintained a high level of habitual activity; indeed, at the age of forty, the ex-athletes were in poorer physical condition than their sedentary colleagues, smoking more, drinking more, and having a larger excess weight. One group that persist with vigorous recreational activity until old age are the cross-country skiers of Sweden and Finland. In the Scandinavian countries, large segments of a town or village will participate in regular twenty-mile cross-country races, and if a comparison is drawn between the active and inactive villagers, those who are active live for some seven years longer than the sedentary members of the same community. This, incidentally, is a much larger gain of life expectancy than could be achieved by giving up smoking (p. 333). Unfortunately, it still fails to prove a causal relationship between activity and cardiovascular health, since those who enjoy exercise may also differ constitutionally from the more sedentary villagers.

Community studies have been initiated in the small United States towns of Framingham (Mass.) and Tecumseh (Mich.). Activity has been assessed by questionnaires, interviews, and simple step tests, and benefit has been shown for those members of the community who lead an active life; even walking has given some protection against ischaemic heart disease. Unfortunately, the general level of activity in the United States is so low that it has been difficult to define active groups; furthermore, as in Scandinavia, there remains the vexing question of the initial equivalence of those who like to walk and those who prefer a sedentary life.

Prospective Evidence. Many investigators have concluded that a carefully-planned prospective study would yield a conclusive answer concerning the effects of physical activity upon cardiovascular health. Ideally, a randomly selected population would be allocated between two groups. One group would undertake regular known amounts of intensive physical exercise, using some type of ergometer, while the second group would remain indolent. There are many practical problems to such an undertaking. Let us make the rather optimistic assumption that exercise reduces the incidence of fresh coronary attacks from two cases per thousand man years to one case per thousand man years. Even if we assembled a group of ten thousand volunteers and followed them meticulously for five years, we should be comparing approximately fifty deaths in the inactive group with twenty-five deaths in the active group. This is barely enough to convince a skeptical statistician. Unfortunately, our experiment is most unlikely to achieve this level of confidence. Firstly, the probable benefit of exercise is less than suggested; we may rather be comparing 1.5 with two deaths per thousand man years. This immediately increases the necessary sample size by a factor of four. Then we are faced with the problem of "dropouts." If we start our programme with an exercise group of five thousand, within a year 50 percent will have defected. Perhaps 20 percent will have moved out of town, others will have suffered minor injuries, and many will have lost interest in the experiment. Formal studies of attrition have been limited to a total of eighteen months. But let us suppose that the loss of subjects continues unchecked. In the fifth year, our sample of five thousand has shrunk to a pitiful 156. Furthermore, these are not a normal group. Some are dogged and devoted subjects, while others are people who have failed to be promoted, or who have had their natural mobility restricted for other reasons. They are men who have escaped from home three nights per week and have built up a fine spirit of camaradie; they have also exchanged advice on smoking, diet, and the healthful life in general, so that even if we can show an apparent benefit in the exercised group, it may be attributable to factors other than to the exercise *per se.*

The United States Public Health Service has recently carried out a number of pilot studies to determine the probable cost of a definitive investigation linking exercise and cardiovascular health. The likely figure seems some $30 million. One way to reduce this exorbitant figure would be to minimize the "drop-out" rate.

The only identifying feature so far discovered by the United States investigators has been a poor credit rating! However, work conducted in this laboratory shows that the "drop-out" is also heavier than his more persistent colleague, smokes more, and is likely to be engaged in a personal programme (such as Cooper's *Aerobics*) rather than a group exercise plan. A second method of reducing the cost of an experiment is to restrict the survey to those who are coronary prone, with extensive business problems, high cigarette consumption, obesity, inactivity, a high blood pressure, high serum cholesterol, and a poor glucose tolerance curve. If the incidence of coronary attacks can be increased tenfold by this approach, then the necessary sample size is decreased by a factor of one hundred. It still remains to be seen whether a manageable project can be devised by such measures, and if so, whether there will be investigators and supporting agencies willing to devote themselves to what could be a lifetime study. Nevertheless, the question is important to the future of modern metropolitan man and deserves resolution.

Mechanisms Whereby Exercise Could Prevent Ischaemic Heart Disease

If there were no obvious mechanisms whereby exercise could protect the myocardium against ischaemic disease, it would be difficult to justify the large and expensive prospective investigation suggested above. But we may suggest several potential ways in which exercise could influence the atherosclerotic process.

Burning of Excess Calories. In animals, forced activity can decrease the extent of atheromatous plaques—particularly if a diet rich in animal fat is given at the same time. The mechanism seems a burning of excess calories. Unfortunately, it is difficult to demonstrate this effect if the animal remains on a normal diet, undertaking the more moderate levels of exercise practical for a presently sedentary man. Nevertheless, studies of primitive populations and of soldiers engaged in long forced marches provide some evidence that man can eat large quantities of animal fat and/or sugar without raising his serum lipids, providing he undertakes sufficient physical activity.

Development of Coronary Collaterals. Many authors have suggested that exercise stimulates the development of collateral vessels within the myocardium. In the event of coronary occlusion, the heart muscle then has an alternative route of blood supply. The initial basis of this hypothesis was the well-known effect of oxygen lack in dilating the coronary arterioles. Studies in both animals subjected to forced exercise and ageing marathon runners have shown some enlargement of the coronary tree relative to sedentary controls; however, this does not prove that collateral vessels have shared in the enlargement of the coronary vasculature. Some authors have claimed an enlargement of collateral vessels in dogs given experimental coronary infarcts and subsequently required to exercise. More recent investigations, while confirming these claims, have shown an equal development of collaterals in sedentary dogs. Relatively few tests have been made in man, since the usual method of visualizing the coronary arteries (the injection of a thick, radio-opaque dye) is itself liable to embarass the myocardial oxygen supply and precipitate ventricular fibrillation. Classical reports that patients can "run through" an anginal attack support the view that exercise produces at least a transient dilatation of collateral vessels. However, there is no conclusive evidence that exercise can bring about a permanent change in the dimensions of the collateral circulation.

Changes in Blood Coagulability. Exercise can modify the coagulability of the blood (p. 237). The acute response is usually an enhancement of clotting, but the more long-term reaction is a favouring of fibrinolysis.

Uniqueness of Exercise. Although it is possible to suggest several mechanisms whereby exercise could exert a beneficial effect on the coronary-prone patient, we should note that not all of these mechanisms are unique to exercise. The tendency to an excessive intake of calories can be controlled, albeit less successfully, by diet rather than by physical activity. The collateral circulation can be improved by surgical operations. The coagulability of the blood can be decreased by drugs. The mood may be improved, with a lowering of blood pressure and a diminished secretion of catecholamines, if the patient is taught suitable techniques of relaxation. Such alternative forms of therapy may also reduce the probability of a coronary attack.

Intensity of Exercise. The intensity of exercise required in

any prophylactic programme depends upon the type of benefit
that is sought. If we believe that heart disease will be controlled
by preventing obesity or providing pleasurable relaxation, then
quite mild effort may suffice. If we seek to reduce the stress of
unanticipated vigorous effort, then the training threshold
(p. 448) must be passed, and if we seek to dilate the coronary
collaterals, then it will be necessary to exercise to the rather
dangerous level where myocardial oxygen lack is induced.

Primary Prophylaxis

Let us now jump forward several steps. We have carried out
a prospective study, and have shown (as we currently suspect)
that exercise reduces the incidence of ischaemic heart disease.
We have further established how exercise produces this effect,
and we have concluded that although a similar response could
be brought about in other ways, exercise is the procedure of
choice. How should the physical educator or the practitioner
of public health seek to change public attitudes and provide
the facilities needed for greater activity?

Attitudes are formed at an early age. The chances of reform-
ing the habitually sedentary adult are poor. Temporary converts
can be bought by intensive advertising that concentrates on
fear of heart attacks (in the male), and on weight reduction and
glamorous facilities (in the female); studies of commercial
gymnasia show the cost is about $40 to $50 per convert. The
enthusiasm of the average novitiate soon wanes. If you operate
a small and cramped gymnasium this may not be too alarming
a trend, but if your concern is public health it is essential to
ensure that interest in physical activity is life-long. The solution
may be more effective instruction within the school system,
with the emphasis upon activities that can be performed as a
family, using a minimum of equipment.

Available space and facilities will be particularly important
if sport again becomes popular. Current facilities in most urban
centres are grossly inadequate, particularly if they are related
to the entire population. The only reason that swimming pools,
ice rinks, tennis courts and the like are not more overcrowded

is that so few of the population take any exercise. Part of the cost of providing more facilities could perhaps be justified in terms of the economic loss attributable to heart disease; in the year 1972, this may well reach $400 per wage earner. Unfortunately, land prices in the major urban conglomerations are now so high that it would cost even more to provide every citizen with the opportunity to participate in formal athletic programmes. On the other hand, if the necessary physical activity was based on walking, jogging, cycling and domestic hobbies, then the cost to government could be minimal.

Secondary Prophylaxis

Benefits of Secondary Prophylaxis

Requests for physical activity programmes come most frequently from those who have already sustained a "coronary" attack. As with primary prophylaxis, there is little "hard" evidence of the value of exercise. Some authors have claimed that attacks recur 50 percent to 70 percent less frequently in their exercise classes than in normal medical practice. Unfortunately, the comparison is invalid, since it ignores the important general benefits conferred on the exercise class—advice on smoking and diet, and the value of a more disciplined approach to life. The main present justification for the coronary exercise class lies not in the survival of members, but in the quality of life they enjoy. It is surely preferable for a "coronary" victim to be restored to four years of full activity, rather than live an unhappy and very restricted life for five years.

Immediate Treatment of the "Coronary" Patient

At one time, it was feared that premature activity might lead to a rupture of the heart at the site of infarction. However, it is now recognized that such occurrences are rare—the main hazards are cardiac failure and the development of an arrhythmia, and if the first twenty-four hours are passed safely, the prognosis rapidly improves.

Unless the patient shows signs of heart failure, shock, intractable pain, or uncontrolled arrhythmia, exercise may be commenced within twenty-four hours. Over the next week, effort is restricted to a maximum of about 2.5 kcal/min. This initially includes such items as sitting at 45° in bed, feeding oneself, and carrying out light physiotherapeutic exercises to individual muscle groups. By the end of the week, the patient is sitting in a chair for three one hour periods per day.

In the second and third weeks, activity is gradually increased to occasional peaks of 3.8 kcal/min. The patient undertakes such tasks as washing and cleaning his teeth, and may engage in light craft work while preparing himself for home care. Walking is commenced in the second week, and by the third week amounts to one hundred feet per trip. Each new stage in the activity programme is tried before rather than after a meal, and the electrocardiographic response is carefully watched for signs of an adverse reaction.

In the fourth week, the patient may be transferred to a convalescent facility, and at this stage he should aim at walking half a mile at a stretch. Within eight weeks, he should reach his previous level of activity, and be prepared for the energy expenditures involved in most forms of industrial work. Thereafter, further progress may be made through specific exercise classes.

Exercise for the "Post-coronary" Patient

Even eight weeks after the acute episode, there is still some risk that acute exercise may precipitate ventricular fibrillation or infarction. This risk is minimized if the exercise tolerance of the patient is assessed by periodic laboratory evaluation. Such evaluation not only enables the physician to monitor accurately the rate of improvement in cardiorespiratory fitness, but also serves to define the level of physical activity at which adverse signs or symptoms may be expected. A patient of average intelligence can be quoted a "safe" pulse reading, and can be trained to measure his immediate postexercise heart rate, holding it below the prescribed level. He can also be trained to recognise extrasystoles, and to halt exercise momentarily should these become frequent. Angina is generally a rather late symptom, and myocardial oxygen lack (as shown by depression of the ST segment of the electrocardiogram) can be diagnosed at an earlier stage; normally, the patient is prescribed a pulse rate intended to restrict his ST depression to 0.2 mV or less.

A physician should undoubtedly be present when the safe limit of exercise is defined or revised. He should also be equipped and prepared to carry out external cardiac message and/or defibrillation should this prove necessary. There is much to commend the idea of the postcoronary patient attending at least one physician-supervised gymnasium session per week. Gymnasium work may include warm-up calisthenics, interval running, and free sporting activity. The calisthenics should avoid movements that involve the sustained support of the body weight by the arms, as this causes an undue rise of blood pressure and cardiac work (p. 66). An interval sequence of jogging and slow walking is better than continuous running, for the same reason. Unfortunately, the total number of coronary victims is so large that it would be impracticable to arrange medically supervised activity more frequently than once per week. The postinfarct patient must thus continue the intervening sessions of his exercise programme under the guidance of a physical educator or even a fellow patient, himself watching for an excessive rise of pulse rate, extrasystoles, and other untoward symptoms.

The majority of patients have a substantial fear of their disease, and are unlikely to exercise too hard; indeed, the problem may be to get them to exercise hard enough, particularly when they are away from medical supervision. The extent of personal activity may be followed by requiring patients to keep a logbook (p. 31) and by observing the response to objective physiological tests. Care must be taken to avoid any spirit of competition; each patient should progress at his own speed, and some slowing of training may be necessary if the weather is warm or business commitments are heavy. Young "coronary" cases can eventually return to very active lives, but men of a "postmenopausal" age sometimes show disappointing response even with several years of conscientious training.

Work Tolerance of the "Postcoronary" Patient

In the past, the majority of patients who have survived a coronary infarction have seriously restricted their subsequent economic activity. However, the recent success of training regimes has shown that such restriction is unnecessary. It certainly makes the patient unhappy, and it may even have an adverse effect upon the incidence and severity of recurrent infarction.

Quite low energy expenditures are involved in most industrial operations. Typical factory work requires an energy usage of less than 4 kcal/min, and it thus falls within the competence of the average patient within a few weeks of infarction. Where there is doubt as to the patient's working capacity, an objective exercise test is invaluable. Some patients are very good at simulating disability, and in one series of "postcoronary" cases there was no more than 70 percent agreement between subjective and physiological evaluations of working capacity. Many large cities now have *work classification units* where patients can be examined by a team of specialists that includes physicians, vocational and social workers, psychologists and physiologists. Such units not only place the coronary cripple in suitable employment, but follow his subsequent progress. Most of those seen are initially unemployed. However, as many as 60 percent are employable. In Boston, 16 percent of employable patients were already active in their previous jobs, and a further 44 percent were able to return to their accustomed work; 10 percent required some adjustment of their duties, and new tasks were found for the remaining 40 percent.

In general, the "coronary" victim is more conscientious that the average worker, and the subsequent employment record of men placed by work classification units is good. The Belle-Vue (New York) unit found 50 percent still working in the post obtained for them after the elapse of one year. The Cleveland unit commented that employment of such patients was dangerous to neither the employee nor his employer, and a study at the Gillette razor factory showed that the "postcoronary" patient was superior to the average worker on a number of objective criteria such as performance, accident rate, absenteeism and earnings of premium payments.

The patient who can exercise without symptoms is usually capable of full employment. If symptoms are occasionally found with vigorous exercise, he should still work full time, but take added rest. Only if symptoms are frequent should employment be restricted. Despite these simple rules, in actual practice motivation, experience, training, and the anxiety of the patient and his family are more important than the disease process in determining the likelihood of a successful return to work.

Medico-legal Considerations

Since there is some evidence that vigorous activity can precipitate a "coronary" attack, there are important medico-legal implications for those who require hard work of an individual, whether this be carried out in a gymnasium, a laboratory or a factory. The courts have commonly assumed that a temporal relationship between activity and a coronary infarction is presumptive evidence of "cause and effect." If there has been a substantial interval of time between the supposed stress and the "coronary" episode, compensation is unlikely to be awarded unless there is a history of "bridging" symptoms.

Exercise and Other Forms of Disease

Convalescence

The general value of graded physical activity during convalescence is well recognised. Prolonged bed rest or inactivity following bone injury is accompanied by a loss of aerobic power, muscle wasting, decalcification of bones, and an increase of subcutaneous fat. All of these defects can be corrected by a suitable progressive training regime (p. 439).

General Health

It is less certain whether exercise has any positive effect upon the level of general health. From the viewpoint of the employer, the main problem of the present day is not major illness, but uncertified minor illness and absenteeism. This can be a physiological problem—the worker may have an aerobic power that is inadequate to meet the demands of both home and an eight-hour day. But frequent absenteeism usually has a psychological basis; often, it is a reaction to the drudgery of modern production-line tasks. Exercise may help to relieve this boredom and provide an outlet where personal achievement and success can be recognised. Absenteeism is infrequent among those holding responsible executive positions; however, even in such individuals exercise could minimise the duration and frequency of major illnesses. It could also increase productivity "on the job" by increasing the level of cortical arousal. An increase of arousal is beneficial in most people, but there are undoubtedly some who remain overaroused throughout a day's work, and in such people exercise may have an adverse effect upon performance.

Specific Medical Problems

Exercise has its advocates in the treatment of a number of specific medical conditions. If the middle-aged and overweight diabetic can be persuaded to undertake regular physical activity, then he will require a smaller dosage of insulin. Exercise may also be helpful in dispelling the anxieties of neurotic patients. Some authors have claimed that training leads to a dramatic improvement in patients suffering from chronic obstructive lung disease; certainly, the duration of slow treadmill walking is greatly extended, but it is less clear whether this is due to an improvement of cardiac status, or whether it merely reflects a lessening of fear and the learning of a more efficient technique of walking. Many patients with chronic disease are in a detrained state due to habitual restriction of physical activity, and it is likely that a proportion of such patients would respond favourably to an increase in their level of training. However, the right heart is already under considerable strain in many cases of chronic obstructive lung disease and it is then more difficult to see how an increase of physical activity could be beneficial.

Other Adverse Effects of Exercise

Our balance sheet would not be complete if adverse effects of exercise were not also briefly discussed. Injuries are a serious hazard in many sports, particularly if competition is intense, and often an injury may be expected after fifty to sixty days of play (Table XXXII).

The possibility of cardiovascular death—whether from infarction, heart failure, or rupture of an aneurysm has already been mentioned (p. 509). To this toll must be added occasional deaths from trauma, drowning, cold exposure, and heat stress.

Serious infective diseases such as poliomyelitis and typhoid fever may be contracted while swimming in infected water. Minor infections of the feet (athlete's foot) and groin (dobie itch) of the eyes and external ear, and of the skin are hazards encountered by all athletes. Again, the swimmer is particularly at risk.

Lastly, exercise can exacerbate a preexisting infection. If the

TABLE XXXII
THE NUMBER OF DAYS PARTICIPATION IN A GIVEN SPORT
BEFORE AN INJURY IS SUSTAINED*

Sport	Number of Days
Wrestling	50
Football	51
Rugger	54
Basketball	107
Soccer	140
Hockey	190
Squash	253
Boxing	375
Swimming	1399
Rowing	7865

* Data obtained by the author and his associates at the University of Toronto; "injuries" were here of sufficient severity to require treatment by the attendant surgeon.

patient has polio virus circulating in the blood stream, the microorganism may localize in the active ventral horn cells (p. 173). If there is a quiescent tuberculous lesion within the lungs, this may be activated by vigorous ventilatory efforts.

Most adverse effects of exercise can be avoided if suitable safety and hygienic measures are adopted. Accidents are much less likely if the players are fairly matched, if rules are rigorously applied, if contests are prohibited when ground conditions are unfavourable, and if safety equipment is carefully sized and correctly worn. Heat deaths are unlikely if attention is paid to environmental conditions (p. 306, 323), the fluid balance of the contestants is maintained (p. 316) and permeable garments are worn. The spread of infection can be checked through preliminary showering and inspection of contestants, control of water quality, and adequate drainage and ventilation of changing areas. Such measures are important if exercise is not to fall into unwarranted disrepute. The problem of the occasional coronary death is more difficult to control, but even here, the chances of survival are greatly increased if a clear plan of procedure has been laid down for all staff of an athletic facility (p. 548–551).

References

Shephard, R.J. (Ed.): International Symposium on Physical Activity and Cardiovascular Health. *Canad Med Ass J, 96*:695–917, 1967.

White, P.D., Rusk, H.A., Lee, P.R., and Williams, B.: *Rehabilitation of the Cardiac Patient,* New York, McGraw Hill, 1958.

Rosenbaum, F.F., and Belknap, E.L.: *Work and the Heart.* New York, Hoeber, 1959.

Likoff, W., and Moyer, J.H.: *Coronary Heart Disease.* New York, Grune & Stratton, 1963.

Raab, W.: *Prevention of Ischemic Heart Disease.* Springfield, Thomas, 1966.

Stamler, J.: *Lectures on Preventive Cardiology.* New York, Grune & Stratton 1967.

Stamler, J., Stamler, R., and Pullman, T.N.: *The Epidemiology of Hypertension.* New York, Grune & Stratton, 1967.

Harrison, T.R., and Reeves, T.J.: *Principles and Problems of Ischemic Heart Disease.* Chicago, Year Book Publishers, 1968.

Evang, K., and Andersen, K.L.: *Physical Activity in Health and Disease.* Baltimore, Williams & Wilkins, 1966.

Karvonen, M.J., and Barry, A.J.: *Physical Activity and the Heart.* Springfield, Thomas, 1967.

Symposium on Cardiovascular Stress Testing. *J Occup Med 10:*627–662, 1968.

Haimevici, H.: Atherosclerosis: Recent Advances. *Ann NY Acad Sci 149:* 585–1068, 1968.

Lenti, G.: Symposium on "Aspects physiologiques et cliniques de la réadaptation du cardiaque." *Mal Cardiovasc 10:*1–476, 1969.

Parmley, L.: Proceedings of the national workshop on exercise in the prevention, in the evaluation, in the treatment of heart disease. *S Carol Med J, 65:* Suppl. 1.

Skrien, T.: Physical activity and injury (Sports injuries at the University of Toronto 1951–1968). M.Sc. Thesis, University of Toronto, 1970.

PART FOUR

SPECIAL TOPICS

18

MECHANICS OF SELECTED ACTIVITIES

The gross energy costs of various industrial and athletic pursuits have been summarized in Tables XXI and XXII. Such data are useful in preparing an exercise prescription. The object of the present chapter is to supplement this basic data with a more detailed discussion of physiological concerns in the performance of specific activities.

Standing

Benedict showed many years ago that a man used at least 9 percent more energy when standing than when in the lying position. The extra energy is spent in the maintenance of posture. Least work is performed if the knee joints are securely locked and a large part of the body weight is transmitted directly through the long bones to the ground. Added effort is required if the centre of gravity is either permanently displaced to one side of equilibrium (as with a slouching posture) or oscillates about a neutral position (as with an excess of muscular tension). The choice of a suitable posture reduces the oxygen cost of many industrial and domestic tasks (p. 209).

Walking

Over the normal range of walking speeds (2–4 miles per hour), a man with a body weight of 70 kg has an energy expenditure E of

$$E = 1.28V + 0.5 \text{ kcal/min}$$

where V is his speed in miles per hour. As with other tasks, the energy expenditure is also a function of body weight, so that at a speed of three miles per hour

$$E = 0.047W + 1.02 \text{ kcal/min}$$

where W is the body weight in kilogrammes. Some authors have found a lower cost per unit weight in women than in men (possibly because women use less exuberant movements).

At moderate speeds, walking is a more efficient mode of progression than running. Margaria has suggested that when walking, a proportion of the potential energy developed in raising the centre of gravity of the body is reconverted to kinetic energy as the body descends. The mechanical efficiency is about 25 percent for positive work (lifting the body weight), and about −120 percent for negative work (the lowering of body weight); the latter figure implies that the energy expenditure during descent is 80 percent of the potential energy that has to be dissipated. The overall mechanical efficiency of level walking is thus 20.7 percent.

> The oxygen costs quoted apply to men traversing ideal surfaces; energy expenditures are much increased by a rough field (as in cross-country running) or by a heavy snowfall. Work is also increased if weather conditions require the wearing of heavy clothing. Repetition of treadmill walking has relatively little influence upon oxygen cost; exceptions to this generalization include rapid walking (where the subject may learn to move his arms less exuberantly) and the maintenance of a fixed position on a steeply sloping treadmill (an unnatural type of exercise).

The oxygen cost of walking rises steeply at speeds above four miles per hour, and a champion who walks at eight miles per hour has an oxygen consumption as great or greater than that of a man running at the same speed (Fig. 94). Ralston has suggested a quadratic formula for estimating the energy expenditure of fast walking. This may be written in the form

$$E = 2.03 + 0.265(V^2) \text{ kcal/min}$$

where V is the speed in miles per hour.

At eight miles per hour, the calculated energy expenditure is 18.9 kcal/min—corresponding quite well with measurements made on an Olympic walker (oxygen consumption 4 litre/min STPD).

> A load such as a soldier's pack is best carried on the back. In this position, the added oxygen cost is slightly less than that of an

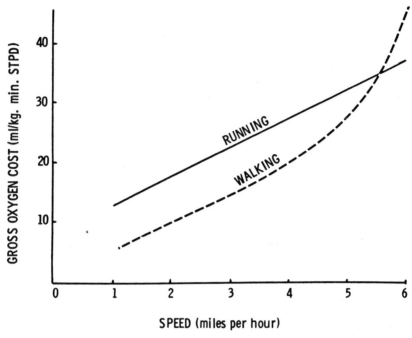

Figure 94. A comparison of the oxygen cost of walking and of running on a level treadmill.

equivalent increase of body weight. A load applied elsewhere (for instance, a pair of heavy boots) is less well tolerated. Efficiency also deteriorates if the load exceeds 30 percent of body weight. Unfortunately, it is sometimes necessary for a soldier to carry much heavier burdens, and considerable thought must thus be given to the weight of personal military equipment.

Stair-climbing

Stair-climbing is one of the few current activities in most Canadian homes. It is also the probable basis of cardiorespiratory health in the London bus conductor (p. 515). The overall efficiency of stepping, as normally calculated, is rather low (about 16 percent, p. 23). However, if account is taken of the cost of descent (about a quarter of the total energy expenditure), then the efficiency of climbing is similar to that of many other tasks (21–22%).

Running

The oxygen cost of treadmill running is linearly related to speed and slope (Fig. 94) and is influenced relatively little by sex and athletic ability. Most subjects are unfamiliar with treadmill running and there is thus a small decrease of energy expenditure (5%–10%) if a run is repeated on successive days.

The optimum stride length increases with speed, from thirty-one to thirty-two inches at 5 mph, to as much as eighty to ninety inches at 18 to 20 mph; the frequency of stride increases less, from 170/min at moderate speeds to 230/min in maximum effort. An experienced runner normally chooses a running pattern close to his optimum. As noted elsewhere (p. 218), stride frequency is limited by the natural frequency of the part. In short distance events, the economy of true ballistic movement may be sacrificed; a sprinter can exceed his natural limb frequency, executing forced movements throughout the range of leg motion. However, if a long-distance runner adopts such tactics, he will be outclassed by competitors with equal aerobic power, but a more economical technique of running.

It is often claimed that the energy cost of travelling a given distance is independent of speed. This concept holds for men walking or running on a treadmill at moderate speeds, but it does not apply to an athlete running on a track at high speed. Under track conditions, wind resistance is a nonlinear function of velocity, and the energy cost of running a given distance varies as the 2.8th power of the speed.

Margaria has measured the mechanical efficiency of running, taking into account both vertical oscillations of the trunk and changes of limb speed as assessed by cinematography. His data indicate the "impossibly" high answer of 40 percent to 45 percent; it may be that as the foot strikes the ground, kinetic energy is absorbed by the contracting leg muscles, to be released during the next stride.

Friction between the foot and the ground limits running speed. The force developed per stride can be resolved (Fig. 95) into a vertical component (proportional to body weight) and a horizontal component (proportional to speed). Slipping is

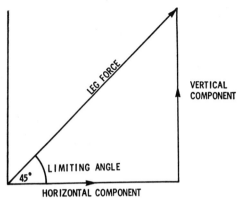

Figure 95. Resolution of forces developed by the leg during running into a vertical component (proportional to body weight) and a horizontal component (proportional to running speed). Slipping occurs if the resultant force operates at an angle of less than 45° to the track.

likely to occur if the resultant of these two forces makes an angle of less than 45° with the track. If friction is reduced by a dusty surface, then the speed must be proportionately reduced; conversely, if friction is increased by spiked shoes, greater speeds are possible. In moon-walking, the running speed is severely restricted by a diminution of effective body weight, and the most effective mode of progression is probably a form of jumping.

Downhill Skiing

Downhill skiing is of interest as an active sport that is gaining popularity in North America. The intensity of exercise depends on the speed that is attained. Measurements on champions have shown oxygen consumptions of 3–4 litre/min, but the normal recreational skier does not approach this figure. Substantial isometric loads are thrown upon the legs, and the champions often have very strong extensor muscles. The intense isometric contractions also lead to large accumulations of blood lactate (100–140 mg/100 ml) even if the total duration of activity is less than a minute. Competitors are under considerable psychic stress during the slalom events, and the coupling of anxiety, a high oxygen consumption and intense isometric activity may yield "supramaximal" pulse rates (p. 51).

Cross-country Skiing

Cross-country skiing is a popular sport in Scandinavia, and it apparently contributes to longevity (p. 516). The required energy expenditure varies with (a) snow conditions (being least when the snow is firmly packed), (b) the speed of travel (Fig. 96), and (c) the weight of any pack that is carried.

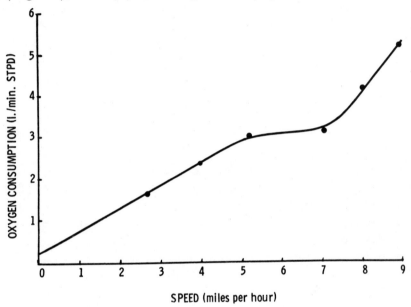

Figure 96. The influence of speed upon the energy cost of cross-country skiing (based on data of Christensen and Hogberg).

Northern armies have traditionally travelled on skis, and military laboratories have thus found it useful to compare the cost of carrying loads on the back and upon a small sleigh. The back is a more economical mode of transport, but the sleigh has advantages for the movement of bulky and awkward objects.

Snowshoes are still used in rural Canada. In general, skis provide a more economical method of travelling, but much depends on snow conditions.

Skating

As with walking and running, the oxygen cost of recreational skating is linearly related to the speed of movement, so that the energy usage is related quite closely to the distance traversed. Although a useful source of activity in the winter months, normal skating cannot be regarded as a strenuous sport. If measurements are extended to the speeds reached by Olympic champions (Fig. 97), the relationship between velocity and

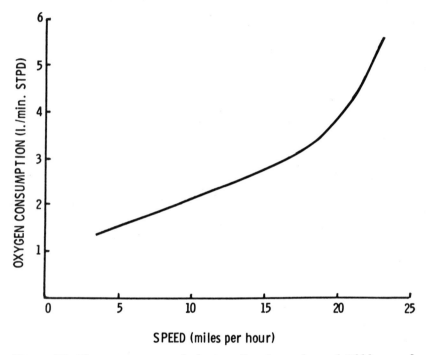

Figure 97. The energy cost of skating. Based on data of Ekblom and associates.

energy expenditure becomes curvilinear. Speed skating can then become a physically demanding activity, and under such conditions, a large part of the total energy loss is attributable to wind resistance.

Swimming

The energy cost of various swimming strokes is illustrated in Fig. 98. The curves refer to skilled swimmers. Much higher costs are encountered if an inexperienced person attempts to move at comparable speeds. Competitive swimming is evidently a very intensive form of activity, and in the shorter

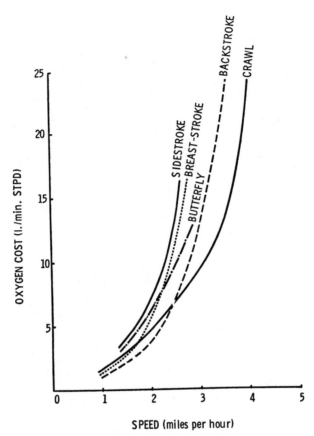

Figure 98. The relationship between swimming speed and energy consumption (based on data of Karpovich and associates; to permit comparison with other modes of activity, 5 kCal of energy cost assumed = 1 litre O_2).

events a large part of the total energy cost must be borne by oxygen debt mechanisms. The oxygen consumption has been measured during endurance events; values have amounted to 80 percent to 100 percent of the maximum oxygen intake as measured by normal laboratory procedures. A person who chooses to exercise in the water faces a number of unusual physiological problems. Adoption of the prone or supine position eliminates postural work. Compression of the limbs and thorax reduces lung gas volumes, increases the pulmonary blood volume, and imposes an external work load upon the chest muscles. Water immersion increases body heat loss, and in consequence skin blood flow and resting pulse rate are diminished, while there is a tendency to shiver if the water temperature is more than 3–4° C below the neutral temperature (33–34° C). Breathing must be coordinated with swimming; one breath is taken per stroke during the crawl (40–70 strokes/min) and two breaths per cycle in the back stroke (32 cycles/min). Lastly, a large part of the total work of swimming is performed by the arm muscles.

In view of these various peculiarities of physiology, it is hardly surprising that the normal sedentary subject fails to develop his full maximal oxygen intake while he is in the water. On the other hand, a trained swimmer with well-developed arm muscles may achieve a higher oxygen consumption while swimming than when he is performing some laboratory exercise that stresses specific and less-well trained leg muscles.

The oxygen cost of swimming is influenced by buoyancy. Short distance swimmers have a normal percentage of body fat, but long distance swimmers are typically more obese than other athletes. The extra fat not only keeps them afloat, but also provides insulation in chill waters. Because of the difference of body configuration between sprint and distance swimmers, Pugh found that the energy expenditure of English cross-channel competitors was only about a half of that shown in Fig. 98. For the same reason, most women spend less energy than men while swimming at a given speed. If the aerobic power of a distance swimmer is expressed in the traditional units (ml/kg min), he often appears rather unfit. However, fat is an advantage rather than a disadvantage to aquatic performance, and it is thus not particularly meangingful to divide maximum oxygen intake by body weight; if expressed in absolute units (litre/min), the distance swimmer has a substantial aerobic power.

The mechanical efficiency of swimming is low. The work performed by a swimmer can be estimated roughly from the force required to drag him through the water at a steady rate. Other causes of energy loss such as acceleration and deceleration of the limbs and alterations in the configuration of the body are ignored with this approach, and the very low value of 2–4 percent efficiency is obtained. This should be compared not with the efficiency of bicycle ergometry (23%), but with that of arm work (18%–20% in the author's laboratory). The drag encountered by a swimmer includes viscous and turbulent water resistance, and effects due to hydroplaning and the creation of a bow wave. At racing speeds, drag increases as the square of water velocity, with a tendency to hydroplaning between 1.3 and 4.5 miles per hour, and the appearance of a bow wave at 4.5 miles per hour. The drag is doubled by the carriage of SCUBA equipment.

A well-performed crawl is the most economical racing stroke (Fig. 98). The "butterfly" rapidly causes fatigue of the back and shoulder muscles, and it only becomes an economical mode of progression at high speeds, where water turbulence is an increasing problem.

Differences in the energy expenditure of recreational swimmers reflect the experience of the individual rather than the type of stroke that he is using. Karpovich has suggested that a poor swimmer spends five times as much energy as a champion performer who is moving at the same speed. Detailed study of movement patterns suggests that the experienced swimmer learns to avoid sudden accelerations and decelerations of the arms (p. 219). The energy cost of moving at moderate speeds is reduced somewhat if fins are worn.

Calisthenics

Many exercise regimes for both school-children and middle-aged adults have a heavy emphasis upon calisthenics. Their effectiveness in improving cardiorespiratory fitness depends upon the cadence that is adopted (p. 448, 456). The average pulse rate attained during a business men's calisthenics class may be no more than ninety to one hundred per minute, but with a firm instructor, the oxygen consumption can rise to a substantial fraction of aerobic power.

Bicycling

Most data refer to the use of a laboratory bicycle ergometer. In recreational cycling, the load is imposed by a combination of frictional resistance, wind resistance and any opposing wind force. Laboratory usage of the bicycle suggests that an average sedentary man can sustain a load of 1200 kgm/min for a few minutes, and perhaps 600 kgm/min over an eight hour day. Let us suppose a speed of 20 km per hour (12.5 mph). Our cyclists covers 0.33 km per minute, and exerts a total force of 1.8–3.6 kg, depending on the duration of effort. The frictional force varies with the weight of the cycle plus rider, the nature of the road surface, and the tyre width, being in the range 0.005–0.030 kg force per kg weight, or assuming a weight of 90 kg and a friction of 0.02 kg/kg a total of 1.8 kg. In the first few minutes of effort, this leaves a margin of 1.8 kg to meet wind resistance and force, but thereafter the cyclist must slow down—particularly if he is riding into the wind. The wind resistance varies as the square of road speed, and in a racing cyclist accounts for a large proportion of the total force exerted. The use of "drop" handlebars is thus valuable, even though it places an abnormal stress on the back muscles.

At recreational loadings, the optimum pedal speed is about 50 rpm; however, competitive cyclists prefer a rate of at least 80 rpm. Under racing conditions, the rate of breathing may become linked with the frequency of pedalling, and this can cause respiratory embarrassment when a steep hill is climbed. A cyclist who has been breathing steadily at forty breaths per minute finds that the rate of pedalling drops from eighty to sixty per/min; he is now inclined to breathe at a rate of sixty breaths per minute, leading to hyperventilation and a serious increase in the work of breathing. The obvious remedy is to dissociate pedalling and breathing, but some cyclists find this hard to achieve.

References

Durnin, J.V.G.A., and Passmore, R.: *Energy, Work, and Leisure.* London, Heinemann, 1967.

Karpovich, P. V.: *Physiology of Muscular Activity,* 6th ed. Philadelphia, Saunders, 1966.

Åstrand, P-O., and Rodahl, K.: *Textbook of Work Physiology.* New York, McGraw Hill, 1970.

Margaria, R.: Current concepts of walking and running. In Shephard, R.J. (Ed.): *Frontiers of Fitness.* Springfield, Thomas, 1971.

Faulkner, J.A.: Physiology of swimming and diving. In Falls, H. (Ed.): *Exercise Physiology.* New York, Academic Press, 1968.

Banister, E.W., and Brown, S.R.: The relative energy requirements of physical activity. In Falls, H. (Ed.): *Exercise Physiology.* New York, Academic Press, 1968.

19

SAFETY AND MEDICO-LEGAL
CONSIDERATIONS

Legal Responsibility

Any person arranging a programme of exercise for a human subject carries a heavy responsibility for the safety of the activities that are proposed. This responsibility is particularly great if the exercise is conceived as part of an experiment. The curiosity of the investigator must be curbed to ensure that the privacy and other rights of the subject are respected, and the individual who is tested should give his free and informed consent to all procedures that are to be carried out. Failure to respect the rights of the citizen can expose the investigator, his associates, and his superiors to charges of assault and heavy claims for damages. It is therefore important that all who work in exercise laboratories and gymnasia should understand the nature and the extent of their responsibilities.

Medical Responsibility

It is anticipated that this book will be read by both medical and paramedical personnel. At a few points, reference has thus been made to matters that are legally the responsibility of a duly qualified and registered medical practitioner. It would not be particularly helpful to specify problems that must be referred to a physician, since (a) the role of paramedical personnel is currently being reviewed in many countries, and (b) the laws governing medical practice vary from one country to another, and even from one province or state to another. The prudent physical educator will sense what lies outside of his competence, but if in doubt, the local situation should be reviewed with the appropriate medical licensing authority.

The division of responsibility between the physician and his assistants is more clearly defined for a routine investigation than for an emergency situation. Persons attending a gymnastics class may well wish to know the results of a fitness test in which they have participated, but in presenting such information, a paramedical investigator should be careful to avoid creating the impression that he is providing a diagnosis. He may have occasion to use an electrocardiograph machine, but he should emphasize that in using such equipment his purpose is to measure the pulse rate accurately and not to report upon the electrical health of the myocardium. While measuring the pulse rate, a physical educator may well recognize some common abnormality such as an arrhythmia or an ST segmental depression induced by exercise, and here lies the biggest potential source of conflict with the physician. The subject should be told that in the opinion of the experimenter the tracing looks atypical, and that a doctor should be consulted regarding this matter.

Let us now suppose that a man of thirty-five suddenly collapses while exercising in a gymnasium. The victim has received permission to exercise from his physician, and to this point has seemed completely healthy. There is no doctor on the premises, and the nearest physician is perhaps ten minutes drive away. The physical educator feels for the carotid pulse, and finds that it is absent. A "heart attack" seems likely. Unless some "medical" treatment is carried out, the patient will die in four minutes or less. If the physical educator in question has received training in external cardiac massage, he would then be justified in applying such treatment even in the absence of a physician. It is also vital that the patient should be admitted as quickly as possible to a coronary care unit. The first telephone call should thus be for an ambulance (preferably fitted with equipment for resuscitation), and the second call to a doctor's office. Paramedical personnel would be unwise to use a defibrillator outside of a hospital (although nurses in some coronary care units are permitted to use such equipment). In the unhappy event that the relatives of the patient initiated a lawsuit, it would be difficult for an inexperienced operator to prove that he had treated rather than caused the fibrillation.

What of medical approval for an exercise regime? If the exercise is required for experimental purposes, the subject should invariably be examined either by his personal physician or by a medically qualified member of the laboratory staff. Furthermore, the details of the proposed procedures should be approved by both a physician and a committee on the ethics of human experimentation (p. 553). No exercise experiment involving human subjects should proceed unless a qualified physician is available in the building where the test is to be carried out. For some procedures, such as maximum effort testing, the physician should be physically present in the laboratory, to observe the condition of the patient under stress and to interpret any electrocardiographic changes that may develop.

A little more latitude is possible when a subject merely volunteers for an exercise class with no prompting from an eager investigator. However, in the best interests of both the patient and the operator of an athletic facility a preliminary medical examination should be recommended to those under the age of thirty, and required of any who are either older, or have suspected disease conditions.

Initial Medical Examination

When an apparently healthy patient consults his physician regarding the desirability of entering an exercise programme, the request may be approved rather lightly. What are the minimum requirements of such an examination?

Much depends upon the age of the individual. If he is under thirty years, there should be a careful physical examination with the emphasis upon the cardiorespiratory system, and a detailed history should also have been taken not earlier than one year previously. If the patient is between thirty and forty years of age, the detailed history should be of more recent origin, and the physical examination should be supplemented by the recording of both resting and exercise electrocardiograms. If the age is more than forty, exercise electrocardiograms should certainly be obtained.

In discussion with the patient, the current level of activity should be established, and reasons why the patient has become interested in fitness should be explored. Regimes may be suggested for the development of endurance, the control of weight, or the building up of the body muscles, as appropriate. Sudden progression to intense competitive effort should be avoided, particularly if the patient is more than forty years of age. Exercise should be halted if there is undue fatigue, breathlessness, sudden chest pain, or other unanticipated symptoms. In the first few weeks of training, effort should be kept to a level that permits rapid and fairly complete recovery, with a heart rate of 100/min or less ten minutes after exertion. The exercise should precede rather than follow a heavy meal, and extremes of hot and cold weather should be avoided (p. 306, 325). An adequate warm-up (p. 190) and warm-down (p. 193) are also important to a trouble-free programme.

Many of the specific contraindications to exercise have been discussed in the section on the cardiovascular system (p. 72). Exercise should be avoided if there is evidence of acute inflammation of the heart muscle ("myocarditis"), a recent myocardial infarction, severe valvular disease—especially narrowing of the aortic valve ("aortic stenosis"), failure of the right ventricle ("congestive failure") secondary to valvular disease or chronic chest disease ("decompensated cor pulmonale"), gross cardiac enlargement without obvious cause, or gross arrhythmia. Other circulatory contraindications include a known aneurysmal swelling of a major blood vessel and a gross uncontrolled increase of systemic blood pressure ("hypertension"). Exercise should be prohibited for patients with uncontrolled diabetes, and recent or suspected lodgement of clots in the pulmonary circulation ("pulmonary embolism").

Relative contraindications to exercise are largely a matter of good medical practice. A patient will require careful supervision if he has the abnormalities of cardiac rhythm and electrocardiogram discussed on page 72; congenital or acquired valvular disease of the heart, coronary atherosclerosis, organic hypertension, intense ischaemic pain in the calf muscles ("intermittent claudication") and inflammation of major veins ("thrombophlebitis") are other cardiovascular indications for a cautious approach. Musculoskeletal disorders that may restrict exercise in specific body regions include fractures, dislocations of joints, tendon and cartilage injuries, inflammation of joints ("arthritis"), and congenital or acquired malfunction of specific muscle groups. Exacerbation of a "disc" injury is a well-recognized problem of repeated treadmill running. Exercise may be contraindicated if a patient is liable to convulsive seizures, or has a history of intracranial bleeding. Acute or chronic lung disease may limit exercise, particularly if there is severe pulmonary insufficiency. Hepatic disease marked by jaundice, or renal disease with acidosis or uraemia are further indications for caution, as are diabetes needing regular insulin, and blood disorders associated with anaemia. Finally, care is necessary in convalescence from acute infections and recent surgery. In many of the conditions cited, mild exercise may be beneficial, but in order to draw up a precise balance sheet of good and harm, regular medical assessment is necessary.

Perhaps the commonest type of patient currently requesting an exercise programme is the man who has sustained a coronary infarction. It may thus be worth quoting some recommendations of the Ontario Heart Foundation concerning the admission of "coronary" patients to a graduated programme of physical training:

1. The training should commence no sooner than three months after infarction.
2. There should be no evidence of heart failure at rest or, on ordinary exertion (walking on level ground or up one flight of stairs).
3. There should be no angina at rest, and any angina of effort should be relieved by a few minutes of rest. Further, there should be no recent increase in the severity and frequency of exertional angina.
4. There should be no serious arrhythmias at rest or after exertion. However, patients with infrequent ventricular ectopic beats or paroxysmal tachycardia may be admitted to an exercise programme if the arrhythmia is not precipitated by exercise.
5. The ECG pattern should be stable, and tracings obtained at successive medical examinations should show no evidence of increasing myocardial ischaemia, either at rest or after mild exercise.
6. There should be no radiological evidence of recent cardiac enlargement (although an enlarged heart shadow would be no contraindication if due to habitual participation in athletic events).

Safety of the Exercise Regime

It is important that all concerned with the exercising of human patients understand the criteria for halting a specific bout of exercise, and for slowing the rate of progression in a graduated training programme.

Acute Indications for the Cessation of Exercise

Postmortem study of patients who have died suddenly in the gymnasium has revealed three main causes of death-coronary insufficiency, rupture of a major blood vessel, and cardiac failure.

Acute Coronary Insufficiency may induce either a fatal abnormality of cardiac rhythm or a coronary infarction. The patient may detect warning ventricular extrasystoles (p. 76) as sudden "thumps" in the chest, but the first symptom is often anginal pain (p. 502). Occasional extrasystoles may ocur prior to exercise, particularly in a nervous subject. However, frequent extrasystoles appearing for the first time during exercise are a sign that the heart muscle is becoming over-irritable, and exercise should be stopped. Myocardial oxygen lack may sometimes lead to marked alterations of atrioventricular or interventricular conduction, and to other dysrhythmias arising at a ventricular or supraventricular level. Coronary insufficiency is also indicated by a horizontal or downward sloping depression of the ST segment of the electrocardiogram. It is unwise to proceed with exercise in the face of increasing angina, rhythm disturbances of the types mentioned, or ST-segment depression of more than 0.2 millivolts. Unfortunately, ECG disturbances often become more marked in the first thirty seconds after effort is stopped. Thus, if there is any doubt as to safety, it is a proper precaution to halt an exercise test.

Normally, both anginal symptoms and ECG abnormalities disappear with rest. If anginal pain persists, a physician may recommend that the patient be given a capsule of *amyl nitrite* (5 mimims, crushed into a handkerchief) a tablet of *nitroglycerine* (0.3–1.2 mg) or a longer acting compound such as *pentaerythritol tetranitrate* (10 mg). Oxygen inhalation is also of value.

If symptoms continue for more than two minutes, a coronary infarction may be suspected. The pain associated with infarction is normally much more intense than in angina, and the patient typically shows signs of collapse. Admission to hospital is urgently required, and pending arrival of an ambulance the patient should lie quietly, breathing *oxygen* if available. The pulse should be monitored, and in the event of cardiac arrest or ventricular fibrillation, staff with the necessary training should give *external cardiac massage.* If a physician is present, he may give up to 20 mg of *morphine* i.m. to relieve pain, and in the event that ventricular fibrillation develops, he may use a d.c. defibrillator to restore a normal heart rhythm. The ECG leads are temporarily disconnected from the recorder, and in an adult of average size a stimulus of 200 watt-sec is applied to electrodes held over the aortic and apical areas of the chest wall. The intensity of successive shocks is increased progressively until fibrillation ceases. If the heart is driven into asystole, the defibrillation is followed by external cardiac massage until a normal rhythm reappears.

Rupture of a Major Blood Vessel. The two commonest sites of rupture are the aorta, and the circle of Willis (an anastomotic connection of blood vessels at the base of the brain). The precipitating cause of a vascular catastrophe is commonly an excessive rise of systemic blood pressure; this may be brought about by anger, anxiety, sustained isometric exercise, or very prolonged and intense rhythmic exercise.

Complete rupture of the aorta is rapidly fatal, and no emergency treatment of this condition is likely to be effective. A slower "leak" may give local pain as blood escapes into the vessel wall, and there will also be more general signs of collapse, including pallor, sweating, and ultimately loss of consciousness. As with haemorrhage from a torn peripheral vessel, a physician may decide to set up an infusion of *plasma or dextran* in an attempt to maintain the cerebral circulation while the patient is being transferred to hospital; a minimum blood pressure is necessary to maintain life, but excessive transfusion may worsen the condition of the damaged vessel.

Rupture of a small "berry" aneurysm in the circle of Willis gives rise to a characteristic ache at the back of the head and stiffness of the neck. The important feature of emergency treatment is to keep the patient still, thus reducing further haemorrhage. Many physicians avoid giving depressants because symptoms are thereby obscured, but some minimise restlessness by giving up to 20 mg morphine i.m. Symptoms are due to a rising intracranial pressure, and in this condition no useful purpose is served by dextrose/saline or other more persistent infusions.

Cardiac Failure. This is unlikely to occur in the absence of some initial cardiac abnormality. A preliminary medical examination should thus establish the patients upon whom a particular watch should be kept. Failure of the left side of the heart presents as an acute shortness of breath ("cardiac asthma"); warning signs are a failure of the blood pressure to rise in the anticipated manner, and a breathlessness that is grossly disproportionate to effort. Failure of the right side of the heart is shown by pain along the right margin of the rib cage, and acute venous congestion. With either left-or right-sided heart failure, the patient should be given immediate rest with the head propped up, and oxygen should be supplied if available. If the signs indicate a predominant failure of the left ventricle, a physician may give an injection of *theophylline/ethylene diamine* (250 mg i.v. or 500 mg i.m. or furosenide (40 mg i.v.) together with atropine (1–2 mg i.m.). If right-sided (congestive) failure predominates, the physician may give digoxin (2–4 ml of solution 0.25 mg/ml i.m.). If a doctor is not available immediately, a first-aid worker can reduce ventricular loading by applying tourniquets to the limbs, thereby carrying out what amounts to a physiological venesection.

Peripheral circulatory failure may occur either during, or immediately following vigorous exercise. Signs include sweating, a cold, ashen-grey pallor or cyanosis, a staggering, poorly coordinated gait, and a confused response to questioning. The main hazard is injury on falling, should consciousness be lost. Exercise should be stopped at the first signs of peripheral failure, and the patient should be supported until he can assume the prone or supine position. Sharp objects must be kept away from the scene of exercise experiments. The incidence of peripheral circulatory failure after exercise is much reduced by an adequate "warm-down" routine.

Other Indications to Halt Exercise. The physician may have other reasons for halting an exercise test, as suggested by the "relative contraindications." (p. 546). In particular, tests should be stopped if there are complaints of fatigue of physical rather than psychological origin, feelings of faintness, or marked intermittent claudication.

General Precautions in Acute Experiments. Normal sterile precautions must be observed at all times. This is particularly important when obtaining blood specimens or carrying out other procedures that involve a breach of the skin surface; nevertheless, sterility is also required in such items as mouthpieces, box-valves, and noseclips. A convenient routine for the disinfection of respiratory equipment includes washing with warm soapy water and drying immediately after use, immersion in 2% Dettol or equivalent twenty-four hours prior to further use, and rinsing in running water immediately before setting up an experiment.

The investigator must guard the subjects from injury due to both stumbling, and excessive activity without proper warm-up (p. 191). He must also be prepared for vasovagal attacks induced by the sight of a needle, blood, or some other "visceral" stimulus. Recovery from a vasovagal attack is rapid if the prone position is assumed.

Indications for Halting or Slowing a Training Programme

Minor musculo-skeletal pains are a common early accompaniment of increased activity. Nevertheless, they are a warning that training has reached the maximum desirable initial level. If discomfort becomes more acute, a temporary reduction in the frequency of exercise may be needed (for instance, the patient may train on three days per week instead of five).

Indications for a complete halt to training and detailed medical reappraisal include the onset of anginal pain, abnormalities of heart rhythm or disproportionate hyperventilation during exercise, light-headedness or collapse during or after exercise, persistent weakness, fatigue, nausea or vomiting after exercise, the development of pain or swelling in the joints, and unexpected loss of weight.

Regulations for "Health Clubs"

At present, any enterprising entrepreneur can establish a "health club." The qualifications of attendant personnel are left to the discretion of the operator, and in some cases the basis of selection seems a good figure, a pleasant smile, and an ability to persuade customers to sign a binding contract. The facilities offered are very variable, and in some instances may consist of little more than steam rooms. Although the term "health club" is used, the programme often does little to improve health. There thus seems a need to specify the conditions under which "health clubs" may operate; appropriate regulations should be drawn up either by the gymnasium operators themselves, or in default by municipal departments of health.

The requirement of initial medical examination has been discussed (p. 545). If a patient has any medical abnormality, he should obtain from his physician a clear statement of limitations to be imposed upon his activity, together with suggestions as to the type of regime best suited to his condition. Clubs using the terms "health" or "fitness" should offer facilities for active exercise such as running, cycling, or swimming; furthermore, the effectiveness of their programme in improving cardiorespiratory fitness should be evaluated by suitably testing the response of individual club members. Personnel should ideally have a degree in physical education and/or applied physiology. It is unrealistic to expect that this can be achieved "overnight," but clubs should move towards an establishment of at least one qualified staff member per five hundred subscribers, and this could perhaps become mandatory in ten years time. Exercise equipment should be tested periodically, and regular checks of electrical wiring, plumbing, and fire hazards should be instituted. Finally, inspection should ensure that municipal bylaws are met with respect to matters of hygiene, particularly water quality in the pool area, availability of showers and soap dispensers, and adequate lighting, ventilation and drainage of locker rooms.

Ethics of Human Experimentation

Review Committees

"Experiments" conducted in concentration camps during World War II shocked many consciences, and in response to this concern, the World Medical Association drafted a code of ethics to be observed by those testing human subjects. More recently, major Universities and granting agencies have approved this code, and set up suitable committees to review the ethics of all proposed experiments on man. A typical review committee includes two scientific peers of the investigator and a representative of the administrative arm of the research institution. The scientists have a working knowledge of the area to be investigated, but are unconnected with the project, while the administrative representative usually has legal training. The committee members meet with the principal investigator to review the proposed study, and satisfy themselves on three points:

1. that the rights and welfare of the individual subject are protected;
2. that the degree of information communicated and the methods used to secure informed consent of the subject are appropriate; and
3. that the risks do not outweigh the potential benefits of the investigation.

Assuming that these criteria are met, the application may be approved, but the committee continues its general surveillance of the project, and the principal investigator is required to discuss with the committee any untoward incidents, and any changes in the procedures to be followed.

Summary of Research

The principal investigator should outline the proposed project to the committee, with particular emphasis upon any minor medical or surgical procedures that are contemplated (for instance, arterial or venous puncture), the dosage and route of administration of any drugs involved, the potential exposure to irradiation, and other possible hazards of the investigation.

Method of Population Sampling

The committee must satisfy itself that all participants in the study are truly volunteers who understand the nature and extent of the risks that they are taking. This largely rules out such popular sources as technicians and students; both groups are inevitably exposed to some coercion and cannot be considered true volunteers. It also makes difficult the use of random sampling; if all risks and hazards are fairly explained to a normal population, it is unlikely that a high percentage will volunteer for testing. The investigator must be content to accept a biassed sample, and to determine the nature of this bias, estimating the effect of it upon his conclusions.

Informed Consent

All volunteers should be asked to complete a witnessed document, agreeing that the nature and risks of the investigation have been duly explained and understood, and giving their free consent to participation in the study. It is helpful if all intended procedures are listed on such a document, together with brief statements of any discomfort or incapacity that may be incurred. If the subject is a patient seeking medical treatment, experimental departures from current medical practice should be clearly specified.

Particular difficulty arises in experiments on children. The consent of both the child and his parent or legal guardian should be obtained, and the parent should be encouraged to accompany the child to the laboratory.

It should be clearly accepted that a patient has the right to withdraw from a test at any point that he chooses. This may be most inconvenient to the investigator, but it is an essential component of volunteer status.

None of these precautions will eliminate all possibility of legal complaint by the occasional litigation-minded citizen. However, the basis of any court proceedings will be a judgment on the professional competence of the investigator rather than a discussion of his violation of the basic rights of the subject.

Confidence

It is often necessary in physiological and psychological testing to obtain confidential information on the movements, background and thoughts of the subjects by means of interviews and questionnaires. Unfortunately, there are circumstances in which this information could be used against a patient. Knowledge of poor health my affect the security of employment, and knowledge of either movements or attitudes could be adduced as evidence in matrimonial cases. It is thus important that the investigator assume full responsibility for the confidence of information received, that he code the subject's name in such a manner that the documents resist a court subpoena, and that all records are destroyed once the legitimate aims of an experiment are attained.

Risks and Benefits

The reviewing committee should assess any risks of the investigation in the light of potential benefit to the community. Even if subjects are prepared to agree to hazardous or heroic procedures, these should not be permitted if the likely benefits of the experiment are few.

References

Cooper, K.H.: Guidelines in the management of the exercising patient. *JAMA, 211:* 1663–1667, 1970.
Shephard, R. T.: Ethical considerations in human experimentation. *J Canad Ass Health Phys Ed Recr, 33:* 13–16, 1967.

GLOSSARY

The use of technical terms and abbreviations can save the expert much space in writing a scientific article. On the other hand, a bewildering array of subscripts, superscripts and other strange hieroglyphs is a potent source of confusion and discouragement to the novitiate in any discipline. It may thus be helpful to summarize some of the more common jargon of the exercise physiologist, showing commonly accepted abbreviations and likely normal values in a sedentary young man. For simplicity, single values have been shown for most variables. However, in interpreting these, due allowance must be made for age, sex, size, and individual variation, as discussed in detail elsewhere in the text. Significance can rarely be attached to a result that departs by less than 20 percent from the normal standard.

Units of Work—kg-m/min; kp-m/min; watts; ft-lb/min; kcal/min

Activity is usually expressed as a rate of performing external work (a power). The units may be mechanical (force $\times$ distance—kg-m/min, ft-lb/min) electrical (watts) or thermal (kcal/min). The mode of expression commonly depends upon the technique of measurement (for instance, a mechanically braked or electrical bicycle ergometer), but the metric units of mechanical work (kg-m/min) have the widest international acceptance.

In unit gravitational field, 1 kg-m/min = 1 kp-m/min (kilopond metre per minute); in view of the small variations in gravity with latitude, and the potential confusion of pound and pond, kg-m/min seems preferable to kp-m/min.

$$427 \text{ kg-m/min} = 427 \text{ kp-m/min} = 71.5 \text{ watts}$$
$$= 3088 \text{ ft-lb/min} = 1 \text{ kcal/min}$$

Aerobic Power—$\dot{V}_{O_{2max}}$, maximum oxygen intake, aerobic capacity

The maximum oxygen intake is often described as the aerobic capacity, but it is strictly a rate of working, or power. Traditionally, it refers to brief periods of maximum effort (5–10 min), and it may be measured directly or predicted from the response to submaximum exercise. Results may be reported either as an absolute rate of gas transfer, or as an oxygen intake per unit of body weight:

$$\dot{V}_{O_2 \ max} = 3 \ litre/min \ STPD \quad \dot{V}_{O_2} \ max/kg = 44 \ ml/kg \ min \ STPD$$

$\dot{V}_{O_2,170}; PWR_{170}; PWC_{170}; W_{170}$

If it is not possible to measure the aerobic power directly, some investigators prefer to state the oxygen consumption ($\dot{V}_{O_2,170}$) or the rate of working (predicted work rate, PWR_{170}, rather than physical working capacity, PWC_{170} or W_{170}) at a closely interpolated pulse rate of 170/min. The task is easy for a younger person, but falls outside the tolerance of an older individual, for whom it is necessary to use the alternative index of PWR_{150}.

$$\dot{V}_{O_2, \ 170} = 2.4 \ litre/min \ STPD; \ PWR_{170} = 1000 \ kg\text{-}m/min;$$

$$PWR_{170}/kg = 13.5 \ kg\text{-}m/kg \ min$$

Leistungspuls Index, LPI, Oxygen Pulse

The LPI is the increase of pulse rate produced by a 60 kg-m/min increase of work load. A specially designed bicycle ergometer allows a progressive increase of loading from zero to 600 kg-m/min. The oxygen pulse is the quantity of oxygen transported per pulse beat. Sometimes the increase of pulse over resting (erholungspuls) is used in the calculation; this naturally gives a larger reading than when the absolute pulse rate is taken.

LPI = 3.5 units O_2 pulse = 12 ml, ΔO_2 pulse = 24 ml
(According to Muller, 1 LPI unit = 8.33 O_2 pulse).

MR, Met

These terms are found in studies of thermal stress. MR is the metabolic rate, and Met is the ratio of observed to basal metabolic rate.

Anaerobic Work—ATP, CP; LA, XL; R, RQ

The anaerobic power of the body is derived from adenosine triphosphate (ATP) and creatine phosphate (CP). The breakdown of one gram molecule of ATP to adenosine diphosphate (ADP) or CP to creatine (C) liberates 10–12 kcal of energy. In some books CP is also described as phosphagen. The present author regards the sum of ATP plus CP as phosphagen.

Anaerobic power is also developed by the incomplete oxidation of glycogen to lactic acid (LA). Concentrations of blood and tissue lactate are expressed in three ways: mg/100 ml of blood, mM/litre and mE/litre. In maximum effort, blood levels are

$$100 \text{ mg LA}/100 \text{ ml} = 11.1 \text{ mM/litre} = 11.1 \text{ mE/litre}$$

Huckabee attaches considerable significance to the excess lactate (XL); however, most other authors do not believe the XL adds to information yielded by measurement of LA.

Anaerobic work results in an increase of the respiratory gas exchange ratio (R). This is the ratio of CO_2 output to O_2 intake, and unlike the respiratory quotient (RQ) is influenced by changes of CO_2 stores during hyperventilation

RQ   normal 0.83   R   normal 0.83
      fat diet 0.7–0.75   maximum effort 1.15–1.20
      carbohydrate diet 0.9–1.0

Static and Dynamic Work—MVC; $\dot{V}_v$; $\dot{W}_v$

Static contractions are commonly expressed as a percentage of maximum voluntary contractions (MVC). A given percentage of MVC has similar haemodynamic consequences for muscles of widely differing strength. Normal values of MVC are given in Table XVII.

When measuring dynamic power, it is sometimes useful to record vertical velocity ($\dot{V}_v$ or vertical work ($\dot{W}_v$) using a flight of steps.

$$\dot{V}_V = 1.5 \text{ m/sec} \qquad \dot{W}_V = 6300 \text{ kg-m/min}$$

Ventilatory Capacity—VC; MC; FRC; TLV; V_T; RV

VC = vital capacity (maximum volume expired after maximal inspiration) = 5.25 litre BTPS (prediction equation p. 112).

MC = pulmonary midcapacity (average lung volume at which ventilation is carried out) = about 4.4 litre BTPS

TLV = TLC = total lung capacity = 6.50 litre BTPS

RV = residual volume = 1.25 litre BTPS (about 22% of TLC

FRC = functional residual capacity (sum of RV plus expiratory reserve, about 2.25 litre BTPS).

V_T = tidal volume, increasing from 500 ml at rest to 2500 ml in vigorous exercise.

Ventilatory Power—MVV_{100}, MBC_{100}; $FEV_{1.0}$; MVV_{40}; PEF, $\dot{V}_{max}$; $\dot{V}_{E\ max}$

MVV_{100} = maximum voluntary ventilation of a resting subject at the breathing rate specified by the subscript; it is measured over a 15 sec period, and is sometimes described as the maximum breathing capacity

$$MVV_{100} = 160 - 200\ \text{litre/min BTPS}$$

$FEV_{1.0}$ = forced expiratory volume, measured over the interval specified by the subscript (usually one second). In a young and healthy person it exceeds 80% of VC (i.e. about 4.2 litre BTPS). MVV_{40} is the indirect maximum voluntary ventilation, calculated by multiplying the $FEV_{0:75}$ by an assumed breathing rate of 40 (i.e. normal value about 120 litre/min).

PEF = peak expiratory flow rate, sometimes written $\dot{V}_{max}$. There is a danger of confusing the latter—an instantaneous velocity—with the maximum expired minute volume sustained during exercise ($\dot{V}_{E\ max}$)

$$PEF = 600\ \text{litre/min BTPS}$$

Gas Conditions—STPD, BTPS, ATPS

Ventilatory capacity and power are expressed in terms of gas volumes at body temperature and pressure, saturated with water vapour (BTPS). However, they are usually measured at atmospheric temperature and pressure, saturated with water vapour (ATPS). Volumes relating to gas transfer (such as aerobic power) are expressed as an equivalent volume of dry gas, measured under standard conditions of temperature and pressure (STPD).

1 litre STPD = approx 1.1 litre ATPS = approx 1.2 litre BTPS

Volumes are interconverted using Boyle's and Charle's Laws. The calculations can be carried out by means of a desk computer, or by reference to tables or nomograms.

Gas Transfer—$\dot{V}_E$; $\dot{V}_A$; $\dot{D}_L$; $\dot{Q}_c$; $\dot{Q}$; λ; $\dot{D}_t$; C_{I,O_2}; F_{I,O_2}; P_{I,O_2}; $\dot{U}_{O_2}$

The terminology developed by respiratory physiologists is used. The dot above a symbol implies a *time derivative*. Thus:

$\dot{V}_E$ is the volume of gas expired per minute (7 litre/min BTPS at rest, up to 120 litre/min BTPS in maximum exercise).

$\dot{V}_A$ is the alveolar ventilation (4.9 litre/min BTPS at rest, up to 90 litre/min BTPS in maximum exercise).

$\dot{D}_L$ is the "diffusing capacity" of the lungs, sometimes described as the transfer factor. Some authors believe the diffusing capacity reaches a maximum at a pulse rate of 120/min, hence the symbols $\dot{D}_{L \cdot CO_{max}}$ and $\dot{D}_{L \cdot CO_{120}}$. However, present indications are that $\dot{D}_L$ increases uniformly from the resting value of 20–25 ml/min/mm Hg STPD (14–18 litre/min)* to the maximum exercise reading of 50–70 ml/min/mm Hg STPD (35–50 litre/min).

$\dot{Q}$ is the cardiac output in litre/min—about 6 litre/min at rest, and 25 litre/min in maximum exercise. $\dot{Q}_c$ is the pulmonary capillary flow, 1%–2% smaller than $\dot{Q}$ due to pulmonary shunts.

λ is the air/blood partition coefficient. This varies in magnitude with the portion of the oxygen dissociation curve that is being used, but is commonly in the range 1.0–1.3.

D_t is the tissue diffusing capacity; this is difficult to esti-

---

* The units of litre/min are compatible with other terms in the process of gas transfer.

mate, but is probably at least 200 litre/min in maximum exercise.

The primary symbol C refers to gas concentration in ml/litre. (the units used in gas transfer equations) or ml/100 ml (the traditional units of the Fick equation, p. 57). F refers to fractional concentration (ml/ml) and P to the partial pressure (mm Hg or Torr).

The first subscript refers to the phase where the measurement is made:

I = inspired gas	a = arterial blood
E = expired gas	v = venous blood
A = alveolar gas	t = tissues

The second subscript specifies the nature of the gas, while a bar above a symbol refers to a mean value.

$$P_{I,O_2} = 150 \text{ mm Hg} \qquad P_{I,CO_2} = 0 \text{ mm Hg}$$
$$P_{E,O_2} = 114 \text{ mm Hg} \qquad P_{E,CO_2} = 28 \text{ mm Hg}$$

	Rest	*Exercise*		*Rest*	*Exercise*
P_{A,O_2}	100	105	P_{A,CO_2}	40	38
P_{a,CO_2}	90	88	P_{a,CO_2}	41	40
$P_{\bar{v},O_2}$	40	20	$P_{\bar{v},CO_2}$	47	65
C_{a,O_2}	19.2	19.0	C_{a,CO_2}	49.0	47.0
$C_{\bar{v},O_2}$	15.0	5.0	$C_{\bar{v},CO_2}$	53.1	61.0

Blood Pressures

Some cardiologists use the symbol Pa, or less correctly P_A to represent the hydrostatic pressure in the pulmonary artery, and Pc to represent the corresponding pressure in the pulmonary capillary. The fact that total pressure is implied can be deduced from the absence of a second subscript.

Systemic blood pressure (rest) 120/80 mm Hg   For the effect of exercise, see Fig. 19.

Pulmonary blood pressure (rest) 25/10 mm Hg

Circulatory Capacity—Q, SV; f_h, F, HR; $\dot{Q}$, $\dot{Q}_{max}$, CO, q; BV; CBV; HV; AVD; THb

The stroke volume (Q,SV) is preferably written in symbols compatible with gas transfer. It increases from 70–80 ml at rest to 120–130 ml in maximum exercise.

The heart rate is preferably shown as f_h, rather than F or HR. It increases from sixty-five to seventy-five at rest to 190 to 200 in maximum exercise.

The cardiac output is preferably shown as $\dot{Q}$ rather than CO or q. It increases from about 6 litre/min at rest to 25 litre/min in maximum exercise.

The blood volume (BV) is about 5 litres. The central blood volume (CBV) of the heart and pulmonary circulation accounts for about 1.5 litres at rest and rather more in exercise.

The heart volume (HV) is proportional to body size, averaging 11–12 ml/kg.

The arteriovenous oxygen difference (AVD) is better shown as $(Cao_2 - C\bar{v},o_2)$; it amounts to 4–5 ml/100 ml at rest and 14–16 ml/100 ml in exercise.

The haemoglobin level is about 15.6 gm/100 ml in men and 13.8 gm/100 ml in women. The total haemoglobin (THb) of a young man is thus some 780 gm.

Heat Transfer—Ts, Tr

Heat transfer is proportional to the thermal gradient from the body core (indicated by such measures as rectal temperature, Tr) to the skin (temperature Ts). Typical gradients are illustrated in Fig. 68.

Obesity

There are as yet no standard symbols. Normal values for a young man are as follows:

Excess weight	0 kg (see Table XV)
Average skinfold thickness	10 mm (see Table XVI)
Percentage body fat	$10\% - 15\%$
Specific gravity	$1.06 - 1.07$
Serum cholesterol	<250 mg/100 ml
Serum triglycerides	$100 - 180$ mg/100 ml

Drugs

A detailed glossary of synonyms for addictive drugs is given on pages 364–367.

Statistical Terms—$\overline{X}$; S.D.; S.E; r; F; t; N,n; P

All of the statistical terms to be defined are estimated values, having limits imposed by the sample size and the assumption of a normal distribution curve.

$\overline{X}$ = mean value
S.D. = standard deviation
S.E. = standard error of the mean
r = coefficient of correlation
F = variance ratio
t = the student's t ratio
N = the number of degrees of statistical freedom
n = the number of subjects or observations
p = probability

References

Pappenheimer, J.: Standardization of definitions and symbols in respiratory physiology. *Fed Proc, 9:*602–605, 1950.

Shephard, R.J.: Glossary of specialized terms and units. *Canad Med Ass J., 96:*912–915, 1967.

Denolin, H., Konig, K., Messin, R., and Degré, S.: L'ergometrie en cardiologie. Boehringer Mannheim GmbH, 1968.

MULTIPLE-CHOICE
SELF-APPRAISAL EXAMINATION

The questions on the following pages are taken from the examination papers of the fourth year BPHE course "Physiology of Physical Activity" offered by the University of Toronto. You should be able to complete all the hundred questions within three hours. Mark your answers very sure (S), fairly sure (F), or guess (G). The correct answers are given on p. 584. Score your paper as follows:

	Correct	Incorrect
Very Sure	4/3	−1/3
Fairly Sure	3/3	0
Guess	2/3	1/3

The minimum pass mark is 50; a "B" standing carries a mark of 66–74, and 75 or over is required for "A" standing.

1. *What was the view of environment put forward by Claude Bernard?*
   a) The external environment is held constant by man's efforts.
   b) The body maintains the constancy of the internal environment.
   c) The external environment has a marked effect on the internal environment.
   d) Claude Bernard was predominantly a theologian, and used environment in a metaphysical sense.

2. *What environmental factor do you think has the least influence on human performance?*
   a) heat
   b) cold
   c) high altitude
   d) solar radiation

3. *Which of the following is not a very practical method of measuring physical activity over a twelve hour period?*
   a) a tape-recording of the electrocardiogram
   b) use of an electrochemical pulse integrator

564

c) periodic measurements of oxygen consumption supplemented by observation
d) a careful record of calorie intake in the food

4. *What is the normal daytime pulse rate of an office worker?*
a) It is rarely greater than 110/min.
b) It varies from 100/min to 140/min, and is often greater than 130/min.
c) It is rarely greater than 80/min.
d) It varies from 80/min to 180/min, and values of 150/min are quite frequent.

5. *If a frog were suddenly cooled by 10°C, what would happen to the rate of chemical reactions in its leg muscles?*
a) It would regulate body temperature so that chemical reactions proceeded as normal.
b) Glycogen and related carbohydrates would be broken down at about twice the normal rate.
c) All chemical reactions would proceed at about four times the normal rate.
d) The rate of all chemical reactions would be some 50% of normal.

6. *A marathon race is conducted at an ambient temperature of 25°C. Towards the end of the event, a runner is checked and a rectal thermometer indicates a body temperature of 38.1°C. What would you advise?*
a) that it is safe to proceed with the race
b) that the measurement be repeated
c) that the runner stop running
d) that immediate hospital admission be arranged

7. *Which of the following is a valid objection to physiological studies on an animal preparation anaesthetized by modern techniques?*
a) Most anaesthetics depress body reflexes.
b) There is no means of judging an appropriate level of ventilation.
c) The commonly used barbiturate anaesthetics cause hypersecretion of bronchial mucus.
d) Massive doses of noradrenaline are released due to struggling of the animal in the early phase of induction.

8. *A test volunteer turns out to be a flighty young girl who is over-excited by the laboratory equipment. What would be the best method of obtaining useful data from this subject?*

a) Give her a heavy dose of tranquillizer and carry out the test in three hours time.
b) Arrange for an initial one hour period of psychotherapy.
c) Carry out the test as quickly as possible, in case her excitement increases.
d) Repeat the observations on two or more successive days.

9. *Which of the following bodily changes is most likely to occur during the acculturation of a primitive Eskimo community?*
   a) increase of carbohydrate intake
   b) increase of total calorie intake
   c) improvement of dental health
   d) increase of cold acclimatization

10. *Campbell is Scottish, and saves money by using a step-test in his laboratory. The subject weighs 70 kg and climbs a flight of two wooden steps each just under ten inches tall, twenty times per minute. What is the approximate work load imposed upon his subject?*
    a) 1400 kgm/min
    b) 14000 kgm/min
    c) 350 kgm/min
    d) 700 kgm/min

11. *Winkelheimer works in Houston, and can afford a bicycle ergometer. This has a flywheel with a radius of ten inches. The tension in the brake belt is indicated by a spring balance. Assuming that his subject can pedal at such a rate that the flywheel turns one hundred times per minute, approximately what setting of the spring balance will impose a load of 600 kgm/min?*
    a) 60 kg
    b) 4 kg
    c) 0.6 kg
    d) 3.1416 kg

12. *Jones works in Toronto, and can obtain money for neither a bicycle nor a step. He wants to estimate the cardiorespiratory fitness of fifty young men. Would you advise*
    a) 12 minute run
    b) 300 yard run
    c) 600 yard run/walk
    d) one minute speed sit-ups

13. *You are given one day to establish the caloric requirements of a party of twenty commandoes. What would be your best approach?*
    a) Measure the total food intake and estimate its caloric value.

b) Deprive the group of food for eight hours and measure the average weight loss.
c) Fit all twenty men with pedometers.
d) Keep a minute by minute diary of activities and measure the O_2 consumption for any unusual tasks.

14. *A miner drinks three pints of 6% beer per night. His total daily caloric needs are 3600 kcal. About how much of his energy needs are supplied by the beer, assuming that the majority of it is oxidized within the body?*
    a) 6%
    b) 16%
    c) 1.6%
    d) 0.6%

15. *Professor Smith has four students collecting data on blood flow at rest and in just sub-maximum exercise. Their results, expressed in ml/100ml of tissue/min, are as follows*

	REST			EXERCISE		
	Muscle	*Skin*	*Kidney*	*Muscle*	*Skin*	*Kidney*
a)	1	1	3	2	2	3
b)	3	2	1	50	2	1
c)	1	1	3	50	30	1
d)	25	20	3	50	40	3

Which student do you suggest made the most accurate observations?

16. *A telemeter is used to transmit the pulse rate of a young man aged twenty-two who is engaged in an important slalom contest. Lab tests have previously shown a maximum heart rate of 195. What would be the highest likely telemeter reading?*
    a) 195
    b) 190
    c) 250
    d) 180

17. *A man of sixty competes in a one-hour cross-country ski-race. What is his likely heart rate in the final five minutes of the race?*
    a) 185
    b) 120
    c) 190
    d) 150

18. *During exercise, an athletic boy of twelve increases his stroke volume from 35 to 70 ml. At the same time, the mean systolic*

pressure increases from 120 to 150 mmHg. How much work does the left ventricle perform in expelling blood during exercise? An extra
a) 100%
b)   25%
c) 150%
d) 210%

19. *Winkelheimer's bicycle is so expensive it can be pedalled by the arms or the legs. Assuming Winkelheimer knows how to measure stroke volume, what would be his likely findings if a man of twenty is exercised at an effort of 700 kgm/min?*

	Stroke Volume During Arm Work	Stroke Volume During Leg Work
a)	100 ml	140 ml
b)	200 ml	140 ml
c)	145 ml	140 ml
d)	60 ml	70 ml

20. *A slightly blue-faced young boy reports to the laboratory for detailed testing. Data is obtained on stroke volume and diastolic volume at three increasing work loads as follows:*

Stroke Volume	End Diastolic Volume
30 ml	75 ml
50 ml	125 ml
45 ml	175 ml

What is the next step?
a) Increase the work load by a further 50%.
b) Stop the test pending cardiological assessment.
c) Continue at the same load for a further five minutes.
d) Repeat the test at a higher load next day.

21. *Which is the least likely explanation of a heart murmur?*
a) polycythaemia
b) roughening of a heart valve
c) anxiety
d) an interventricular septal defect

22. *Cardiac catheterization data is collected on a normal young man at rest and in maximum effort. Indicate the likely values of oxygen content in blood drawn from the pulmonary artery and coronary sinus (ml/litre).*

	REST		EXERCISE	
	P.A.	C.S.	P.A.	C.S.
a)	150	15	30	30
b)	150	15	30	10
c)	50	50	30	30
d)	50	150	10	30

23. *Quantitative measurements are made on the V leads of a resting electrocardiogram. In Lead V_1, the S wave measures 2mV, and in Lead V_5 the R wave measures 3mV. The pulse rate is 35/min. What is the likely explanation?*
    a) The subject has suffered a recent coronary infarction.
    b) The heart is lying rather horizontally within the chest.
    c) The heart is unusually vertical in position.
    d) There is considerable hypertrophy of the left ventricle.

24. *Electrocardiograms are obtained on three subjects. One is normal, one is being resuscitated from fresh-water drowning, and one is recovering from salt-water drowning. Indicate the correct set of data for the PR interval (seconds).*

	Normal	Salt-water	Fresh-water
a)	0.11	0.16	0.26
b)	0.16	0.11	0.26
c)	0.26	0.16	0.11
d)	0.11	0.11	0.16

25. *What is a single Master's test?*
    a) a period of $1\frac{1}{2}$ min exercise using a flight of two nine-inch steps
    b) a period of 3 min exercise using a single nine-inch step
    c) a period of 3 min exercise using a single eighteen-inch step
    d) a single trip backwards and forwards over a flight of two steps

26. *What is the main criticism of the single Master's test?*
    a) The intensity of exercise is dangerously great.
    b) The task is unfamiliar to the average person.
    c) The terminology is confusing.
    d) The intensity of stress is too low for the average subject.

27. *What is the significance of a horizontal 0.1mV depression of the ST segment of the exercise electrocardiogram?*
    a) It is unequivocal evidence of coronary occlusion.
    b) It can only arise when the heart muscle is short of oxygen.
    c) It is usually due to digitalis poisoning.
    d) It indicates a slowing of the myocardial sodium pump.

28. *The factors contributing to the late continuing increase of heart rate in exercise include*
    a) a hypothalamic response to increasing body temperature
    b) a conditioned reflex from the highest centres of the brain
    c) irradiation of impulses from the motor cortex
    d) stimulation of mechanoreceptors in the limbs

29. *Which of the following factors is least likely to contribute to the syndrome of "shock"?*
    a) entry of microorganisms into the circulation
    b) a sustained increase of systemic blood pressure
    c) exhaustion of the adrenal glands
    d) death of the large intestine

30. *Which of the following factors is unlikely to increase exudation of fluid from the capillaries?*
    a) prolonged physical activity
    b) reduction of capillary hydrostatic pressure
    c) starvation
    d) heart failure

31. *Measurements of inspiratory and expiratory reserve volumes are made at rest and during vigorous exercise. Which values seem appropriate for a normal healthy young woman?*

	REST		EXERCISE	
	Insp Reserve	*Exp Reserve*	*Insp Reserve*	*Exp Reserve*
a)	2900	1000	1400	800
b)	1000	2900	800	1400
c)	3500	1500	1400	800
d)	1500	3500	800	1400

32. *How would you explain "second wind"?*
    a) Ventilation increases as body temperature is raised by exercise.
    b) The metabolic efficiency of the heart increases after several minutes of sustained work.
    c) Ventilation decreases as lactate is eliminated from the body.
    d) Spasm of the diaphragm is reversed as body temperature rises.

33. *Some people find it easier to breathe out hard when they purse their lips. Why is this?*
    a) It is a subjective phenomenon; in fact, expiration is more difficult.
    b) The nasal passages are opened up, and air flows through the nose.
    c) With slower expiration, more muscles can be used in the breathing process.
    d) The speed of expiration is reduced, and the "equal pressure" point is not reached until air is flowing through the major bronchi.

34. *How would you demonstrate to a class of school children the effect that smoking a cigarette had upon your airway resistance?*

a) measure airway resistances with a body plethysmograph
b) estimate residual volumes by helium dilution
c) measure peak expiratory flow rates with a vane anemometer
d) estimate intraoesophageal pressures before and after smoking

35. *Which factor is unlikely to cause a worsening of dead space/tidal volume ratio in exercise?*
a) enlargement of the bronchial tree
b) decrease of gas mixing time
c) worsening of ventilation/perfusion inequalities
d) expansion of the respiratory bronchioles

36. *Susan has trouble with her damping ratio. The valves on her SCUBA set have an annoying rattle in use. Four different salesmen suggest*
a) the problem will be helped by use of helium
b) the problem will disappear at depth
c) the problem will disappear if the resistance of the circuit can be diminished
d) the problem will be helped if the capacity of the system is minimized
Which salesman should Susan believe?

37. *An Eastern University suggested that a slow breathing pattern gave swimmers a large pulmonary diffusing capacity. What is the appropriate comment to this suggestion?*
a) They are quite right. Go east and learn some more exercise physiology.
b) They are quite wrong. Sampling of alveolar carbon monoxide is a problem when breathing slowly.
c) They may be right. Go south and test a much larger sample of swimmers.
d) They may be wrong. Measurements should have been made by a carbon monoxide breathing method. Go west to Los Angeles and get some carbon monoxide.

38. *An athlete asks your advice on drinking a small dose of sodium bicarbonate three hours before a race. What should you suggest?*
a) The timing is optimal to improve physical performance.
b) The buffers will likely be restored to normal before the race begins.
c) The sensitivity of the respiratory centres to CO_2 will be improved, but lactate tolerance will remain unchanged.
d) Both lactate tolerance and respiratory centre sensitivity can be improved by bicarbonate, but it must be taken one hour before a contest.

39. *Much has been written on oxygen poisoning. How long can a young man at sea level breathe 100% oxygen before serious symptoms are encountered?*
   a) 10 min
   b) one hour
   c) one day
   d) one month

40. *What is the approximate volume of oxygen that can be stored in the body if an athlete inhales oxygen until fifteen seconds before a race?*
   a) 150 litre
   b) 1.5 ml
   c) 1.5 litre
   d) 150 ml

41. *Smoking increases the risk of many diseases. Which of the following is an* unlikely *hazard to the habitual smoker?*
   a) thromboangitis obiterans
   b) cancer of the mouth
   c) cancer of the intestine
   d) cancer of the bladder

42. *You are working at a smoking withdrawal clinic, testing the carboxyhaemoglobin level in the blood. The first patient you test claims to have given up smoking, but has a 7% carboxyhaemoglobin level. What is the longest period for which he could have given up smoking?*
   a) two hours
   b) twelve hours
   c) two days
   d) about one week

43. *Which of the following is the* least *likely explanation of the resting tachycardia induced by smoking?*
   a) Smoking produces an increase of airway resistance, thus increasing the work of breathing.
   b) Nicotine stimulates chemosensitive tissue in the carotid body.
   c) Nor-adrenaline is released locally in the cardiac pacemaker.
   d) The output of noradrenaline from the adrenal cortex is increased.

44. *Which of the following statements about alcohol and health is* correct?

a) Alcohol is a toxic substance that produces cirrhosis of the liver by poisoning specific —SH enzyme systems.

b) Alcohol in small doses increases confidence but impairs skill and judgment.

c) Alcohol makes the body feel warm because the skin vessels are constricted and elimination of heat becomes difficult.

d) A drinker tends to lose weight because alcohol has a poor calorie content.

45. *You are making physiological tests on four athletes and you happen to know that each normally has a blood pressure of 120/80 mm Hg with a skin blood flow of 2 ml/min/100 ml of tissue. Which of the four would you suspect of taking amphetamines?*

	Blood pressure	Blood flow
a)	120/90 mm Hg	3 ml/min/100 ml
b)	100/60 mm Hg	3 ml/min/100 ml
c)	100/60 mm Hg	1 ml/min/100 ml
d)	140/95 mm Hg	1 ml/min/100 ml

46. *Attempts to improve performance by changing the buffering systems of the body are not normally very successful. Which seems the* least *reasonable explanation of this phenomenon?*

a) Even in brief activity (10–30 seconds), oxygen transport is the main factor limiting performance, and O_2 transport is not modified by an alteration of blood buffers.

b) The alkalies that are given are usually eliminated rapidly by the kidney.

c) Many of the investigators concerned have not tested organic buffers such as "T.H.A.M." (trishydroxymethylaminomethane)

d) An increase of buffering capacity may lower the sensitivity of the respiratory centres.

47. *Which of the following tests would provide the* best *information on the developmental age of a child born eleven years ago.*

a) the determination of K^{40}, using a whole body counter

b) the measurement of standing height

c) a radiograph of the wrist

d) the measurement of triceps, subscapular and suprailiac skinfolds

48. *Height bears some relationship to social class in children. Which set of figures gives the most likely indication of this trend in boys aged 11?*

Height of Child (cm)

	Year 1870		Year 1970	
	Father a Doctor	Father a Construction Worker	Father a Doctor	Father a Construction Worker
a)	120	110	138	135
b)	113	110	138	135
c)	138	135	138	135
d)	120	110	145	135

49. *What sort of haemoglobin readings might be anticipated in a survey of Toronto school children? All values are gm/100 ml blood.*

	Age 10		Age 17	
	Boys	Girls	Boys	Girls
a)	15.6	15.6	15.6	15.6
b)	15.6	13.8	15.6	13.8
c)	13.8	13.8	15.6	13.8
d)	13.8	12.0	15.6	13.8

50. *Which of the following is* unlikely *to occur as a man ages?*
    a) increase of the arterial lactate concentration in maximum effort from $60 \rightarrow 100$ mg/100 ml of blood
    b) decrease of maximum oxygen intake 3 litre/min $\rightarrow$ 2 litre/min
    c) rather constantly maintained haemoglobin level
    d) increase in the ratio residual volume/total lung capacity $22\% \rightarrow 35\%$

51. *Coronary disease is often said to be helped by an exercise rehabilitation programme. Which of the following is* unlikely *to provide a physiological basis for the observed improvement?*
    a) development of collateral vessels to supply ischaemic myocardium
    b) a relaxation of "capacity" blood vessels, shifting excess blood away from the heart and lungs
    c) a decreased secretion of catecholamines in response to a given load
    d) a late enhancement of fibrinolysis

52. *Epidemiological evidence that coronary disease can be minimized by physical activity was sought in a group of bus company employees. There were certain limitations to this data. Which of the following is the* least *valid objection?*
    a) Bus drivers are initially fatter than conductors.
    b) Bus conductors have as much coronary atheroma as drivers, and indeed have a higher incidence of angina pectoris.
    c) Bus conductors do not do much more physical work than drivers.

d) Different constitutional types may decide to become drivers and conductors.

53. *If a man aged sixty has an aerobic power of 2 litre/min, what would be a reasonable limit to suggest for his energy expenditure during the working day?*
a) 2.5 kcal/min
b) 15 kcal/min
c) 10 kcal/min
d) 5 kcal/min

54. *Obesity carries several hazards to health. Select the* least *likely hazard from the following list:*
a) increased risk of hypotension and related vascular problems
b) impaired glucose tolerance
c) increased liability to chronic gall bladder disease
d) increased risk of surgical procedures

55. *A man exercises at a load of 900 kgm/min and has a pulse rate of 150/min. He then exercises at 1080 kgm/min and has a pulse rate of 180/min. What is his PWC_{170}?*
a) 990 Kgm/min
b) 1020 Kgm/min
c) 6 PWC units
d) 109140 PWC units

56. *A man aged twenty-five and weighing 70 kg has an oxygen consumption of 1.7 litre/min while pedalling a bicycle erogometer; his pulse rate is 128 beats per minute. What is his approximate maximum oxygen intake?*
a) 37 ml/kg min
b) 42 ml/kg min
c) 49 ml/kg min
d) 34 ml/kg min

57. *What would be the likely discrepancy between an estimate of maximum oxygen intake, made as in question (56), and the directly measured reading?*
a) 10%
b) 2%
c) 0.5%
d) 0.2%

58. *If a patient is anxious, what will happen to the maximum oxygen intake as predicted from the Åstrand nomogram?*
a) It will remain unchanged, because the respiratory and cardiac changes induced by anxiety operate in opposing directions.
b) The prediction will underestimate the true value.

c) The prediction will overestimate the true value.

d) The patient will exceed his anticipated maximum heart rate, and this will make it impossible to use the nomogram.

59. *A middle-aged and overweight business man wants a fair statement of the risks of a twelve minute submaximum exercise test. What incidence of ventricular fibrillation should you have in your mind as you discuss the question with him?*
    a) 1 in 15,000
    b) 1 in ·3,000
    c) 1 in 100,000
    d) 1 in 1,000,000

60. *What are the predominant characteristics of the ectomorph?*
    a) long arms and legs with generally thin build
    b) well developed thigh and chest musculature
    c) thick-set, broad-necked "John Bull" appearance
    d) protruberant abdomen and general obesity

61. *Which would be an* inappropriate *method of assessing body fat?*
    a) Measurement of triceps, subscapular and suprailiac skinfolds.
    b) Soft tissue radiographs of selected regions of the body.
    c) Hydrostatic weighing.
    d) Calculation of the index $W/3\sqrt{H}$

62. *What would be your main objection to the use of a performance test battery to evaluate the fitness of a group of school children?*
    a) The tests are complicated, and require very skilled personnel to administer.
    b) The results depend mainly on the size of individual participants.
    c) Some of the tests in the proposed batteries are dangerous to the children.
    d) There are no adequate normal standards for purposes of comparison.

63. *Which item of the Kraus-Weber test battery do many children fail?*
    a) Shuttle run
    b) Forward bend
    c) Trunk lift
    d) Sit-ups

64. *What is your assessment of breath-holding as a test of fitness?*
    a) It may have a role in assessing suitability for specific sports such as underwater swimming.

b) It is meaningful unless the subject is allowed to watch the second hand of a clock.

c) It is useful mainly in assessing suitability for endurance-type effort.

d) It has never been suggested as a fitness test.

65. *Patient A complains that he feels faint on standing. Patient B has no complaints relating to his cardiovascular system. Patient C has persistent headaches which his doctor told him were related to his blood pressure. Patient D is commended by his physician as being very fit. What are their respective systemic blood pressures?*

	Patient A	Patient B	Patient C	Patient D
a)	160/100	130/70	120/80	100/60
b)	100/60	120/80	130/70	160/100
c)	100/60	120/80	160/100	130/70
d)	160/100	100/60	130/70	120/80

66. *A student measures the knee extension strength with a cable tensiometer and obtains a reading that is only 50 percent of normal. What could have produced this result?*

a) The subject has become habituated to the test through several practice attempts.

b) The cable harness has been attached too close to the knee joint.

c) The tensiometer cable has been attached at 90° to the long axis of the leg.

d) The knee joint has not been at the correct angulation.

67. *The mechanical efficiency of effort is commonly quoted as 25 percent. A student measures the energy cost of lifting thirty pound boxes from the floor into a truck, and finds an efficiency of only 4 percent. What is the most likely primary reason for this?*

a) Much of the energy is still stored as potential energy in the elevation of the boxes; this could later be recovered if the boxes were lowered by the same subject.

b) The boxes are raised much higher than the truck during lifting, thereby increasing the work performed.

c) The cost of effort is increased by movements of the centre of gravity of the body, while efficiency is decreased by a restriction of blood flow to the arm muscles.

d) The unmeasured energy cost involved in acceleration and deceleration of the boxes accounts for the discrepancy.

68. *What is the likely relation between energy cost of working and the height of working surface?*

	26 Inches	*36 Inches*	*64 Inches*
a)	2.8 kcal/min	3.1 kcal/min	4.1 kcal/min
b)	4.1	3.1	2.8
c)	2.8	2.8	2.8
d)	4.1	2.8	3.1

69. *Measurements of muscle blood flow are made during isometric contraction. Which set of data is correct?*

Blood Flow at Stated Force (% Maximum Strength)

	0 (rest)	10%	50%	80%
a)	2 ml/min/100 ml	15 ml/min/100 ml	8 ml/min/100 ml	0 ml/min/100 ml
b)	2	8	15	30
c)	2	15	65	120
d)	2	8	8	8

70. *Which of the following receptors contribute the least information towards the regulation of posture?*
    a) the eyes
    b) the cochlea
    c) the muscle spindles
    d) pressure receptors in the feet

71. *What would be likely to set a physiological limit to the frequency of stride for a runner?*
    a) the natural frequency of the legs.
    b) the power of the leg muscles
    c) the time taken for transmission of impulses through the γ loop.
    d) the duration of twitch of a white muscle.

72. *West has divided the lungs into three zones, based on the relationships of alveolar pressure P_A, pulmonary arterial pressure P_a and pulmonary venous pressure P_v. How would you describe these relationships?*

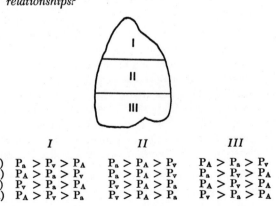

	I	*II*	*III*
a)	$P_a > P_v > P_A$	$P_a > P_A > P_v$	$P_A > P_a > P_v$
b)	$P_A > P_a > P_v$	$P_a > P_A > P_v$	$P_a > P_v > P_A$
c)	$P_v > P_a > P_A$	$P_v > P_A > P_a$	$P_A > P_v > P_A$
d)	$P_A > P_v > P_a$	$P_v > P_A > P_a$	$P_v > P_a > P_A$

73. A businessman complains that his shoes are tight after he has engaged in a prolonged jogging/walking programme. What is the most likely explanation?
   a) He has sprained his ankle due to unaccustomed exertion.
   b) Sweating of the feet is very marked and this has led to a thickening of his socks.
   c) The fluid content of the muscles and related tissues has been increased by 20%.
   d) The sensory receptors of the feet are temporarily reporting inaccurate information to his cerebral cortex.

74. Which statement about "warm up" is most correct?
   a) Warm-up is more closely related to core temperature than to to local muscle temperature.
   b) Warm-up decreases the internal viscous work of the active muscles.
   c) Few of the effects of warm-up can be achieved by local heating of the part.
   d) The benefits of warm-up are independent of recent learning and the benefits of a familiar ritual.

75. The diagram shows the metabolic pathways of glucose utilization. What are the yields of A.T.P. per mole of glucose at points W, X, Y, and Z?

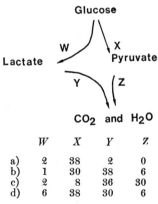

	W	*X*	*Y*	*Z*
a)	2	38	2	0
b)	1	30	38	6
c)	2	8	36	30
d)	6	38	30	6

76. Two men A and B perform equal and intensive interval work on a bicycle ergometer. A has a pattern 10 sec work 30 sec rest, while B has a pattern of 60 sec work 180 sec rest. What will be the lactate levels achieved?
   a) Neither will accumulate lactic acid.
   b) Both will accumulate lactate equally.
   c) A will accumulate more than B.
   d) B will accumulate more than A.

77. *What will happen to the muscle glycogen three days after a bout of strenuous and prolonged exercise?*
    a) It will rise unless the man has a high carbohydrate diet.
    b) It will fall particularly if he is given supplementary insulin and glucose.
    c) It will not yet have recovered from the effects of exercise.
    d) It will be 50% to 100% above the initial resting level.

78. *Jones has a resting R.Q. of 0.71, while Smith has an R.Q. of 0.72. What would you infer about their diet?*
    a) Jones has a high sugar consumption relative to Smith.
    b) Both Jones and Smith eat mainly fat.
    c) Smith has a high sugar consumption relative to Jones.
    d) Both Jones and Smith eat mainly carbohydrate.

79. *In a hot, dry climate, a major part of the body heat is lost by which of the following mechanisms?*
    a) radiation
    b) convection
    c) evaporation of sweat
    d) conduction

80. *What programme would you recommend for producing dynamic muscle strength?*
    a) "isotonic" exercise with overloading of the muscles
    b) isometric contractions at 70% of maximum strnegth for 6 sec per day
    c) "isotonic" exercise with underloading of the muscles
    d) isometric contractions at 45% of maximum strength for 6 sec per day

81. *What factors would concern you most in planning an endurance training programme?*
    a) the length and frequency of training sessions
    b) the intensity of exercise and fitness of the subjects
    c) the length and intensity of exercise
    d) the frequency of exercise and the fitness of the subjects

82. *Upon exposure to cold a number of physiology adaptations occur. Indicate the first adaptation.*
    a) shivering
    b) vasoconstriction
    c) sweating
    d) an increase of heart rate

83. *Why does a professional weight-lifter use the technique of "clean and jerk."*

a) Inertial work is minimized by moving weights briskly.
b) The simultaneous activity of all motor units can only be sustained for a brief period.
c) The incidence of back-injuries is reduced by the jerking motion.
d) The γ reflexes from the stretch receptors are stimulated by the jerking motion.

84. *When can a muscle develop maximum isometric tension?*
    a) when it is slightly shorter than its resting length
    b) when it is elongated by 50% to 100% of its resting length
    c) when it is under slight tension
    d) when it is forcibly compressed by 30% to 40% of its normal length

85. *When does a muscle perform the most external work?*
    a) when it contracts isometrically
    b) when it contracts isotonically with zero load
    c) when it contracts at maximum velocity of shortening
    d) when it contracts isotonically at about 60% of maximum isometric strength

86. *Which of the following factors has little influence on skill?*
    a) the sensitivity of the semicircular canals
    b) the strength of the active muscles.
    c) the coordination of eye and muscle movements
    d) muscle tension

87. *Roughly what length of time can activity be sustained by breakdown of the A.T.P. stored in muscle?*
    a) 0.5 sec
    b) 30 sec
    c) 5 min
    d) 15 min

88. *A diver ascending from work at one hundred feet must never exceed a critical ratio between tissue pressure and mouth pressure. What is this critical ratio?*
    a) 4:1
    b) 3:1
    c) 2:1
    d) 1.25:1

89. *What is the significance of the pressure ratio of question 88?*
    a) avoidance of decompression sickness
    b) avoidance of thoracic squeeze
    c) avoidance of lung rupture
    d) avoidance of oxygen poisoning

90. *What is the* least *desirable aspect of helium breathing for the diver?*
    a) the density of helium alters the work of breathing
    b) the replacement of nitrogen by helium modifies the incidence of high pressure narcosis
    c) the Reynolds number of the breathing mixture is changed
    d) heat elimination is altered

91. *Why does the recovery pulse not correspond very closely with the exercise reading?*
    a) A large part of the exercise pulse response is attributable to elevation of deep body temperature.
    b) The neural drive to the vasoregulatory centres of the medulla differs from one person to another, and is rapidly lost on stopping exercise.
    c) Individuals differ widely in the efficiency of glycogen resynthesis during the recovery period.
    d) The size of the oxygen debt can be three to four times greater in an athlete than in a sedentary individual.

92. *When a muscle is stimulated via its motor nerve, the maximum tension is not developed immediately. What is the main reason for this?*
    a) The series elastic elements must be stretched.
    b) There is a long transmission delay at the neuromuscular junction.
    c) The breakdown of ATP is a relatively slow reaction.
    d) Time is required for activation of the muscle spindles and γ loop.

93. *Three subjects exercise for ten minutes at 80% of aerobic power. One performs on the treadmill, one on the bicycle, and one on a step test. What are the final arterial lactate readings?*

	Treadmill	Bicycle	Step
a)	120 mg/100 ml	110 mg/100 ml	105 mg/100 ml
b)	30 mg/100 ml	50 mg/100 ml	25 mg/100 ml
c)	30 mg/100 ml	25 mg/100 ml	50 mg/100 ml
d)	105 mg/100 ml	120 mg/100 ml	110 mg/100 ml

94. *What is the main cause of "high altitude deterioration" in a mountain climber?*
    a) Increasing lethargy, with much of the day spent sleeping.
    b) An excessive calorie intake in an attempt to counteract the cold.
    c) Progressive dehydration.
    d) Prolonged acclimatization at moderate altitudes.

95. *Why is the benefit gained from altitude training rapidly lost?*
   a) Most of the increased red cell count is dissipated in a few weeks.
   b. The greater maximum oxygen intake is attributable mainly to the lower gas density while at altitude.
   c) The body rapidly reduces blood and tissue bicarbonate levels on return to sea level.
   d) The control of ventilation passes mainly to the carotid body chemoreceptors after a few days at sea level.

96. *What is the best definition of coronary thrombosis?*
   a) a sudden depression of the ST segment of the electrocardiogram
   b) a sudden pain in the chest or left arm lasting less than one minute
   c) death of an area of tissue in the heart wall
   d) a sudden occlusion of one of the coronary arteries

97. *If a nonathletic person runs as fast as he can for thirty minutes every day, what will happen?*
   a) His endurance time on a treadmill test will increase in proportion to his maximum oxygen intake.
   b) His endurance time will increase several times more than the percentage increase in his maximum oxygen intake.
   c) The maximum oxygen intake will increase more than endurance time.
   d) The maximum oxygen intake will not increase unless he exercises for longer than thirty minutes per day.

98. *If you were buying a defibrillator for a fitness unit, what type would you choose?*
   a) a d.c. defibrillator giving a discharge of up to 350 watt sec
   b) an a.c. defibrillator developing a potential of 5000 volts
   c) an a.c. defibrillator developing a potential of 50 volts
   d) a simple unit involving a push-button timed impulse from the domestic electricity supply

99. *Many middle-aged men take exercise in the form of golf. What would be the likely energy expenditure if they walk around the course carrying their clubs?*
   a) 1.5–2.0 kcal/min
   b) 4–5 kcal/min
   c) 9–10 kcal/min
   d) 10–15 kcal/min

100. *What is the main objection to the proposition that CO_2 accumulation regulates breathing in maximum exercise?*

a) The alveolar CO_2 tension oscillates markedly during exercise.
b) The shape of the oscillations of alveolar CO_2 are modified by exercise.
c) There are very adequate alternative explanations of respiratory regulation in exercise.
d) The arterial CO_2 tension is less than normal in maximum exercise.

ANSWERS TO MULTIPLE-CHOICE
SELF-APPRAISAL EXAMINATION

1 B	11 B	21 A	31 A	41 C
2 D	12 A	22 B	32 C	42 A
3 D	13 D	23 D	33 D	43 A
4 A	14 B	24 B	34 C	44 B
5 D	15 C	25 A	35 C	45 D
6 B	16 C	26 D	36 A	46 A
7 A	17 D	27 D	37 B	47 C
8 D	18 C	28 A	38 B	48 A
9 A	19 A	29 B	39 C	49 C
10 D	20 B	30 B	40 D	50 A
51 B	61 D	71 A	81 B	91 B
52 C	62 B	72 B	82 B	92 A
53 D	63 B	73 C	83 B	93 B
54 A	64 A	74 B	84 C	94 C
55 B	65 C	75 C	85 D	95 A
56 C	66 D	76 D	86 B	96 D
57 A	67 C	77 D	87 A	97 B
58 B	68 D	78 B	88 C	98 A
59 A	69 A	79 C	89 A	99 B
60 A	70 B	80 A	90 D	100 D

Reference

Rothman, A.I.: Confidence testing: An extension of multiple choice testing. *Brit J Med Educ*, 3:237–239, 1969.

INDEX

THE LIBRARY
ST. MARY'S COLLEGE OF MARYLAND
ST. MARY'S CITY, MARYLAND 20686

081158

QP
301
.S47

Shephard, R.J.
Alive man!

081158

78

DATE DUE			
MAR 1 1983			
MY 19 '86			
DEC 18 1989			

Library of St. Mary's College of Maryland
St. Mary's City, Maryland 20686